Edited by
MICHELE TANSELLA
GRAHAM THORNICROFT

Mental Health Outcome Measures

Second edition

GASKELL

First edition published by Springer-Verlag (Berlin, Heidelberg), 1996
© First edition, 1996 individual contributors
© Second edition, 2001 The Royal College of Psychiatrists

Gaskell is an imprint and registered trade mark of the Royal College of Psychiatrists, 17 Belgrave Square, London SW1X 8PG

British Library Cataloguing-in-Publication Data
A catalogue record for this book is available from the British Library.
ISBN 1-901242-55-2

Distributed in North America
by American Psychiatric Press, Inc.

Printed in Great Britain by Bell & Bain Limited, Glasgow.

Contents

Contributors

Annibale Biggeri, Associate Professor of Medical Statistics, University of Florence, Florence, Italy

Giulia Bisoffi, Statistician, Department of Medicine and Public Health, Section of Psychiatry, University of Verona (WHO Collaborating Centre for Research and Training in Mental Health and Service Evaluation), Verona, Italy

Traolach S. Brugha, Professor of Psychiatry and Head of the Section of Social and Epidemiological Psychiatry, Department of Psychiatry, University of Leicester, UK

Graham Dunn, Professor of Biomedical Statistics, Biostatistics Group, School of Epidemiology and Health Sciences, University of Manchester, UK

Gail M. Gamache, Project Director, Homeless Veterans Dental Program, Veterans Administration Medical Center (VAMC), MIRECC, Building 12 (Upper), Leeds, MA 01053-9764, USA

David Goldberg, Emeritus Professor of Psychiatry, Institute of Psychiatry, King's College London, De Crespigny Park, Denmark Hill, London SE5 8AF, UK

Howard Goldman, Department of Psychiatry, University of Maryland, School of Medicine, Baltimore, Maryland, USA

Aleksandar Janca, Department of Psychiatry and Behavioural Science, University of Western Australia, Perth, Australia

Rachel Jenkins, Institute of Psychiatry, King's College London, De Crespigny Park, Denmark Hill, London SE5 8AF, UK

Sonia Johnson, Department of Psychiatry and Behavioural Sciences, Royal Free and University College Medical Schools, Wolfson Building, 48 Riding House Street, London W1N 8AA, UK

Ronald C. Kessler, Office of the Director, National Institute of Mental Health, 9000 Rockville Pike, Building 31, Room 4A52, Bethesda, MD 20892-2475, USA

Anthony F. Lehman, Department of Psychiatry, University of Maryland, Center for Mental Health Services Research, Baltimore, Maryland, USA

Fiona Lindsay, Section of Social and Epidemiological Psychiatry, Department of Psychiatry, University of Leicester, UK

Paul McCrone, Senior Lecturer in Health Economics, Section of Community Psychiatry, Institute of Psychiatry, King's College London, De Crespigny Park, London SE5 8AF, UK

William E. Narrow, Visiting Scientist, American Psychiatric Institute for Research and Education, Washington, DC, USA

Michael Phelan, Charing Cross Hospital, London, UK

Darrel A. Regier, Director, American Psychiatric Institute for Research and Education and Office of Research, Washington, DC, USA

Paola Rucci, Statistician, Department of Medicine and Public Health, Section of Psychiatry, University of Verona (WHO Collaborating Centre for Research and Training in Mental Health and Service Evaluation), Verona, Italy and Western Psychiatric Institute and Clinic, University of Pittsburg, Pittsburgh, PA, USA

Mirella Ruggeri, Associate Professor of Psychiatry, Department of Medicine and Public Health, Section of Psychiatry, University of Verona (WHO Collaborating Centre for Research and Training in Mental Health and Service Evaluation), Verona, Italy

D. Salas, Psychologist, PROMI Foundation, Cabra (Córdoba), Spain

L. Salvador-Carulla, Professor of Psychiatry, Department of Neurosciences, University of Cadiz, Spain

Norman Sartorius, Department of Psychiatry, University of Geneva, Switzerland

Aart H. Schene, Professor of Psychiatry, Academic Medical Center, University of Amsterdam, PO Box 22700, 1100 DE Amsterdam, The Netherlands

Bruce Singh, Department of Psychiatry, University of Melbourne, Melbourne, Victoria 3050, Australia

Michael Slade, Section of Community Psychiatry, Health Services Research Department, Institute of Psychiatry, King's College London, De Crespigny Park, London SE5 8AF, UK

Michele Tansella, Professor of Psychiatry and Director of the Department of Medicine and Public Health, University of Verona; Director of the WHO Collaborating Centre for Research and Training in Mental Health and Service Evaluation, Verona, Italy

Ruth Taylor, Section of Epidemiology and General Practice, Institute of Psychiatry, King's College London, De Crespigny Park, London SE5 8AF, UK

Richard C. Tessler, Professor in Sociology, Social and Demographic Research Institute, W-35 Machmer Hall, University of Massachusetts, Amherst, Massachusetts 01003, USA

Graham Thornicroft, Professor of Community Psychiatry, Health Service Research Department, Institute of Psychiatry, King's College London, De Crespigny Park, London SE5 8AF, UK

Bedirhan Üstün, Scientist, Division of Mental Health, WHO, Avenue Appix 20, CH-1211 Geneva 27, Switzerland.

Scott Weich, Royal Free and University College Medical School, University College London, UK

Durk Wiersma, Department of Social Psychiatry, University Hospital, Groningen, The Netherlands

Bob van Wijngaarden, Research Associate, Netherlands Institute of Mental Health and Addiction, PO Box 725, 3500 AS Utrecht, The Netherlands

John K. Wing, c/o Royal College of Psychiatrists' Research Unit, 6th Floor, 83 Victoria Street, London SW1H 0HW

Hans-Ulrich Wittchen, Professor of Clinical Psychology and Psychotherapy, Technical Univeristy of Dresden, and Head of Clinical Psychology and Epidemiology, Clinical Psychology, Max Planck Institue of Psychiatry, Kraeplinstrasse 2–10, D-80804 Munich 40, Germany

Til Wykes, Institute of Psychiatry, King's College London, De Crespigny Park, London SE5 8AF, UK

Foreword

Mental health services across Europe are in a state of ferment. It is essential that researchers use replicable measures to assess those developments that are desirable, as well as those forms of service that can be shown to be cost-effective. The appearance of this book is timely, since it brings together a set of influential papers on the measurement of outcome. There is therefore an opportunity for investigators in different countries to use measures and procedures that are comparable with one another. At present we do not have a single set of measures that can be confidently recommended; however, the various contributions should allow researchers to make an informed choice.

This book brings together two sets of articles written for special issues *of Social Psychiatry and Psychiatric Epidemiology* (vol. 29, no. 5; vol. 31, no. 2) with five articles especially written for this volume. Chapter 11, by Taylor and Thornicroft, considers the limitations of randomised controlled trials (RCTs) in the evaluation of mental health services, which are numerous and real, despite the obvious theoretical appeal of such designs. All of the famous RCTs excluded patients who were homicidal, and many excluded patients who had no home to go to. This is important, since planners of services have tended to generalise the results of such studies, with the result that, in England at least, too many beds have been closed in the name of community care. It may be concluded that other, naturalistic designs should be used in the evaluation of complex services. The RCT should be reserved for situations in which prospective randomisation is feasible, and in which specifiable outcomes are likely to follow the treatment to which subjects are being randomised. However, naturalistic studies also have their shortcomings, so that investigators tend to use unsatisfactory compromises between the two designs. An alternative approach is to use multi-dimensional assessments of outcome, as described by Biggeri *et al* in Chapter 15. At present, such approaches are in their early stages and serve to generate hypotheses about possible relationships between variables.

A consensus is beginning to emerge on methods of evaluation; this would indicate that progress has been made. We hope that this book will contribute to the understanding that is developing between investigators working in very different settings. In the conclusion of this volume, Rachel Jenkins and Bruce Singh emphasise the pre-occupation of previous studies with input and process variables, and welcome the present emphasis on outcome variables. At present, investigators tend to use separate measures of symptom loss, user and carer satisfaction with services, quality of life, and various measures of need that are reviewed in this book. It is evident that we are still picking our way across a minefield. The chapters that follow offer the reader a state-of-the-art map of the territory and point out the various hazards that lie ahead.

Professor Sir David Goldberg
London

1 A prospectus for mental health outcome measures

GRAHAM THORNICROFT and MICHELE TANSELLA

That this second edition of *Mental Health Outcome Measures* should follow its predecessor after only four years (Thornicroft & Tansella, 1996) reflects the pace of change in this field. Until recently we were used to hearing input or process changes (such as service investment or length of stay) described *as if* they indicated the outcomes of care, as the account by Brugha & Lindsay shows (Chapter 7). But during the 1990s the construction of valid and reliable outcome measures has prompted an acceleration in their use, at least in research settings.

To put outcome measures in context, there is a need for an overall conceptual framework. We have proposed such a framework, the Matrix Model, which uses two dimensions, the *geographical* (country, local and patient levels, identified by the numbers 1, 2 and 3) and the *temporal* (input, process and outcome phases, referred to by the letters A, B and C) (Thornicroft & Tansella, 1999). Using these two dimensions, a 3 × 3 matrix with nine cells can be constructed to bring into focus critical issues for mental health service practice and research, and the overall scheme is illustrated in Table 1.1.

TABLE 1.1
Overview of the matrix model

Geographical dimension	Temporal dimension		
	(A) Input phase	*(B) Process phase*	*(C) Outcome phase*
(1) Country/regional level	1A	1B	1C
(2) Local level (catchment area)	2A	2B	2C
(3) Patient level	3A	3B	3C

This book provides a series of authoritative reviews in the most important outcome domains in psychiatric patient-level research (cell 3C) and in the evaluation of mental health services (cell 2C). Each chapter has been revised to ensure that the reviews remain both up to date and comprehensive.

While an airline pilot would not consider flying without an altimeter that had been very carefully calibrated, assessments without established psychometric properties are still common in psychiatric research. Some of the contributions in this book therefore assess the psychometric adequacy of commonly used measures, as discussed by Salvador-Carulla & Salas (Chapter 14), and propose how they should be further developed.

Until recently the measurement of the outcomes of mental health treatment and care was directed almost entirely towards two issues: psychopathology (e.g. symptom severity) and service utilisation (e.g. number of admissions). Those involved in mental health research increasingly recognise the limitations of this approach; indeed, relatively few innovative services in the field of community mental health have yielded benefits in terms of symptom improvement or reduced bed usage.

Over the last decade a wider perspective has been adopted in relation to research design and data analysis. With respect to research design, for example, Taylor & Thornicroft (Chapter 11) set out the advantages of randomised controlled trials for medical research, in addition to the limitations in their application to mental health service research. The difficulties inherent in the interpretation of data in complex human service systems and the need for refined and innovative statistical methods are discussed in detail by Dunn (Chapter 2) and Biggeri and colleagues (Chapter 15).

In terms of domains of measurement that go beyond symptoms, Phelan *et al* (Chapter 3) show that global rating scales are conceptually attractive, but extremely difficult to operate well. There is also a lack of conceptual clarity about the subjective perspective of users in rating outcomes, as Johnson and colleagues argue in relation to needs assessment (Chapter 16). Patient satisfaction is another case in point and, as Ruggeri (Chapter 4) makes clear, satisfaction must be considered in relation both to expectations and to the wider cultural context of health practices and beliefs. Moreover, in order to be valid, measures of satisfaction must be sufficiently detailed and comprehensive and cannot rely on global questions alone. Furthermore, as the need for mental health service research extends into community settings, the importance of the interactions between patients and their families gain prominence, as discussed by Schene and colleagues (Chapter 5).

The contributions in this book also show that care is needed in establishing new measurement scales. As detailed by Wing & Brugha (Chapter 9), both the ninth edition of the Present State Examination (PSE–9) and the Schedules for Clinical Assessment in Neuropsychiatry (SCAN) were developed over 10 years and are part of the wider family of scales developed within the framework of the World Health Organization, which are elaborated by Sartorius & Janca (Chapter 12). A further example of the careful development of a scale suitable for widespread international use is the Composite International Diagnostic Interview (CIDI), described here by Wittchen *et al* (Chapter 13).

In addition to the recent emphasis on community-orientated mental health services, there is an increasing interest in three further research areas. With respect to therapeutic, planning and political aspects, cost evaluation has become of paramount interest, as detailed by McCrone & Weich (Chapter 10). Indeed, cost analyses have revealed that service use is more often associated with disability than symptom levels. Wiersma's review (Chapter 8) considers both the conceptual and the operational aspects of social disability. Finally, as Lehman argues (Chapter 6), the quality of patients' lives and the quality of the care they receive are important considerations, in that differences are often detected between treatment settings and service models, and because they are seen as important by the people who use mental health services.

Research instruments are the basic tools of health service evaluation. These tools must be well designed and used only by trained research and clinical staff. The recurring themes in this book are the care that is required in designing these tools, and the importance of standardising their use in different reference groups, including primary-care populations, as Narrow & Regier persuasively argue (Chapter 17). The stringent requirements for their use in different languages, for example, can be met within multi-site collaborative frameworks, such as the European Network for Mental Health Service Evaluation[1] (ENMESH). These are exacting conditions, but for optimal results such precise instruments and rigorous methods need to be further developed. As Jenkins & Singh show (Chapter 18), the consolidation of outcome measures is necessary for the extension of an evidence base that can inform improved mental health practice and mental health policy (Department of Health, 1999).

---

1. Details from Professor Aart Schene, Secretary of the ENMESH Executive Committee, Academisch Medisch Centrum, Polikliniek Psychiatrie, 9, 1105 AZ, Amsterdam, (ZO), The Netherlands (fax +31 20 56 6440).

References

DEPARTMENT OF HEALTH (1999) *The National Service Framework for Mental Health. Modern Standards and Service Models.* London: Department of Health.

THORNICROFT, G. & TANSELLA, M. (1996) *Mental Health Outcome Measures.* Heidelberg: Springer-Verlag.

—— & —— (1999) *The Mental Health Matrix. A Manual to Improve Services.* Cambridge: Cambridge University Press.

2 Statistical methods for measuring outcomes

GRAHAM DUNN

The aim of this book is to promote the routine use of outcome measures in clinical practice; the purpose of this chapter, however, is to warn care providers to think very, very carefully before routinely using such measures. Just what are the benefits of their use? What are the outcome measures intended to demonstrate? In order to try to convince the reader that there may be real difficulties in the interpretation of the results, the main body of the paper concentrates on the difficulties in the interpretation of data from a structured research project that has been specifically designed to evaluate an innovation in mental health care provision. The difficulties of interpreting haphazardly collected data as part of routine clinical or administrative practice will be far greater. One of the main purposes of an evaluation exercise is comparison: which approach to service provision is the better? If care providers really want to be involved in mental health service evaluation, then their time would be much better spent in taking part in a large, multi-centre trial.

Outcome measures in routine clinical practice

The title of this chapter might have been better formulated as "Statistical problems in the interpretation of outcomes". The main aim of the chapter is to point out the great difficulties in the analysis and interpretation of routinely collected but unstructured clinical outcome data. But it will make this point by discussing the design and analysis of research programmes, on the assumption that if readers can be convinced of the difficulties of doing worthwhile research, then they may realise how difficult it can be to make sense of data collected as part of routine clinical practice. The collection of outcome data has a cost, however well hidden that cost might be.

In the context of a research study, there are staff specifically employed to collect the data. It is a very time-consuming and expensive activity. Given the cost of collecting, recording and analysing the resulting data, one must ask whether the benefits of the exercise are worthwhile. Just what are the intended benefits? What are the data meant to show, and to whom?

It is not the intention of the present author to try to prevent the introduction of outcome measures into routine clinical practice; rather, it is to stop clinicians and other care providers from enthusiastically rushing to collect data without giving very careful thought to the costs and the potential benefits of the exercise. Much routinely collected data will be unanalysable because it is unstructured, full of holes (missing values) and laden with subjective biases. The last are likely to arise because the outcomes are generally measured by the clinicians themselves rather than by neutral observers. It is for the same reasons that many data collected as part of the exercise of medical audit also have such limited value.

The author's conclusion is that anyone really wishing to evaluate the clinical services he or she is instrumental in providing should get involved in some sort of formal and appropriately planned evaluation exercise, that is, some sort of controlled health care trial. The rest of this chapter will be concerned with statistical approaches to the design and analysis of such a trial, partly to underline the enormous difficulties in drawing inferences from outcome data, and partly to convince the reader of the benefits of multi-centre evaluations involving cluster randomisation. We start by explaining what is meant by a health care trial.

What is a health care trial?

We will assume that all clinicians are familiar with the concept of a controlled clinical trial in which the investigator assesses the relative effectiveness of competing treatments (typically, chemotherapies). Arguments in favour of the controlled trial will not be rehearsed here. According to Spitzer *et al* (1975), "The research strategy of the controlled clinical trial has been a powerful scientific tool that can avoid or minimize the errors produced either by the fashions of authoritarian pronouncement or by the oversimplifications of socio-political zealotry" (p. 161). The randomised controlled trial is the 'gold standard' (in terms of methodological rigour) against which other forms of evaluation are to be assessed.

In a traditional clinical trial, the experimental conditions are usually competing therapies and the experimental subjects are individual patients. In a health care trial, the experimental conditions are competing ways of providing a health care service and the experimental subjects may be patients but are not necessarily so. They may, for example, be care providers, managers or units of health care provision (e.g. clinics, wards or hospitals). Spitzer *et al* (1975) distinguish two types of health care trial: a health service trial, in which one assesses the mechanisms (or records) of health care provision, and a patient care trial, in which one assesses conventional therapies but the clinical outcome variables are augmented by sociopersonal data. The patient care trial is distinguished from the traditional clinical trial through the use of the non-clinical outcome measures. The latter may include the use of medical and other services, administrative problems, family burden, days of confinement to bed and absence from work or school. They may also include estimates of cost. The health service trial may include sociopersonal data among the variables under assessment, but not always.

Experiment, quasi-experiment or survey?

In his discussion on the methodology of clinical trials in psychiatry, Johnson (1989) starts with a quotation from one of the founders of clinical trial methodology, Sir Austin Bradford Hill. He describes a clinical trial as a carefully, and ethically, designed experiment with the aim of answering some precisely framed question. In its most rigorous form it demands equivalent groups of patients concurrently treated in different ways. These groups are constructed by the random allocation of patients to one or other treatment. In some instances, patients may form their own controls, different treatment being applied to them in random order and the effect compared. In principle, the method is applicable to any disease and any treatment (Hill, 1955).

The key component of a trial of this type is the random allocation of patients (or clusters of patients) to treatments. Randomisation serves three important roles. First, it is an impartial method of allocation of patients to the competing treatments. Second, it will tend to balance the treatment groups in terms of the effects of extraneous variables that may influence the outcome of treatment. One might argue that it would be more effective to match or stratify on the basis of the extraneous variables. Stratification can be an important component of trial design, but it cannot cope with the extraneous variable(s) that no one has thought of. A stratified trial should still have random allocation within the strata. The third role of randomisation is that it guarantees the validity of a subsequent statistical test of significance. If there are no treatment effects (i.e. the null hypothesis is true) then, apart from unforeseen or uncontrolled biases, the observed treatment differences must be the result of randomisation (chance). One can simply ask "What is the probability that the results have arisen solely as a result of randomisation?" and decide whether the data are consistent with the null hypothesis.

Returning to the problem of health care evaluation, randomised controlled trials of the type described by Johnson (1989) and Hill (1955) cannot always be conducted, for a variety of reasons, including logistics, ethics, cost or public opinion (Spitzer *et al*, 1975). The allocation of services to patients is often beyond the control of the evaluator. He or she simply has to act as a neutral observer of someone else's innovation. That someone else could be a clinician, a health service administrator or manager, or a politician. This does not preclude evaluation, but it does considerably weaken the validity of any conclusions arising from it.

The type of evaluative experiment that, for whatever reason, cannot include random allocation of experimental subjects to the competing treatments or services has often been called a 'quasi-experiment' (Cook & Campbell, 1979). Spitzer *et al* (1975) talk of 'health care surveys'. Cochran (1983) uses the term 'observational study', and this will be used here. We illustrate the idea of an observational study by reference to two simple alternative designs, one using historical controls and the other using concurrent ones.

In the first type of observational study, we first assess the outcome of care for a cohort of patients before the introduction of the innovation. We then introduce the innovation (e.g. a reorganisation of the clinical services or the introduction of a case-management service) and monitor the outcome for a new cohort of patients receiving it. Comparison of the outcomes for these two cohorts will, we hope, given us an estimate of the effect of the innovation.

In the second example of an observational study, we might be planning to introduce a new service in one particular clinic, hospital or health district. Before its introduction, however, we search for another clinic, hospital or district that is as similar as possible to ours – except that there are no immediate plans to change its health care services. The latter centre provides us with a concurrent control. Observation of the outcomes for a cohort of patients exposed to the innovation in one centre can be compared with the outcomes for the other cohort, in the centre in which the innovation has not been introduced. Again, comparison of the outcomes for the two cohorts of patients will, we hope, give us an estimate of the impact of the introduction of the innovation.

The weaknesses in both of the above designs are the very weaknesses that randomisation helps to rectify. First, there may be differences between the patients in the two arms of the study. Referral patterns may have inadvertently changed at about the same time as the introduction of the innovation, for example. There may be other differences between the innovative and the control arms of the trial. Innovation is usually managed by a newly appointed enthusiast (or even an evangelist) with commitment, drive and lots of energy. In the control situation there may be a run-down service managed by an ageing sceptic who is looking forward to early retirement. As Buck & Donner (1982) point out, in many health care experiments the placebo effect falls upon the providers rather than the recipients of care. The estimate of the effectiveness is likely to be biased – that is, overoptimistic: the effect of the innovation *per se* is likely to be confounded with inherent patient differences, environmental and staff differences and non-specific effects of the introduction of an innovative service (the Hawthorne effect).

Finally, we have more subtle problems of statistical inference. In the absence of randomisation we have to build in more assumptions for our significance tests, and so on. We usually pretend, quite unrealistically, for example, that the innovation and control groups have been randomly selected from a much larger population of potential treatment groups. We then ask "What is the probability of selecting by chance two groups that are as different as these two?"

Now, the above weaknesses of observational studies have not been pointed out in an attempt to stop people carrying them out, but to point out the care that is needed in drawing valid inferences from the results. We have to try to avoid biases by carefully matching centres, for example, or by ensuring that the care staff are equally well organised and motivated, with equal access to appropriate facilities in both arms of the trial. We also have to think more carefully about the use of various methods of statistical analysis (e.g. covariate adjustment) to attempt to eliminate or reduce the impact of potential sources of bias. Cochran (1983, p. 14) gives the following advice:

> "Control can usually be attempted on only a few of many variables that influence outcome; that control is likely to be only partially effective on these variables. Thus the investigator might do well to suppose that, in general, estimates from an observational study are likely to be biased. It is therefore worthwhile to think hard about what biases are most likely, and to think seriously about their sources, directions, and even their plausible magnitudes."

In the following section we continue to discuss potential problems in the interpretation of the results of an evaluation, and return again to randomisation of experimental units to the different arms of a trial. We suggest that the experimental unit should be a group (cluster) of patients, however, rather than the individuals themselves.

What are the experimental units?

In the interpretation of the outcome of an innovation we are concerned with two possible threats to the validity of our inferences. These are threats to the internal validity of our evaluation (has the change seen really arisen as the result of the innovation, or via some unintended mechanism?) and to the external validity (can we generalise our findings to other settings or services?). Interesting analogies can be drawn with the outcome of the clinical psychiatrist's well-controlled single-case study and with that of a controlled clinical trial. In the single-case study, the quality of the design of the experiment might be such that it is very safe to conclude that the therapy or management given was indeed the cause of the resulting changes to the patient. But what about other patients? One cannot safely use statistical inference to predict the behaviour of future patients from this one, possibly very atypical patient, however well controlled the study was shown to be. We need an evaluation involving several patients to find out how patients in general respond to treatment or management. The single-case study may have near-perfect internal validity, but we cannot safely generalise from it – it has very limited or even no external validity.

The above arguments apply equally cogently to the evaluation of, say, a new clinic or clinical service. Can we infer anything about clinics in general from our knowledge of this one? Do we want to? We may simply want to show that our unique clinic works very effectively and be quite happy to leave others to evaluate their own services. If, however, we wish to generalise from our evaluation to other clinics, then either we have to acknowledge that statistical inference does not play a part in this generalisation (a rather unsatisfactory option), or we need to observe the behaviour of several similar clinics and compare it with that of a control group of services. It is vital that the correct unit of observation is identified at all stages of the evaluation: in the design, in the analysis of the results and in the interpretation of the findings.

Now consider a related but slightly more subtle problem. In both qualitative and quantitative approaches to evaluation, one has to be very wary of the pitfalls of what Manly (1992), after Hurlbert (1984), called "pseudoreplication". This arises when the units of measurement (patients, clinics, districts) are not independent replicates.

Patients within a clinic will tend to have similar experiences of service provision, they share facilities and care staff, and may talk to each other and influence each other's views; they will have relatively similar outcomes (as compared with patients from different clinics), and so on. Patients, to some extent, will exhibit within-clinic or within-group correlations and they will thus not provide statistically independent items of information. The data obtained, whether qualitative or quantitative, should not be treated as if they had been obtained from a group of completely independent patients. The evaluator is not obtaining as much information as he or she may naively think! The problem is particularly acute in group-based therapies or activities. The group as a whole might do well, or it might fail. In either case the experience of the patients within the group is likely to exhibit a fairly high within-group correlation. Evaluators often treat the individual patient as the unit for their analysis when, in fact, it should be the group, clinic, and so on. What is needed is replication of groups, not replication of individual units within the group.

The above provides reasons why we may wish to summarise and interpret the outcomes at the level of groups or, in a more sophisticated analysis, simultaneously analyse variation at the level of the group as well as at the level of the individual. There are also reasons why one may wish to allocate clusters of patients rather than individual patients to the competing arms of a health care trial, that is, to change the design of the trial. One reason is the rather obvious administrative and managerial one: it is often impossible to introduce an innovative service or change in administration to only part of a service and leave the rest as it is. These changes are usually all or nothing. The cost of having two competing services within a single district, for example, may be prohibitive. Sometimes it would simply be impossible not to introduce the changes at the level of the cluster rather than the individual. Outside the mental health field, one simply needs to think of the evaluation of the fluoridation of drinking water or the introduction of car seatbelt legislation to realise that there are often overriding practical difficulties concerning the introduction of change at the level of the individual.

Another powerful argument in favour of cluster allocation is the fact that patients within a cluster are not isolated individuals (see the point about pseudoreplication, above). However, as well as correlation within groups receiving the same service, there may also be contamination between the competing arms of the trial if they are both present within a cluster. If a trial involves the evaluation of some sort of educational activity (either at the level of the patient or at that of the service providers or clinicians), then there will be contamination through 'cross-talk'. Patients may try to compensate for the perceived deficiencies in their service and may even attempt to change sides. Patient knowledge ("lack of blindness") is likely to contribute to a placebo effect, and there is also the possibility of patient resentment if one of the competing services is perceived to be better than the other. If the innovations occur at the level of clinic, hospital or district, on the other hand, all the patients within the same cluster get the same service. They do not necessarily know that there is an alternative service being offered in a different location – there will usually be no need to inform the patients that they are part of a trial, and there may be no need to seek informed consent.

The problem of informed consent, however, does need careful thought. If a trial will add an active ingredient to the traditional service – personal counselling or case management, for example – will it be necessary to consider whether it is unethical for the control groups to be aware of what they are missing? Is it ethically justified randomly to allocate this extra service at the level of the individual patient? Buck & Donner (1982) considered this problem and decided that the situation should not be regarded as analogous to the traditional drug trial. They concluded that "if group unawareness is ethically permissible in certain kinds of intervention and health care trials, it offers a means of achieving subject blindness which is attractively congruent with the method of randomisation".

The literature on trials involving randomisation of clusters has been reviewed by Donner *et al* (1990). Let us assume that we are to allocate clusters of patients (clinics, districts, and so on) randomly to the alternative services, rather than randomly allocating the individual patients themselves. One of the major concerns of the clinical trial designer is that of statistical power: how many patients are required to ensure a sufficiently high probability of finding a statistically significant effect? This requires a knowledge of patient variability and a fairly clear idea of the likely difference between the effects of the competing therapies (including expert judgement on what would constitute a *clinically* significant difference between the groups). Readers who are unfamiliar with power calculations are referred to Lachin (1981), Pocock (1983) or to Day & Graham (1991).

Once we acknowledge that the cluster is the unit of randomisation, rather than the individual patient, we then have to take this into account in our power calculations. The total number of patients entering the trial is the product of the number of clusters and the number of patients within each cluster (assuming for simplicity that the latter is constant). Cornfield (1978) provides a method for estimating sample size when large clusters, such as districts or hospitals, are being randomised, while Donner *et al* (1981) deal primarily with the case of small clusters, such as families.

The design of a trial involving cluster randomisation can involve completely randomised clusters, stratification of clusters before randomisation or, as a special case of stratification, matched pairs of clusters. Outcome could be assessed using an interval-scaled measurement, or it could be binary (e.g. well versus ill). Sample-size formulae for intervention studies involving all these possibilities are provided by Hsieh (1988). Shipley *et al* (1989) also discuss power considerations for matched-pair studies. One of the aims of stratification of clusters before randomisation is to reduce the probability of lack of comparability of patients in the two (or more) arms of the trial. Stratification can be based on the demographic characteristics of the clusters' patients, geographical and social differences between the areas within which the clusters are embedded, various administrative characteristics of the clusters, and so on. Further issues concerning cluster randomisation in large public health trials are discussed by Duffy *et al* (1992).

Returning to power calculations for trials involving complete randomisation (i.e. no stratification or matching), what is the effect on required sample sizes of randomising at the level of the cluster rather than the individual patient? It should be obvious from the discussion of the problem of pseudoreplication that we need more patients in the trial, but how many more? Basically, the size of the trial (number of patients in each arm of the trial) should be increased by a factor calculated as:

$$[1 + (m - 1)\rho] \tag{1}$$

where ρ is the intra-class correlation (the within-cluster or within-group correlation or dependence) and m the number of patients per cluster (Buck & Donner 1982). Increasing the sample size by this factor will achieve the same statistical power as would be obtained under a design with no clustering. The intra-class correlation would typically be estimated from pilot data in which several patients from a sample of clusters were assessed and the results subjected to a one-way analysis of variance (i.e. outcome measure by cluster membership) – see, for example, Dunn (1989). This analysis of variance will yield a between-cluster mean square (BMS) and a within-cluster mean square (WMS). The required estimate of the intra-class correlation is then given by:

$$\rho = (\text{BMS} - \text{WMS}) / [\text{BMS} + (m - 1)\text{WMS}] \tag{2}$$

where, as before, m is the number of patients per cluster.

The estimation of intra-class correlation coefficients is further discussed below.

Evaluation of outcome measures

Before we proceed to evaluate outcome, we need to assess the quality of the outcome measures themselves. We need to be assured that we have adequate tools for the job in hand. The discussion will not include the development of outcome measures – for this the reader is referred to Streiner & Norman (1989) and Wright & Feinstein (1992) – nor will we be concerned with validity, this being more of a substantive problem than a statistical one. Instead, we will primarily be concerned with reliability estimation, and even then with the most simple of situations. More complex examples can be found elsewhere (Dunn, 1989, 1992).

Perhaps the most important aspects of the planning of a health care trial is to check the consistency of the raters or interviewers who are to assess the outcome of the innovation(s). Typically, two or more raters will be asked to co-rate the problems or symptoms of a pilot sample of patients. We assume that all raters have assessed each of the sample of patients once and we wish to estimate a measure of agreement between these raters. For both quantitative and binary (yes/no) assessments we can carry out a two-way analysis of variance (outcome by rater and subject) and use the resulting mean squares to estimate a form of the intra-class correlation coefficient:

$$\hat{\rho}= n(\text{PMS} - \text{EMS})/[n.\text{PMS} + m.\text{RMS} + (nm - n - m)\text{EMS}] \qquad (3)$$

where n is the number of patients and m the number of raters. PMS is the patient mean square, RMS is the rater mean square and EMS is the error, or residual mean square. The dots (.) in this expression indicate multiplication. The derivation of this expression is beyond the scope of this article, but is based on the assumption that we are looking at the performance of a random selection of raters selected from a potentially much larger population of potential raters (the so-called random effects model) – see, for example, Fleiss (1987), Dunn (1989) or Streiner & Norman (1989). This intra-class correlation is a measure of reliability. In the case of a binary assessment it is also equivalent to the well known kappa coefficient; in the case of an ordinal measure of outcome, it is equivalent to the form of a weighted kappa coefficient (using quadratic weights) – see, for example, Dunn (1989) or Streiner & Norman (1989).

If the reliability exercise involved, say, the use of only one rater who replicated his or her assessment of each patient m times (a simple replication study, usually with m equal to 2), then the appropriate analysis would be a one-way analysis of variance followed by an estimation of an intra-class correlation using Equation 2 – but in this case the BMS would be the between-patient mean square and the WMS the within-patient mean square. Again, this intra-class correlation provides an estimate of reliability.

Be wary of depending on reliability coefficients provided in the literature or test manuals. They are only estimates (often based on inadequate sample sizes) and they are not fixed characteristics of a particular outcome measure. They are a measure of the proportion of the variability in the outcome measure that is explained by differences among the patients. They will vary as the heterogeneity of the patients changes and also as the heterogeneity (inconsistency) of the raters varies. That is, the reliability will depend on raters using the outcome measure and on the population of patients being assessed.

What is good reliability? Basically, the higher the better, but there is no magic threshold for reliability above which you can relax. The key problem in the context of a health care trial is the power of the trial. Power can be increased by increasing the number of subjects or by decreasing the variability of the measures (i.e. by increasing their precision or by using a more homogeneous group of patients), or both. The precision of the outcome measures will be improved by multiple assessments of each patient, but then the investigator needs to ask whether this is feasible and more cost-effective than simply increasing the number of patients in the trial. The final answer is bound to be a balance between the two.

Analysis of outcomes

This section will be very brief. The statistical analysis of large health care trials is no more the province of amateurs than the analysis of clinical trial data. We will briefly illustrate, however, the problems that the analysis needs to address. Typically, there will be a need to adjust for potentially confounding variables. This will involve some sort of analysis of covariance (either for quantitative outcome measures or for binary ones). This will be particularly true for observational studies in which we are trying to convince the sceptic that we have allowed for sources of bias (Cook & Campbell, 1979; Cochran, 1983). It may also be true for randomised trials. Here, the aim is usually to improve precision, although covariate adjustment may also cope with lack of balance that has arisen by chance in the randomisation. In the analysis of a randomised clinical trial it is an illogical and pointless exercise to carry out significance tests for differences between baseline measures. Unless someone has been cheating, you know that the results have arisen by chance. Important prognostic factors should be included as covariates, whether or not there are statistically significant differences on these variables across groups. If the analysis is being carried out on data arising from cluster randomisation, then the covariates can be measured either at the level of the individual patient, or at the level of the cluster, or both, and the analysis will need to take this into account (Goldstein, 1999).

In recent years there has been considerable stress laid on the reporting of confidence intervals in the medical literature (Gardner & Altman, 1989). The construction of confidence intervals for effect measures arising from cluster randomisation trials is described by Donner & Klar (1993). More complex statistical analyses of cluster-randomised trials will involve modelling of outcome data in which it is explicitly acknowledged that there are different levels of random variation in the measurements. There will be random variation of measurement errors among replications within patients, random variation between patients within clusters and random variations between clusters. Some form of random-effects model will be needed for the data. Readers are referred to Goldstein (1999) for a general discussion, and to Collett (1991, pp. 279–280) for a description of random effects models for binary outcome measures.

Conclusions

It should be clear from the above that the author has a lot of misgivings about the design of many research studies to demonstrate the impact of innovations in the provision of health care. What about the use of outcome measures in routine clinical practice? It would clearly be much more difficult to defend any particular interpretation put on the results. If it is so difficult to interpret the results of a carefully designed research study, of what possible use could they be in the haphazard world of routine clinical practice? The present author is clearly putting himself in the position of the devil's advocate and is accordingly putting forward a particularly strong view against the clinician routinely collecting outcome data. Nevertheless, it would be prudent of the clinician to answer this question convincingly before committing valuable resources to such an exercise.

Lest the reader is inclined to dismiss the author as a sceptical armchair theorist, he has been involved in several trials, including, for example, a trial to evaluate the effects of case management after severe head injury (Greenwood *et al*, 1994). It was a trial that exhibited many of the problems detailed in this article and also illustrates some of the technical solutions. The trial involved the comparison of the outcomes of care of patients from six hospitals in north London. Three of these hospitals were provided with the services of a case manager, three acted as controls. The whole point of the evaluation was comparison. The case managers were convinced that they were doing a good job and none of the outcome measures would have led them to doubt their beliefs. If there had been no control group of hospitals, there would have been no reason to doubt the effectiveness of their service. Comparison of the outcomes for case-managed patients with those of the controls, however, failed to demonstrate any benefits of case management. Case management led to an increase in rates of referrals to specialist clinical services, but this did not appear to lead to any demonstrable benefits to the patients. Note that it is not the collection of outcome data as such that is important to the evaluation of a clinical service. On their own the data are of very limited use. Only when they are used for comparison, and only then if that comparison is suitably controlled, do outcome data really become useful.

In conclusion, the present author has serious doubts about the benefits of routinely collected outcome data, but is convinced that there is a need for large multi-centre evaluations of mental health care services, possibly using cluster randomisation as described by Donner *et al* (1990). In this way, care providers who wish to evaluate their services can do so within the context of a carefully controlled and properly resourced research study. Unfortunately, none of the trials reviewed by Donner *et al* concerned mental health care services (although one or two involved patients from mental hospitals and others were concerned with health education), and it is, therefore, difficult to direct the reader to successful examples!

References

BUCK, C. & DONNER, A. (1982) The design of controlled experiments in the evaluation of non-therapeutic interventions. *Journal of Chronic Disorders*, **35**, 531–538.

COCHRAN, W. G. (1983) *Planning and Analysis of Observational Studies*. Chichester: Wiley.

COLLETT, D. (1991) *Modelling Binary Data*. London: Chapman and Hall.

COOK, T. D. & CAMPBELL, T. D. (1979) *Quasi-experimentation: Design and Analysis Issues for Field Settings*. Boston: Houghton-Mifflin.

CORNFIELD, J. (1978) Randomization by group: a formal analysis. *American Journal of Epidemiology*, **108**, 100–102.

DAY, S. J. & GRAHAM, D. F. (1991) Sample size estimation for comparing two or more treatment groups in clinical trials. *Statistics in Medicine*, **10**, 33–43.

DONNER, A., BIRKETT, N. & BUCK, C. (1981) Randomization by cluster – sample size requirements and analysis. *American Journal of Epidemiology*, **114**, 906–914.

——, BROWN, K. S. & BRASHER, P. (1990) A methodological review of non-therapeutic intervention trials employing cluster randomization, 1979–1989. *International Journal of Epidemiology*, **19**, 795–800.

—— & KLAR, N. (1993) Confidence interval construction for effect measures arising from cluster randomization trials. *Journal of Clinical Epidemiology*, **46**, 123–131.

DUFFY, S. W., SOUTH, M. C. & DAY, N. E. (1992) Cluster randomization in large public health trials: the importance of antecedent data. *Statistics in Medicine*, **11**, 307–316.

DUNN, G. (1989) *Design and Analysis of Reliability Studies: The Statistical Evaluation of Measurement Errors*. London: Edward Arnold.

—— (1992) Design and analysis of reliability studies. *Statistical Methods in Medical Research*, **1**, 123–157.

FLEISS, J. L. (1987) *Design and Analysis of Clinical Experiments*. Chichester: Wiley.

GARDNER, M. J. & ALTMAN, D. G. (1989) *Statistics with Confidence*. London: BMJ.

GOLDSTEIN, H. (1999) *Multilevel Statistical Models* (2nd end). London: Arnold.

GREENWOOD, R. J., MACMILLAN, T. M., BROOKS, D. N., *et al* (1994) An investigation into the effects of case management after severe head injury. *British Medical Journal*, **308**, 1199–1205.

HILL, A. B. (1955) *Introduction to Medical Statistics* (5th edn). London: Lancet.

HSIEH, F. Y. (1988) Sample size formulae for intervention studies with the cluster as unit of randomization. *Statistics in Medicine*, **8**, 1195–1201.

HURLBERT, S. H. (1984) Pseudoreplication in the design of ecological field experiments. *Ecological Monographs*, **54**, 187–211.

JOHNSON, A. L. (1989) Methodology of clinical trials in psychiatry. In *Research Methods in Psychiatry* (eds C. Freeman & P. Tyrer), pp. 12–45. London: Gaskell.

LACHIN, J. M. (1981) Introduction to sample size determination and power analysis for clinical trials. *Controlled Clinical Trials*, **2**, 93–113.

MANLY, B. F. J. (1992) *The Design and Analysis of Research Studies*. Cambridge: Cambridge University Press.

POCOCK, S. (1983) *Clinical Trials: A Practical Approach*. Chichester: Wiley.

SHIPLEY, M. J., SMITH, P. G & DRAMAIX, M. (1989) Calculation of power for matched pair studies when randomization is by group. *International Journal of Epidemiology*, **18**, 457–461.

SPITZER, W. O., FEINSTEIN, A. R. & SACKETT, D. L. (1975) What is a health care trial? *Journal of the American Medical Association*, **233**, 161–163.

STREINER, D. L. & NORMAN, G. R. (1989) *Health Measurement Scales: A Practical Guide to Their Development and Use*. Oxford: Oxford University Press.

WRIGHT, J. G. & FEINSTEIN, A. R. (1992) A comparative contrast of clinimetric and psychometric methods for constructing indexes and rating scales. *Journal of Clinical Epidemiology*, **45**, 1201–1218.

3 Global functioning scales

MICHAEL PHELAN, TIL WYKES and HOWARD GOLDMAN

Global functioning is a rather vague and abstract concept that tries to encompass a broad canvas of behaviour and abilities. In this chapter, assessment schedules that try to provide a measure of a person's level of functioning in all or nearly all areas of life are reviewed. The schedules vary in their approaches. Instrumental behaviours, which encompass the various prerequisite activities for an independent social life, feature strongly, along with impaired performance in major social roles, living skills and overall level of disability (Wykes, 1992).

There is a close and complex relationship between mental illness and impairment of global functioning. At times, impaired functioning such as poor self-care will be the only visible sign of mental illness and may be the most distressing feature for the sufferer. The level of support and care needed by a person is likely to be closely correlated with the level of functioning. Although impairment of functioning is usually viewed as a consequence of mental illness, it may at times be a significant causal or maintaining factor in specific disorders.

The differing uses of schedules measuring levels of function in mental health research and practice have been reviewed by Kane *et al* (1985). They suggested three divisions: epidemiological studies that compare levels of functioning among those with and without mental disorders and within similar diagnostic groups; longitudinal studies that examine the effects of mental illness on levels of functioning; and case-finding studies, especially in primary care. In addition, a measure of global functioning is a useful outcome measure for mental health clinicians. Such measures are important predictors of service use and can provide important information for service planners.

Before examining individual schedules, it is important to consider the tensions inherent in trying to measure global functioning. The majority of the scales reviewed in this chapter are concerned with measuring levels of functioning that are below normal, and in general ignore higher than average levels of functioning. Underpinning this practical approach there is an assumption that "normal" functioning can be defined as recording no problems on a schedule. Clearly, any such norms may be dependent on individual factors such as age and culture, and may vary over time. In terms of social roles, normality is particularly difficult to define, with, for example, the changing role of women in Western societies and the different roles given to older people in Western and non-Western cultures.

A second difficulty facing those designing measures of functioning is whether to include psychiatric symptoms. The distinction between impairments of functioning and psychiatric symptoms is often blurred. Some impairments of functioning, such as poor concentration, may be viewed as psychiatric symptoms in their own right. It is also important to distinguish between overt and covert symptoms, and to consider their relationship to impairment of functioning. Overt symptoms, such as pressure of speech, will usually impinge on functioning. In contrast, covert symptoms, such as a fixed delusional belief, may not directly affect functioning, but may have an indirect effect, for instance if the person talks to others about an abnormal belief. Authors vary in their approach to this dilemma, although in most of the scales there is at least some reference to overt symptoms.

The third area of difficulty is the establishment of validity. To ensure content validity for a schedule measuring a concept as broad as global functioning requires that a large number of areas be included, but this has to be balanced with the need to keep the schedule to a practical length. The lack of any 'gold standard' measure of functioning poses problems in determining concurrent validity. Authors frequently compare scores with levels of service utilisation as a broad confirmation of validity. The danger behind this approach is that the level of service utilisation may have been one of the factors considered by the original rater when deciding the final score. Finally, when considering the construct validity of global functioning it is important to consider the interactions between the many diverse factors that contribute to the concept, such as personality, intelligence, physical abilities, social environment, the level of support received from others, the perception of potential abilities by others and rewards obtained.

The characteristics of the *ideal* scale for measuring functioning are similar to those of any other scale in the field of mental health: applicable to patients with disabilities of differing severity and aetiology, as well as to patients from a wide range of cultural backgrounds; reliable, valid and sensitive to change; and usable by staff during the course of routine work. In addition, the perfect global functioning scale would produce a total rating that would accurately and equally reflect all aspects of a patient's functioning. The schedules reviewed in this chapter all have their strengths, but none could be said to be ideal. Their main characteristics are summarised in Table 3.1. We have included the small number of schedules that attempt to summarise all aspects of a patient's functioning with a single rating, as well as 'social functioning' scales that are broad enough in their coverage to be considered as global measures of functioning.

Global rating scales

The earliest-published global rating scale is the Health Sickness Rating Scale (HSRS; Luborsky, 1962). It was intended as a simple measure of change over time in the condition of psychotherapy patients. During the development of this scale the author concluded that there were seven key factors that should be incorporated into a global rating of health: ability to function autonomously, symptom severity, degree of discomfort, effect upon the environment, utilisation of abilities, quality of interpersonal relationships, and breadth and depth of interests. A scale of 0–100 was used, with eight anchor points, ranging from "an ideal state of complete functioning, integration, resiliency in the face of stress, and social effectiveness" to "any condition which, if unattended, would quickly result in the patient's death, but not necessarily by his own hand". In addition, 30 pre-rated case vignettes were provided for extra guidance.

Twelve years after the HSRS was first published, a review of 18 published studies conducted on a wide range of patient groups concluded that when used by experienced clinicians the scale is a reliable measure of mental health and correlates with a variety of more time-consuming scales (Luborsky & Bachrach, 1974). The authors concluded that reliability is correlated with the comprehensiveness of the information available to the raters, and have interpreted the finding that patients within any diagnostic category have a range of scores as indicating that the score is important additional information for the clinician.

Attempts to improve upon the HSRS resulted in the development of the Global Assessment Scale (GAS; Endicott *et al*, 1976). While maintaining the same basic structure, the authors introduced a number of changes in an attempt to simplify the scale. The number of anchor points was increased from eight to ten. Any reference to diagnostic categories was removed; instead, the anchor points rely on

TABLE 3.1
Summary of schedules suitable for the assessment of global functioning

Schedule	Description	Strengths/weaknesses	Uses
Global Assessment Scale (GAS; Endicott *et al*, 1976)	Single rating on 0–100 scale. Modified version used for DSM–IV	Quick and easy to administer, and widely used; combines symptoms and functioning in single scale; limited reliability amongst practising clinicians	Clinical and research
Disabilities Assessment Schedule (DAS; WHO, 1988)	11-item scale, covering social roles and disabilities	Appears to be valid and reliable, but only a few published studies describing its use; difficult for untrained staff	Clinical and research; but users need training
Denver Community Mental Health Questionnaire (Ciarlo & Riehman, 1977)	61-item schedule, with emphasis on substance abuse and patient satisfaction	Suitable for a wide range of patients; limited coverage of specific behaviours	Only of use in specific situations due to limited coverage
Psychiatric Status Schedule (PSS; Spitzer *et al*, 1970); Psychiatric Evaluation Form (PEF; Endicott & Spitzer, 1972*a*); Current and Past Psychopathology Scale (CAPPS; Endicott & Spitzer, 1972*b*)	Developed in tandem; PSS (321 items) administered to patient, PEF (28 items), and CAPPS (130 items) completed by clinician	Suitable for wide range of patients; limited coverage of social roles	Too long for routine clinical use, suitable for research
Morningside Rehabilitation Status Scale (MRSS; Affleck & McGuire, 1984)	4 individual areas rated on 8-point scale	Easy to use for staff who know patient well; established reliability but validity unclear	More suitable for clinical use than research

TABLE 3.1 (contd...)

Schedule	Description	Strengths/weaknesses	Uses
Social Behaviour Schedule (SBS; Wykes & Sturt, 1986)	21-item schedule; emphasis on observable behaviours	Easy to use, no training; good reliability and validity; suitable for more severely ill patients	Clinical and research
REHAB (Baker & Hall, 1988)	23-item schedule, covering general and deviant behaviour	Easy to use; impressive psychometric properties; only suitable for patients in residential or hospital setting	Clinical and research
Life Skills Profile (LSP; Rosen *et al*, 1989)	39-item schedule covering disability and functioning	Easy to use; free of jargon; currently few published studies	Clinical and research
Social Functioning Scale (Birchwood *et al*, 1990)	7 areas of social functioning covered; designed originally for family intervention studies	Appears to have good psychometric properties, and to be acceptable to patients	Clinical and research
Health of the Nation Outcome Scales (HoNOS; Wing *et al*, 1998)	12 domains covering clinical and social areas	Extensive trials and routine use in recent years. Quick to use, and suitable for wide range of patients	Clinical and research
Social Functioning Schedule (SFS; Remmington & Tyrer, 1979); Social Maladjustment Schedule (SMS; Clare & Cairns, 1978)	12-item (SFS) and 48-item (SMS) schedules; designed specifically for people with non-psychotic illness	Few published studies; only limited psychometric data for both scales	Due to length SMS suitable for research, SFS suitable for both

a combination of specific behavioural characteristics and symptoms. In addition, the authors did not believe it necessary to provide case vignettes, used when completing the HSRS, but did provide guidelines on difficult rating decisions, such as when the level of functioning varies during the evaluation period. The authors have shown that low GAS scores are positively correlated with readmission rates in former in-patients. In five separate studies, the interrater reliability ranged from 0.61 to 0.91. The lowest reliability was among practising clinicians, as opposed to researchers, a worrying finding that has been described by others (Clark & Friedman, 1983; Plakun *et al*, 1987). Systematic training with periodic refresher courses appears to improve reliability among clinical staff (Dworkin *et al*, 1990).

Diagnostic and Statistical Manual (DSM)

As part of the multi-axial approach of DSM–III (American Psychiatric Association, 1980), axis V was introduced as a global measure of "adaptive functioning". A seven-point scale, ranging from superior to grossly impaired, was used. During DSM–III field trials of axis V ratings, intra-class correlation coefficients for interrater and test–retest reliability were 0.80 and 0.69, respectively (Spitzer & Forman, 1979). However, when the scale was used by a group of multi-disciplinary clinical workers, reliability was as low as 0.49 (Fernando *et al*, 1986). When case summaries of adolescents were rated, a slightly higher reliability of 0.57 was reported (Rey *et al*, 1988). Overall, the published studies are limited, and although reliability for axis V was found to be higher than for axis IV, the reliability demonstrated has never been especially good (Rey *et al*, 1987).

A variety of approaches were taken to examine the validity of DSM–III axis V ratings. A number of studies compared the ratings between people in different diagnostic groups (Mezzich *et al*, 1987; Skodol *et al*, 1988; Westermeyer, 1988). Together these findings indicated that people with a psychotic disorder score lower than those with a neurotic disorder, who in turn score lower than those with no diagnosis. One study (Schrader *et al*, 1986), however, found no difference between psychotic, organic and non-psychotic patient groups.

Concurrent validity has been examined by comparing ratings with other measures of adaptive functioning. Low ratings have been found to be positively correlated with low social and occupational functioning scores on the Psychiatric Epidemiology Research Interview (Skodol *et al*, 1988) and negatively correlated with ratings of social networks (Westermeyer & Neider, 1988).

With the advent of DSM–III–R (American Psychiatric Association, 1987), the Global Assessment of Functioning Scale (GAF) was introduced to replace the seven-point scale of DSM–III, with the hope that it would increase the usefulness of the axis. The stated aim was that axis V would be a measure of "a person's psychological, social, and occupational functioning", and that ratings should generally reflect the current need for treatment or care. The GAF itself is a modified version of the GAS (see above), with some minor changes in the wording of the anchor points. The other significant change was that both the highest level of functioning during the previous year and the current level of functioning are recorded, whereas the GAS rates only the lowest level of functioning during the previous week.

The major limitation of all of the above scales is that symptoms and functioning are combined to produce a single rating. There were proposals (see Goldman *et al*, 1992) that these two factors should be rated separately for DSM–IV (American Psychiatric Association, 1994). When this approach gained routine use by mental health practitioners, satisfactory reliability was obtained for the total GAF score and for the separate symptom and disability measures. Jones *et al* (1995) demonstrated differences in the relationships between the three scores and medication and support needs, indicating the usefulness of this separation.

In DSM–IV the GAF is still included as the major axis V assessment. However, an alternative assessment is also included – the Social and Occupational Functioning Assessment Scale (SOFAS), which is similar to the GAF, but with no mention of psychiatric symptoms. It is suggested that SOFAS may be useful in certain settings to monitor social and occupational disability independent of the severity of psychological symptoms, but doubt has been cast on its validity (Roy-Byrne *et al*, 1996).

Disabilities Assessment Schedule

The Disabilities Assessment Schedule (DAS; Schubert *et al*, 1986; World Health Organization, 1988) has been proposed as a measure of global disabilities for ICD–10 (World Health Organization, 1992). Ratings for the DAS are based on information from the person who has had the most contact with the patient over the previous month. There are 11 items, mostly rated on an eight-point scale. Seven of the items are specifically concerned with roles, while the others cover social withdrawal, self-care, social contacts and interests and information. In contrast to the GAF, symptoms are not directly included.

Interrater reliability appears to be high, with kappa coefficients ranging from 0.82 to 0.85 for the different items. Some degree of validity has been established by demonstrating a correlation of 0.79 between the scale, the GAS score and the independent ratings of psychiatrists. However, the schedule has been criticised for being ambiguous in phrasing and being liable to cause difficulty for untrained raters (Rosen *et al*, 1989).

Social functioning scales

Social functioning scales are concerned with three broad areas of human life: social attainment, social role performance and instrumental behaviour (Wykes & Hurry, 1991; Wykes, 1992). In this review, scales that assess only social attainment, such as the Psychiatric Epidemiology Research Interview (Dohrenwend *et al*, 1981), have been excluded. Such scales have the advantage of being easily completed, and are suited to large-scale epidemiological studies. However, social attainment is greatly influenced by social conditions and local culture, and does not provide an accurate guide to individual global functioning. Similar limitations apply to schedules that are limited to assessing social roles, such as the MRC Social Role Performance Schedule (Hurry & Sturt, 1981). Although greater precision is possible when assessing roles rather than attainments, again cultural differences mean that individual functioning cannot be accurately gauged from role performance alone. Thus, we have considered only those social functioning scales that measure instrumental behaviour either alone or in combination with social attainment and roles. Additionally, we have included only those schedules that are sufficiently broad to be considered global measures, are reasonably quick and easy to administer and have robust psychometric properties. For more detailed surveys of social functioning scales the comprehensive reviews by Weissman *et al* (1981) and Wallace (1986) are recommended.

Denver Community Mental Health Questionnaire

The Denver Community Mental Health Questionnaire (DCMHQ; Ciarlo & Riehman, 1977) was designed to assess the wide range of people presenting at a community mental health centre, and is suitable for people with a wide range of mental health disorders. It comprises 61 items, and takes between 30 and 60 minutes to administer. Twelve areas are covered: psychological distress, interpersonal isolation from friends, interpersonal isolation from family, productivity at work, productivity at home, dependency on public agencies, alcohol abuse, soft drug use, hard drug use, client satisfaction with services, interpersonal aggression with friends, and legal difficulties. The time frame is between 24 hours and the last month. Reported interrater reliabilities range from 0.85 to 1.0 for 10 of the 12 areas (two were not tested). Internal consistency reliabilities range from 0.52 to 0.96. Significant differences in all the areas, except interpersonal aggression, have been found between patients and a random sample of Denver residents. The DCMHQ is distinctive for its emphasis on substance abuse (32 of the items) and the inclusion of service satisfaction. However, as a consequence it is limited in its coverage of instrumental behaviours.

Psychiatric Status Schedule

The Psychiatric Status Schedule (PSS; Spitzer *et al*, 1970) is a 321-item schedule covering 15 areas of psychopathology and five social roles (wage earner, housekeeper, student or trainee, spouse and parent). The interview takes between 30 and 50 minutes. The time frame is the last week for psychopathology items and the last month for role items. Interrater reliability coefficients range from 0.57 to 0.99. Scores discriminate between in-patients, out-patients and non-patients, and are correlated with other measures of psychopathology such as the Brief Psychiatric Rating Scale and the Beck Depression Inventory. The roles in the PSS will not be relevant to more disabled patients.

Psychiatric Evaluation Form

The Psychiatric Evaluation Form (PEF; Endicott & Spitzer, 1972*a*) is a 28-item schedule that was designed in tandem with the PSS, and there is considerable overlap in their content. The PEF is designed to be completed by experienced clinicians using information from a variety of sources, rather than from a direct patient interview. Ratings are on a six-point scale, and overall scores for severity of illness and role performance are obtained.

The Current and Past Psychopathology Scale (CAPPS; Endicott & Spitzer, 1972*b*) is a longer version of the PEF and includes an additional 13 psychopathology items and 130 items concerning previous social adjustment, psychopathology and personality characteristics from the age of 12 years to 1 month before completion. Interrater reliabilities range from 0.68 to 1.0 for individual items, and total scores discriminate between different diagnostic groups of patients. As with the PSS, the CAPPS is more appropriate for less disabled patients.

Morningside Rehabilitation Status Scale

This is a brief scale designed to measure the "main areas of change relevant to the rehabilitation of psychiatric patients" (Affleck & McGuire, 1984). Four areas (dependency, occupation and leisure activity, social isolation, and current symptoms) are measured on an eight-point scale. The time taken will vary from a few minutes to half an hour, depending on how well the rater knows the patient. The time frame is the last month. Interrater reliability for the four areas ranges from 0.68 to 0.90.

Social Behaviour Scale

The Social Behaviour Schedule (SBS; Wykes & Sturt, 1986) is designed to measure the functioning of people with severe and long-lasting disabilities, and in particular to identify behaviours that result in dependence on psychiatric care. It is based on the Wing Ward Behaviour Scale, which was published over 30 years ago. It is a 21-item schedule, with most items rated on a five-point scale. The scores discriminate between patients living in accommodation with differing levels of support. Reliability studies have provided data on interrater and test–retest reliability for different settings and informants, with kappa coefficients ranging from 0.67 to 0.94. Internal consistency for the two total problem scores is 0.71 and 0.75. It has been used in numerous studies on patients in institutions and in the community, as well as across different cultures.

REHAB

This is a schedule specifically designed to assess people with long-term or disabling psychiatric handicap who at the time of assessment are "living in, or attending, a residential or day care institutional setting" (Baker & Hall, 1988). One of the aims of the authors was to design a scale that could correctly identify patients who have the potential for living outside hospital. There are 23 items, 7 covering deviant behaviour and 16 covering general behaviour. Each item is measured along a visual analogue scale. The psychometric properties have been extensively studied, and norms for over 800 patients are available. Interrater reliability of the individual items ranges from 0.61 to 0.92, and total scores discriminate day-hospital patients, long-stay in-patients and in-patients selected for a predischarge training programme (Baker & Hall, 1983). The REHAB is easy to use, is suitable for patients with a high level of disability, and provides a broad measure of behaviour. It is particularly suitable as a repeated measure during the routine evaluation of a treatment plan. A user's guide and other training material are available.

Life Skills Profile

The Life Skills Profile (LSP; Rosen *et al*, 1989) is a measure of disability and function designed specifically for people with schizophrenia. Five areas are addressed (self-care, non-turbulence, social contact, communication and responsibility) with 39 individual items that are rated on a four-point scale. It does not contain any functioning measures directly related to symptoms. Reported internal consistency ranges from 0.67 to 0.88, and the mean interrater reliability coefficient is 0.68. This is a carefully developed schedule, which, although specifically designed from people with schizophrenia, can be used in a range of serious psychiatric disorders. It is suitable for routine use by a range of professional staff.

Social Functioning Scale

The Social Functioning Scale (Birchwood *et al*, 1990) was devised to be a measure of social functioning in patients with schizophrenia. The original purpose of the scale was to measure the efficacy of family interventions. The scale covers seven areas: social engagement/withdrawal; interpersonal behaviour; pro-social activities; recreation; independence–competence; independence–performance; and employment/occupation. The authors of the scale have shown its reliability, validity and sensitivity, among people with schizophrenia, and state that it is acceptable to patients and their families, and requires little time to complete. There are no reasons why use of the scale need be limited to the evaluation of family interventions.

Health of the Nation Outcome Scales

The Health of the Nation Outcome Scales (HoNOS) were developed with the aim of finding a simple measure of mental health and social functioning, which would be suitable for routine clinical use. The HoNOS comprise 12 domains, which are rated on a five-point scale, from 0 (no problem) to 4 (severe or very severe problem), and the sum of the ratings is the total score. Eight of the items concern mental state, and potentially dangerous behaviour (including drug and alcohol use), and are related to social activities and situation. The HoNOS are quick to use, and the reliability and validity were established during development (Wing *et al*, 1998). There are versions for children and elderly people. Subsequent use in routine practice has indicated that, as with so many other scales, reliability is less good when completed by clinical staff (Bebbington *et al*, 1999) and that although routine use is feasible, the information obtained is of limited value for care planning (Sharma *et al*, 1999).

Instruments for non-psychotic patients

Social Functioning Schedule

The Social Functioning Schedule (SFS; Remington & Tyrer, 1979) is primarily designed to measure the level of social functioning in people with a non-psychotic psychiatric disorder. Twelve main areas of functioning are included, and these are rated along a 10 cm visual analogue scale. Symptoms are not included. The time frame is the last month. Interrater reliability for the different sections ranges from 0.45 to 0.81 (mean 0.62) when audiotaped interviews are used, and from 0.5 to 0.8 with independent interviews. The scale discriminates between people with personality disorders and those with other psychiatric disorders.

Social Maladjustment Schedule

The Social Maladjustment Schedule (SMS; Clare & Cairns, 1978) was designed to assess social maladjustment and dysfunction in six main areas: housing, occupation and social role, economic situation, leisure and social activities, family and domestic relationships, and marital relationships. Answers are rated on a four-point response scale, and total scores for objective conditions, instrumental performance, satisfaction and overall maladjustment are produced. It was designed for use with patients with chronic neurotic disorders. A 45-minute structured interview is required with either the patient or an informant. The authors have reported interrater reliability data for 17 of the 48 items, with weighted kappas ranging from 0.62 to 0.94 (there were insufficient data for other items).

Conclusions

The scales reviewed in this paper illustrate the difficulties in trying to measure global functioning in people with severe mental illness, and the different approaches to the problem. During the development of these instruments, psychometric properties are often not fully explored. Reliability studies are often limited in their scope, and unsophisticated statistics, such as correlations, used for analysis. Validity studies are frequently limited to examining associations with diagnosis and service utilisation. A tendency for ratings to be influenced by the type of care received, for instance attendance at a day hospital, may, in particular, reduce sensitivity to change in the most disabled patients. In this same group, many of the social roles incorporated into some of the scales will be inappropriate, and undue weight may be given to the patients' behaviour and symptoms.

Despite these reservations, global functioning scales play an important role in mental health service evaluative research, as well as routine clinical work. Although outcome assessments clearly need to focus on a wide range of areas, functioning should be identified as a critical domain within batteries of outcome measures. The actual functioning measure that is selected will depend on the precise situation. For instance, for large, population-based surveys, a quick measure such as the GAF may be suitable. Research studies aimed at specific groups of patients can select more comprehensive measures suitable for the population studied and the resources available.

Within routine clinical work there is a great demand for a simple measure of functioning, and it is essential that the limitations of such measures are appreciated. The common finding that reliability improves with rater training indicates the need for regular training. In addition, staff must be encouraged to interpret the results with caution, and not view them in isolation from other outcome measures.

References

AFFLECK, J. W. & McGUIRE, R. J. (1984) The measurement of psychiatric rehabilitation status: a review of the needs and a new scale. *British Journal of Psychiatry*, **145**, 517–525.

AMERICAN PSYCHIATRIC ASSOCIATION (1980) *Diagnostic and Statistical Manual of Mental Disorders* (3rd edn) (DSM–III). Washington, DC: APA.

—— (1987) *Diagnostic and Statistical Manual of Mental Disorders* (3rd edn, revised) (DSM–III–R). Washington, DC: APA.

—— (1994) *Diagnostic and Statistical Manual of Mental Disorders* (4th edn) (DSM–IV). Washington, DC: APA.

BAKER, R. & HALL, J. N. (1983) *Rehabilitation Evaluation of Hall and Baker (REHAB)*. Aberdeen: Vine Publishing.

—— & —— (1988) REHAB: a new assessment instrument for chronic psychiatric patients. *Schizophrenia Bulletin*, **14**, 95–113.

BEBBINGTON, P., BRUGHA, T., HILL, T., *et al* (1999) Validation of the Health of the Nation Outcome Scales (HoNOS). *British Journal of Psychiatry*, **174**, 389–394.

BIRCHWOOD, M., SMITH, J., COCHRANE, R., *et al* (1990) The Social Functioning Scale. The development and validation of a new scale of social adjustment for use in family intervention programmes with schizophrenic patients. *British Journal of Psychiatry*, **157**, 853–859.

CIARLO, J. A. & RIEHMAN, J. (1977) The Denver Community Mental Health Questionnaire: development of a multidimensional program evaluation. In *Program Evaluation for Mental Health: Methods, Strategies and Participants* (eds R. D. Coursey, G. A. Specter, S. A. Murrell & B. Hunt), pp. 131–167. New York: Grune and Stratton.

CLARE, A. W. & CAIRNS, V. E. (1978) Design, development and use of a standardised interview to assess social maladjustment and dysfunction in community studies. *Psychological Medicine*, **8**, 589–604.

CLARK, A. & FRIEDMAN, M. J. (1983) Nine standardised scales for evaluating treatment outcomes in a mental health clinic. *Journal of Clinical Psychology*, **39**, 939–950.

DOHRENWEND, B. S., COOK, D. & DOHRENWEND, B. P. (1981) Measurement of social functioning in community populations. In *What Is a Case?* (eds J. K. Wing, P. Bebbington & L. Robbins), pp. 183–201. London: Grant McIntyre.

DWORKIN, R. J., FRIEDMAN, L. C., TELSCHOW, R. L., *et al* (1990) The longitudinal use of the Global Assessment Scale in multiple-rater situations. *Community Mental Health Journal*, **26**, 335–344.

ENDICOTT, J. & SPITZER, R. L. (1972*a*) What another rating scale? The Psychiatric Evaluation Form. *Journal of Nervous and Mental Disorders*, **154**, 88–104.

—— & —— (1972*b*) Current and Past Psychopathology Scales (CAPPS): rationale, reliability, and validity. *Archives of General Psychiatry*, **27**, 678–687.

——, ——, FLEISS, J. L., *et al* (1976) The Global Assessment Scale. *Archives of General Psychiatry*, **33**, 766–771.

FERNANDO, T., MELLSOP, G., NELSON, K., *et al* (1986) The reliability of axis V of DSM–III. *American Journal of Psychiatry*, **143**, 752–755.

GOLDMAN, H. H., SKODOL, A. E. & LAVE, T. R. (1992) Revising axis V for DSM–IV: a review of measures of social functioning. *American Journal of Psychiatry*, **149**, 1148–1156.

HURRY, J. & STURT, E. (1981) Social performance in a population sample: relation to psychiatric symptoms. In *What Is a Case?* (eds J. K. Wing, P. Bebbington & L. Robbins) pp. 202–213. London: Grant McIntyre.

JONES, S. H., THORNICROFT, G., COFFEY, M. *et al* (1995) A brief mental health outcome scale. Reliability and validity of the Global Assessment of Functioning (GAF). *British Journal of Psychiatry*, **166**, 654–659.

KANE, R. A., KANE, R. L. & ARNOLD, S. (1985) *Measuring Social Functioning in Mental Health Studies: Concepts and Instruments*. Mental Health Service System Reports, Series DN No.5 NMH. Washington DC: US Government Printing Office.

LUBORSKY, L. (1962) Clinicians' judgements of mental health. A proposed scale. *Archives of General Psychiatry*, **7**, 407–417.

—— & BACHRACH, H. (1974) Factors influencing clinician's judgements of mental health. *Archives of General Psychiatry*, **31**, 292–299.

MEZZICH, J. E., FABREGA, H., JR & COFFMAN, G. A. (1987) Multiaxial characterisation of depressive patients. *Journal of Nervous and Mental Disorders*, **175**, 339–346.

PLAKUN, E. M., MULLER, J. P. & BURKHARDT, P. E. (1987) The significance of borderline and schizotypal overlap. *Hillside Journal of Clinical Psychiatry*, **9**, 47–54.

REMMINGTON, M. & TYRER, P. (1979) The Social Functioning Schedule – a brief semi-structured interview. *Social Psychiatry*, **14**, 151–157.

REY, J. M., PLAPP, J. M., STEWARD, G. W., *et al* (1987) Reliability of the psychosocial axis of DSM–III in an adolescent population. *British Journal of Psychiatry*, **150**, 228–234.

——, STEWARD, G. W., PLAPP, J. M., *et al* (1988) Validity of axis V of DSM–III and other measures of adaptive functioning. *Acta Psychiatrica Scandinavica*, **77**, 534–542.

ROSEN, A., HADZI-PAVLOVIC, D. & PARKER, G. (1989) The Life Skills Profile: a measure assessing function and disability in schizophrenia. *Schizophrenia Bulletin*, **15**, 325–337.

ROY-BYRNE, P., DAGADAKIS, C., UNUTZER, J., *et al* (1996) Evidence for limited validity of the revised global assessment of functioning scale. *Psychiatric Services*, **47**, 864–866.

SCHRADER, G., GORDON, M. & HARCOURT, R. (1986) The usefulness of DSM–III axis IV and V assessments. *American Journal of Psychiatry*, **143**, 904–907.

SCHUBERT, C., KRUMM, B., BIEHL, H., *et al* (1986) Measurement of social disability in a schizophrenic patient group: definition, assessment and outcome over two years in a cohort of schizophrenic patients of recent onset. *Social Psychiatry*, **21**, 1–9.

SHARMA, V. K., WILKINSON, G. & FEAR, S. (1999) Health of the Nation Outcome Scales. A case study in general psychiatry. *British Journal of Psychiatry*, **174**, 395–398.

SKODOL, A. E., LINK, B. G., SHROUT, P. E., *et al* (1988) Toward construct validity for DSM III axis V. *Psychiatry Research*, **24**, 13–23.

SPITZER, R. L., ENDICOTT, J., FLEISS, J. L., *et al* (1970) The Psychiatric Status Schedule: a technique for evaluating psychopathology and impairment in role functioning. *Archives of General Psychiatry*, **23**, 41–55.

—— & FORMAN, J. B. W. (1979) DSM–III field trials, II: initial experience with the multiaxial system. *American Journal of Psychiatry*, **136**, 818–820.

WALLACE, C. J. (1986) Functional assessment in rehabilitation. *Schizophrenia Bulletin*, **12**, 604–624.

WEISSMAN, M. M., SHOLOMSKAS, D. & JOHN, K. (1981) The assessment of social adjustment: an update. *Archives of General Psychiatry*, **38**, 1250–1258.

WESTERMEYER, J. (1988) DSM–III psychiatric disorders among Hmong refugees in the United States. A point prevalence study. *American Journal of Psychiatry*, **145**, 197–202.

—— & NEIDER, J. (1988) Social networks and psychopathology among substance abusers. *American Journal of Psychiatry*, **145**, 1265–1269.

WING, J. K., BEEVOR, A. S., CURTIS, R. H., *et al* (1998) Health of the Nation Outcome Scales: research and development. *British Journal of Psychiatry*, **172**, 11–18.

WORLD HEALTH ORGANIZATION (1988) *WHO Psychiatric Disability Assessment Scale (WHO/DAS)*. Geneva: WHO.

—— (1992) *International Classification of Diseases* (10th edn) (ICD–10). Geneva: WHO.

WYKES, T. (1992) The assessment of severely disabled psychiatric patients for rehabilitation. In *Schizophrenia: An Overview and Practical Handbook* (ed. D. Kavanaugh), pp. 221–238. London: Chapman and Hall.

—— & STURT, E. (1986) The measurement of social behaviour in psychiatric patients: an assessment of the reliability and validity of the SBS schedule. *British Journal of Psychiatry*, **148**, 1–11.

—— & HURRY, J. (1991) Social behaviour and psychiatric disorders. In *Social Psychiatry: Theory, Methodology and Practice* (ed. P. Bebbington), pp. 183–207. New Brunswick: Transactional Publishers.

4 Measuring satisfaction with psychiatric services: towards a multi-dimensional, multi-axial assessment of outcome

MIRELLA RUGGERI

Satisfaction with services has been given increasing attention in the field of mental health services research and evaluation. In the United States, large-scale studies on satisfaction have been performed since the early 1960s, both in medicine and in psychiatry, following the principles of "consumerism" (Attkisson & Pascoe, 1983). In Europe, the interest in satisfaction with services grew later, and attained a widespread diffusion in psychiatry only in the second half of the 1990s. More than from consumerism, this interest derives from developments in social psychiatry and specifically from the attempt to define an agreed model for the assessment of the outcome of psychiatric care useful in both research and clinical routine.

The need for a comprehensive and sophisticated model of outcome measurement started to emerge at the beginning of the 1990s (Jenkins, 1990; Mirin & Namerow, 1991; Attkisson *et al*, 1992; Ruggeri & Tansella, 1995; Smith *et al*, 1997). In the light of current knowledge, in order to be valid, reliable and useful in programme planning, outcome studies should combine optimal measures of both the 'service level' and the 'patient level' (Thornicroft & Tansella, 1999). At the patient level, they should consider an intervention's effect on various *dimensions*, including severity and course of symptoms, social functioning, social support, quality of life, met and unmet needs, family burden and satisfaction with services. Moreover, the assessment should consider simultaneously various *axes*. In fact, in psychiatric settings, professionals, paraprofessionals, patients and relatives all participate in care and should be considered legitimate judges of an intervention's effectiveness, albeit from differing perspectives. The fact that their views may markedly differ (Mayer & Rosenblatt, 1974; Dowds & Fontana, 1977; Andrews *et al*, 1986; Garrard *et al*, 1988; Gunkel & Priebe, 1993) only confirms that integrating their views is a necessary step in outcome studies.

Thus, *multi-dimensionality* and *multi-axiality* are key components of outcome assessment. In both cases, satisfaction with services plays a role, being a major dimension of outcome, one that may involve multiple axes, contributing to a fuller depiction of the performance of a system of care. This chapter should be read as a supplement to the detailed review chapter by Ruggeri (1996), which appeared in the first edition of this book, and which summarised the psychometric properties of satisfaction rating scales published until 1993 and discussed their methodological limitations.

The role of satisfaction in service evaluation

As early as 1966, Donabedian stated that "the effectiveness of care in achieving and producing health and satisfaction, as defined for its individual members by a particular society or subculture, is the ultimate validator of the quality of care" (Donabedian, 1966). Later, Locker & Dunt (1978) suggested that, particularly with long-term care: "quality of care can become synonymous with quality of life and satisfaction with care an important component of life satisfaction". Patients' and relatives' satisfaction with services thus seems to be particularly salient and appropriate as a measure of both outcome and quality; in service evaluation, satisfaction may be viewed both as a measure of outcome and quality *per se* and as a factor in the process of care.

Clients' satisfaction with services is at the same time a dependent and an independent variable. As a dependent variable, satisfaction has been hypothesised to be the effect of various factors, such as the subject's expectations with services, attitudes towards life, self-esteem, illness behaviour and previous experience with services. Conflicting results have been obtained with regard to the characteristics of patients correlated with satisfaction. No clear relationship has been found between patient satisfaction and age, education, family size, income, marital status, occupation, race, religion, sex, social class or diagnosis (Lebow, 1983*a*). Lehman & Zastowny (1983), in a meta-analysis of the literature on satisfaction with mental health services, found that chronic patients tend to express less satisfaction with their treatment than non-chronic patients. The mood of patients seems to affect other self-rated variables, such as quality of life, but has a minor effect on satisfaction with services (Atkinson & Caldwell, 1997). Some characteristics of the intervention seem to be correlated with satisfaction: for example, Lehman & Zastowny (1983) found that innovative programmes tend to be viewed more positively than conventional ones; no differences were found in rates of patient satisfaction between in-patient and out-patient programmes.

As an *independent* variable, satisfaction can influence various behaviours of consumers, such as compliance and service utilisation. According to Ware & Davies (1983), satisfaction influences care-seeking behaviour (e.g. whether consumers seek care during an illness episode and the number of visits), adherence behaviour (whether patients do the things they are supposed to do while in care, for example adherence to regimens, compliance with follow-up visits and referrals) and reactive behaviour (actions initiated by consumers specifically to express their satisfaction or dissatisfaction, such as recommendations in favour or against a particular provider or facility, changing providers and registering formal complaints). They found that differences in patient satisfaction were a significant predictor of changes in both doctor and health insurance schemes, and that relatively small differences in satisfaction ratings have noteworthy consequences for patient behaviour.

Service satisfaction seems to be a key variable both in determining the efficacy of interventions and in understanding the effect of interventions from the patient's perspective. It has been shown that patients with a more negative assessment of treatment tend to have less improvement of psychopathology and longer duration of hospitalization, both in the short and in the long term run (Gunkel & Priebe, 1993; Priebe & Bröker, 1999). Various findings highlight the relevance of the subjective view of users in understanding treatment effectiveness. In fact, when users are given a role as 'consumers', as opposed to passive service recipients, a disparity between the intended purposes of various treatments and the results as described by patients themselves may emerge and greatly enlighten data based on professionals' evaluations alone. As early as the 1980s, some findings pointed to a strong relationship between clients' assessment of satisfaction and their global reports of outcome; a less strong relationship was found between reported satisfaction and outcome as rated by therapists (Lebow, 1983*b*).

More recent studies have confirmed the relevance of the subjective perspective of users in assessing treatment outcome (Dean *et al*, 1993; Dincin *et al*, 1993; Gomez Carrion *et al*, 1993; Diamond & Factor, 1994). The finding that users' satisfaction is the most sensitive discriminator between community psychiatric nursing and traditional out-patient care (Paykel *et al*, 1982), and the most sensitive and long-lasting indicator of differences between an experimental community-based service and traditional hospital-based psychiatric care (Audini *et al*, 1994; Marks *et al*, 1994), is of great interest. Moreover, this result has been confirmed by comparing traditional, hospital-based care with routine community care (Henderson *et al*, 1999).

The study of the correlation between satisfaction with services and other outcome variables is promising but still at an early stage. A six-month follow-up study on the outcome of care in the South-Verona community-based psychiatric service used 'graphical chain models' (a new technique that enables researchers to assess the relationship between two variables after controlling for the effect of antecedent and intervening variables – see Chapter 15) has assessed the relationship of satisfaction with services to psychopathology, disability, functioning and quality of life (Ruggeri *et al*, 1998*a*). Results of this study show that higher satisfaction is predicted by low disability at baseline but also by improvement in global functioning over the following six months. Service satisfaction has been shown to be closely related to quality of life and to be its only predictor. This finding confirms a statement made by Locker & Dunt (1978) and quoted at the beginning of this section; if further confirmed in other studies, it opens up the appealing prospect of improving patients' quality of life by providing adequate and individualised care.

Service satisfaction and clinical routine

Clinicians tend to ignore the views of users about their own treatment. 'Transference distortions', 'manipulative behaviour', 'aggressivity', 'secondary advantages from illness' and 'defence mechanisms' are the reasons professionals commonly give for users' dissatisfaction (if they perceive it). Prejudice against psychiatric patients not being capable of judging the care they receive plays a major role in nourishing such a narrow view of the doctor–patient relationship.

On the other hand, especially with severely ill psychiatric patients, awareness of their problems may be incomplete and their capacity to judge reliably the care they receive is not guaranteed. Moreover, a careful analysis of the components of care that may be properly assessed by users is needed (for a discussion of the perceptions of users of technical and non-technical components of care, see Hornstra & Lubin, 1974; Brody *et al*, 1989; Salmon *et al*, 1994). But, despite these difficulties, assessing the subjective perspective of users is an opportunity not to be missed in service evaluation and in routine clinical practice.

Overall, empirical data disconfirm the prejudice that patients are incapable of judging the care they receive. Andrews *et al* (1986) have shown that most requests for a change of therapist in an out-patient psychotherapy service result from patient–therapist mismatch and the majority of patients who changed therapists remained in treatment with the new therapist and reported being satisfied with the change. Various studies have found that patients are sensitive to verbal and non-verbal elements of the health care process, fairly accurate in distinguishing the quality of provider behaviours, such as courtesy and competence, and that they base their satisfaction ratings on these discriminations. The satisfaction ratings of patients have also been found to correspond to criteria for the skills of doctors customarily used by health providers, such as more years of training, positive motivation towards patients and peer supervision (for a review of these data see Lebow, 1983a). Sheppard (1993) has correlated patients' satisfaction with the nature of intervention and the quality of some skills used by practitioners in extended interventions in a community mental health centre. Considerable differences were identified between satisfied and dissatisfied clients in the service received and their perceptions; satisfaction was clearly related to the use of interpersonal skills such as communication, empathy, listening, openness and genuineness. This paper both indicates that the concept of satisfaction does meaningfully represent the client's experience and provides considerable support for the fundamental importance of the acquisition and use of these skills in practice.

When considering the effect of satisfaction on care, short-term and long-term dissatisfaction should be differentiated. It is obvious that there may be times when fulfilling clients' requests may prove too difficult or too costly to meet, or may not be clinically indicated. Short-term dissatisfaction in some cases can be legitimately considered a side-effect of a therapeutic intervention that changes the patient perspective (e.g. a shift from institutional to community care, or pursuing a change in the relationship of the patient with significant others); apart from the risk of early drop-out from treatment, dissatisfaction itself may not be worrying in such circumstances.

Greater relevance should, instead, be attached to consumers' dissatisfaction in the long term. Long-term dissatisfaction, in fact, may indicate that the planned change did not contribute to an improvement in the client's life: in this case the utility of such interventions should be seriously reconsidered. It may also indicate that clients do not have enough personal resources to appreciate the advantages of that intervention: in this case, if not a change in the therapeutic strategy, at least an improvement in communication between clients and professionals is necessary.

Short-term dissatisfaction can easily become satisfaction in the long run if professionals perceive it correctly, communicate their perception to the consumer, and discuss the problems. Moreover, it should be stressed that different perspectives do not necessarily result in dissatisfaction. In fact, when consumers feel that their viewpoint has been taken into account and an acceptable therapeutic management plan has been worked out through a process of mutual negotiation, they may still feel satisfied even if their initial requests are not fully met.

Methodological issues in measuring satisfaction

That the issue of patient satisfaction has elicited contradictory data and radically divergent opinions among experts is a fact. What has not been stated clearly enough is that most divergences arise from poor quality of the research in the field. Major shortcomings are found in study designs and in the development and validation of instruments. To give more attention to methodological issues in satisfaction measurement is the only way of improving our knowledge, to initiate a more valuable, scientifically based debate.

Efforts to measure satisfaction with services have varied widely in method, and systematic knowledge within the area has been scattered (Ruggeri, 1994). Inadequacy of the study design or implementation and, specifically, lack of confidentiality play a major role in producing flattened responses from patients. But the major problem in the field of satisfaction research is the inadequacy of the instruments used in the vast majority of studies. Although the importance of showing that an instrument has good psychometric properties is widely recognised, psychometric analyses have too often been neglected in the field of users' satisfaction. Acceptability, sensitivity, validity and reliability of the instruments used have been rarely, if ever, reported. Thus, most satisfaction surveys suffer from an incorrect measurement of satisfaction rather than from intrinsic limits on the measurement of satisfaction. Many studies report high overall satisfaction irrespective of the kind of care provided; this may not necessarily be due to passivity on the part of the patient, as is often assumed. At least three methodological aspects should be considered first. First, was confidentiality guaranteed? Second, was the instrument sufficiently sensitive to dissatisfaction? And third, had the instrument good content validity with respect to the setting? Unfortunately, these requirements are seldom fulfilled (Ruggeri, 1994).

Users' views have often been solicited using qualitative methods, such as records of their spontaneous reports, but studies on the sensitivity of this kind of approach have not been implemented. Few studies have compared the psychometric properties of qualitative and quantitative assessment methods in the measurement of satisfaction.

In the validation study of the Verona Service Satisfaction Scale (VSSS; Ruggeri *et al*, 1994), spontaneous reports on dissatisfaction were elicited in 30 subjects by means of an unstructured interview (UI) and recorded before the administration of the VSSS, an 82-item questionnaire which covers various dimensions of satisfaction (see below for further details). The results showed that the vast majority of problems spontaneously mentioned in the UI received a rating of 'terrible' or 'mostly dissatisfactory' in the questionnaire. The opposite was not true: in fact, in the questionnaire, subjects reported dissatisfaction with aspects not previously mentioned in the UI. When considering the totality of reasons for dissatisfaction that emerged in this enquiry, more than 90% were detected by the questionnaire and only about 20% by the UI. Further, subjects who, in the UI, declared that they had had "no dissatisfaction", subsequently, answering the questionnaire, reported considerable dissatisfaction. Thus, it may be hypothesised that subjects' difficulty in analysing, in the absence of prompting stimuli, their interactions with the service, or in expressing it, reduces the sensitivity of unstructured interviews. This work demonstrates that qualitative methods lack sensitivity and that a multi-dimensional questionnaire, when well developed, may be much more sensitive than spontaneous reports in measuring service satisfaction.

So, it seems that the use of spontaneous reports of users, instead of questionnaires, will not usually be the approach of choice in measuring satisfaction. Still, qualitative methods may be essential tools in the early stages of development of quantitative instruments, for example in order to improve a questionnaire's acceptability and content validity (Ruggeri *et al*, 1994). The preference for quantitative methods, preceded by a phase of instrument development and validation when qualitative methods are also employed, is becoming a general trend in assessing the more complex dimensions of outcome, such as quality of life, family burden and needs for care (Becker *et al*, 1999). A combination of quantitative and qualitative methods can also be useful for a deeper understanding of the reasons for dissatisfaction (Everett & Boydell, 1994), but definitely cannot be conceived as a substitute for quantitative assessments.

When quantitative methods are used in satisfaction research, researchers commonly adopt questionnaires composed of either a few broad questions about satisfaction or unstandardised, single-item subscales that tap reactions to one or two dimensions. This happens notwithstanding the fact that the majority of findings available in the literature support the idea that satisfaction is a multi-dimensional concept that includes, for example, professionals' skills and behaviour, access, information, efficacy and type of interventions (Ware & Snyder, 1976; Ware *et al*, 1983; Attkisson & Greenfield, 1994). Thus, enquiries based on overall satisfaction not only may fail to detect dissatisfaction but are also inherently destined *not* to detect the reasons for dissatisfaction. No wonder such measures give highly skewed distributions with little variance.

Scales for measuring satisfaction with services

Researchers conducting satisfaction studies have tended to develop their own instruments; therefore there are very few widely used instruments. In the last decade the need for research that develops and refines measures of client satisfaction and establishes their psychometric properties has been considered a priority in service evaluation (Steinwachs *et al*, 1992; Ruggeri, 1994). In spite of this, in the mental health field, very few validated instruments for measuring satisfaction are currently available.

Some scales were developed in the 1970s and the 1980s for assessing psychiatric out-patient treatment (Love *et al*, 1979; Deiker *et al*, 1981; Slater *et al*, 1981). Several excellent scales are also available that assess satisfaction with medical care (Hulka *et al*, 1970; Ware & Snyder, 1976) and these could readily be adapted to assess mental health treatment. But the former instruments have rarely been used in the last decade and the latter ones have rarely been adapted to psychiatric settings.

A major contribution in this field was made by Attkisson and Greenfield and their colleagues at the University of California at San Francisco (Attkisson & Greenfield, 1994). They first developed the Client Satisfaction Questionnaire (CSQ; Larsen *et al*, 1979). The CSQ, which, in its 31- and 8-item versions, assesses a general satisfaction factor, uses a four-point Likert scale, and has been developed through a careful sequential process to enhance reliability and validity. It is the only instrument for measuring patients' satisfaction that has had widespread use in many types of service setting, including mental health services (Dyck & Azim, 1983; Greenfield, 1983; Azim & Joyce, 1986; Sishta *et al*, 1986; Huxley & Warner, 1992), and that has been translated into other languages, specifically Spanish, Dutch and French (de Brey, 1983; Roberts *et al*, 1984; Sabourin *et al*, 1987). However, the mono-dimensionality of the CSQ constitutes a limit to its sensitivity and content validity other than as a global measure.

Based on the experience with the CSQ, Greenfield & Attkisson (1989) developed another instrument, the Service Satisfaction Scale (SSS–30), specifically designed as a multi-dimensional scale, which, on a five-point Likert scale, assesses several components of satisfaction with either health or mental health out-patient services (practitioner manner and skill, perceived outcome, office procedures and access), and has been used in a range of service settings (Attkisson & Greenfield, 1994).

The SSS-30 can be considered an excellent instrument for cross-setting studies or studies in general practice but, despite being a substantial improvement on previous questionnaires, it still lacks of validity for specifically mental health settings. The Verona Service Satisfaction Scale (VSSS) is an attempt to combine cross-setting and setting-specific items for measuring satisfaction with community-based mental health services. The VSSS covers seven dimensions (overall satisfaction, professionals skills and behaviours, information, access, efficacy, type of intervention, relative's involvement). Its first version consisted of 82 items, rated on the same five-point Likert scale used in the SSS–30. Of these items, 36 had been adapted from the SSS–30 and derivative scales (Ruggeri & Greenfield, 1995); they cover aspects assessed by items reported to be relevant across a broad array of both medical and psychiatric settings. Forty-six items were newly developed; these concern service aspects reported to be relevant specifically in psychiatric settings, particularly in community-based settings, such as social skills and types of intervention. The test–retest reliability (Ruggeri & Dall'Agnola, 1993), acceptability, sensitivity and content validity (Ruggeri *et al*, 1994) of the VSSS-82 have been studied and have proved to be good. Based on results from the validation study and subsequent factor analysis, reduced versions suitable for routine clinical use have been developed: the VSSS–54 and VSSS–32 (Ruggeri *et al*, 1996).

To date, the VSSS-54 and -32 have been translated into English, French, Spanish, Portuguese, German, Dutch, Danish, Greek and Japanese. In the wider frame of the EPSILON Study of Schizophrenia, the European version of the VSSS has been translated, adapted to each cultural context and validated for use in various European countries (Becker *et al*, 1999). Besides use by its authors, the VSSS is currently being used in an increasing number of studies in many countries of the world, some of which have already been published (Tonelli & Merini, 1995; Cozza *et al*, 1997; Parkman *et al*, 1997; Leese *et al*, 1998; Boardman *et al*, 1999; Clarkson *et al*, 1999; Merinder *et al*, 1999).

Conclusions

The process of evaluating mental health services is a timely, long-term and complex process, and different strategies, as well as various techniques, need to be used (Tansella, 1989, 1991; Ruggeri *et al*, 1998*a*; Thornicroft & Tansella, 1999). Developing a comprehensive model for the assessment of the outcome of psychiatric care is a great challenge for service evaluators.

Modelling the concept of outcome in psychiatry has come a long way, from the use of morbidity and mortality rates as indicators of outcome, to the use of data on service utilisation, to the inclusion of social variables in the assessment. Now it is urgent to combine all these contributions and to move towards routine multi-dimensional and multi-axial outcome assessment that considers both subjective and objective variables, and includes clinical and social variables, as well as the characteristics of the user's interaction with a service. Integration of data coming from randomised trials, which assess the efficacy or potential of a treatment under experimental conditions, and naturalistic studies, which assess the effectiveness or result of treatment as provided in the 'real world', should be encouraged. Survey studies in community settings having as their main objective the multi-dimensional measurement of the outcome of mental health interventions, which includes the use of standardised instruments, administered as part of the routine clinical activities within community-based psychiatric services, should be planned.

The South-Verona Outcome Project (Ruggeri *et al*, 1998*a,b*) is an attempt to standardise information that clinicians collect and record, in periodic reviews of cases in treatment in their everyday clinical practice, and to employ for service evaluation the same professionals involved in the clinical work. Variables belonging to six main dimensions are considered: global functioning (with the Global Assessment of Functioning), psychopathology (with the Brief Psychiatric Rating Scale, "expanded version"), social disability (with eight items from the WHO Disability Assessment Scale), needs for care (with the Camberwell Assessment of Needs), quality of life (with the Lancashire Quality of Life Profile) and satisfaction with service (with the VSSS). These data are integrated with data on service utilisation and costs. Most assessments are actually completed, after brief training, by the clinicians themselves; some assessments are made by the patients, with the help of research workers. Standardised assessments take place twice a year: from April to June (wave A) and from October to December (wave B). During these periods both first-ever patients and patients already in contact with the service are assessed at the first or, at latest, second time they are seen. Finally, data are put in the clinical records and are available on-line to clinicians. The project started in 1994. The mean time used by the professionals for the assessment was 26.9 minutes for each patient, with a wide range (8–70 minutes), depending on the type of patient and on the severity of the condition. Results obtained so far confirm both the feasibility of this kind of study and its contribution to service evaluation and planning (Ruggeri *et al*, 1998a).

A long-term objective of outcome assessment is to compare multi-dimensional outcomes of patients in different health care settings using the same tools. In this perspective, users' satisfaction plays an important role and is one of the areas which will require sustained attention. Considerable effort is needed in spreading the use of well-validated instruments and discouraging continual recourse to *ad hoc* measures. Content validity in veridically capturing the users' views, acceptability to the users, established psychometric properties and a norm base should be the rule with all measures. Comparability between studies should be pursued more vigorously, in order both to allow the refinement of existing instruments and to push forward our theoretical and substantive understanding of satisfaction with psychiatric services and its relationships with care provided and with the other indicators of outcome.

References

ANDREWS, S., LEAVY, A., DeCHILLO, N., *et al* (1986) Patient–therapist mismatch: we would rather switch than fight. *Hospital and Community Psychiatry*, **37**, 918–922.

ATKINSON, M. J. & CALDWELL, L. (1997) The differential effects of mood on patients' ratings of life quality and satisfaction with their care. *Journal of Affective Disorders*, **44**, 169–175.

ATTKISSON, C. C. & PASCOE, G. C. (eds) (1983) Patient satisfaction in health and mental health services. *Evaluation and Program Planning*, **6** (special issue).

——, COOK, J., KARNO, M., *et al* (1992) Clinical services research. *Schizophrenia Bulletin*, **18**, 627–668,

—— & GREENFIELD, T. K. (1994) The Client Satisfaction Questionnaire–8 and the Service Satisfaction Questionnaire–30. In *Psychological Testing: Treatment Planning and Outcome Assessment* (ed. M. Maruish), pp. 223–235. San Francisco: Lawrence Erlbaum Associates.

AUDINI, B., MARKS, I. M., LAWRENCE, R. E., *et al* (1994) Home-based versus out-patient/in-patient care for people with serious mental illness. Phase II of a controlled study. *British Journal of Psychiatry*, **165**, 204–210.

AZIM, H. F. A. & JOYCE, A. S. (1986) The impact of data-based program modifications on the satisfaction of outpatients in group psychotherapy. *Canadian Journal of Psychiatry*, **31**, 119–122.

BECKER, T., KNAPP, M., KNUDSEN, H. C., *et al* (1999) The EPSILON study of schizophrenia in five European countries. Design and methodology for standardising outcome measures and comparing patterns of care and service costs. *British Journal of Psychiatry*, **175**, 514–521.

BOARDMAN, A. P., HODGSON, R. E., LEWIS, M., *et al* (1999) North Staffordshire Community Beds Study: longitudinal evaluation of psychiatric in-patient units attached to community mental health centres. *British Journal of Psychiatry*, **175**, 70–78.

BRODY, D. S., MILLER, S. M., LERMAN, C. E., *et al* (1989) The relationship between patients' satisfaction with their physicians and perceptions about interventions they desired and received. *Medical Care*, **27**, 1027–1035.

CLARKSON, P., McCRONE, P., SUTHERBY, K., *et al* (1999) Outcomes and costs of a community support worker service for the severely mentally ill. *Acta Psychiatrica Scandinavica*, **99**, 196–206.

COZZA, M., AMARA, M., BUTERA, N., *et al* (1997) La soddisfazione dei pazienti e dei familiari nei confronti di un Dipartimento di Salute Mentale di Roma. *Epidemiologia e Psichiatria Sociale*, **6**, 173–183.

DEAN, C., PHILIPPS, J., GADD, E. M., *et al* (1993) Comparison of community based service with hospital based service for people with acute, severe psychiatric illness. *British Medical Journal*, **307**, 473–476.

DE BREY, H. (1983) A cross-national validation of the client satisfaction questionnaire: the Dutch experience. *Evaluation and Program Planning*, **6**, 395–400.

DEIKER, T., OSBORN, S. M., DISTEFANO, M. R., *et al* (1981) Consumer accreditation: development of a quality assurance patient evaluation scale. *Hospital and Community Psychiatry*, **32**, 565–567.

DIAMOND, R. J. & FACTOR, R. M. (1994) Taking issue. Treatment-resistant patients or a treatment-resistant system? *Hospital and Community Psychiatry*, **45**, 197.

DINCIN, J., WASMER, D., WITHERIDGE, T. F., *et al* (1993) Impact of assertive community treatment on the use of state hospital inpatient bed-days. *Hospital and Community Psychiatry*, **44**, 833–838.

DONABEDIAN, A. (1966) Evaluating the quality of medical care. *Milbank Memorial Fund Quarterly*, **44**, 166–203.

DOWDS, B. & FONTANA, A. (1977) Patients' and therapists' expectations and evaluations of hospital treatment. *Comprehensive Psychiatry*, **18**, 295–300.

DYCK, R. J. & AZIM, H. F. (1983) Patient satisfaction in a psychiatric walk-in clinic. *Canadian Journal of Psychiatry*, **28**, 30–33.

EVERETT, B. & BOYDELL, K. (1994) A methodology for including consumers' opinions in mental health evaluation research. *Hospital and Community Psychiatry*, **45**, 76–78.

GARRARD, J., HAUSMAN, W., MANSFIELD, E., *et al* (1988) Educational priorities in mental health professions: do educators and consumers agree? *Medical Education*, **22**, 60–66.

GOMEZ CARRION, P., SWANN, A., KELLERT-CECIL, H., *et al* (1993) Compliance with clinic attendance by outpatients with schizophrenia. *Hospital and Community Psychiatry*, **44**, 764–767.

GREENFIELD, T. K. (1983) The role of client satisfaction in evaluating university counselling services. *Evaluation and Program Planning*, **6**, 315–327.

—— & ATTKISSON, C. C. (1989) Steps toward a multifactorial satisfaction scale for primary care and mental health services. *Evaluation and Program Planning*, **12**, 271–278.

GUNKEL, S. & PRIEBE, S. (1993) Different perspectives of short-term changes in the rehabilitation of schizophrenic patients. *Comprehensive Psychiatry*, **34**, 352–359.

HENDERSON, C., PHELAN, M., LOFTUS, L., *et al* (1999) Comparison of patients' satisfaction with community-based vs. hospital psychiatric services. *Acta Psychiatrica Scandinavica*, **99**, 188–195.

HORNSTRA, R. K. & LUBIN, B. (1974) Relationship of outcome of treatment to agreement about treatment assignment by patients and professionals. *Journal of Nervous and Mental Disease*, **158**, 420–423.

HULKA, B., ZYZANSKY, L., CASSEL, J., *et al* (1970) Scale for the measurement of attitudes toward physicians and primary health care. *Medical Care*, **8**, 429–430.

HUXLEY, P. & WARNER, R. (1992) Case management, quality of life, and satisfaction with services of long-term psychiatric patients. *Hospital and Community Psychiatry*, **43**, 799–803.

JENKINS, R. (1990) Toward a system of outcome indicators for mental health care. *British Journal of Psychiatry*, **157**, 500–514.

LARSEN, D., ATTKISSON, C. C., HARGREAVES, W., *et al* (1979) Assessment of client/patient satisfaction: development of a general scale. *Evaluation and Program Planning*, **2**, 197–207.

Lebow, J. L. (1983*a*) Research assessing consumer satisfaction with mental health treatment: a review of findings. *Evaluation and Program Planning*, **6**, 211–236.

—— (1983*b*) Client satisfaction with mental health treatment: methodological considerations in assessment. *Evaluation Review*, **7**, 729–752.

Leese, M., Johnson, S., Slade, M., *et al* (1998) User perspective on needs and satisfaction with mental health services. *British Journal of Psychiatry*, **173**, 409–415.

Lehman, A. F. & Zastowny, T. R. (1983) Patient satisfaction with mental health services: a meta-analysis to establish norms. *Evaluation and Program Planning*, **6**, 265–274.

Linder-Pelz, S. (1982*a*) Toward a theory of patient satisfaction. *Social Science and Medicine*, **16**, 577–582.

Locker, D. & Dunt, D. (1978) Theoretical and methodological issues in sociological studies of consumer satisfaction with medical care. *Social Science and Medicine*, **12**, 283–292.

Love, R. E., Caid, C. D. & Davis, A. (1979) The User Satisfaction Survey: consumer evaluation of an inner city community mental health center. *Evaluation and the Health Profession*, **2**, 42–54.

Marks, I. M., Connolly, J., Muijen, M., *et al* (1994) Home-based versus hospital-based care for people with serious mental illness. *British Journal of Psychiatry*, **165**, 179–194.

Mayer, J. & Rosenblatt, A. (1974) Clash in perspective between mental patients and staff. *American Journal of Orthopsychiatry*, **44**, 432–441.

Merinder, L. B., Viuff, A. G., Laugesen, H. D., *et al* (1999) Patient and relative education in community psychiatry: a randomized controlled trial regarding its effectiveness. *Social Psychiatry and Psychiatric Epidemiology*, **34**, 287–294.

Mirin, S. M. & Namerow, M. J. (1991) Why study treatment outcome? *Hospital and Community Psychiatry*, **42**, 1007–1013.

Parkman, S., Davies, S., Leese, M., *et al* (1997) Ethnic differences in satisfaction with mental health services among representative people with psychosis in South London: PRISM Study 4. *British Journal of Psychiatry*, **171**, 260–264.

Paykel, E. S., Mangen, S. P., Griffith, J. H., *et al* (1982) Community psychiatric nursing for neurotic patients: a controlled trial. *British Journal of Psychiatry*, **140**, 573–581.

Priebe, S. & Bröker, M. (1999) Prediction of hospitalizations by schizophrenia patients' assessment of treatment: an expanded study. *Journal of Psychiatric Research*, **33**, 113–119.

Roberts, R., Attkisson, C. & Mendias, R. M. (1984) Assessing the Client Satisfaction Questionnaire in English and Spanish. *Hispanic Journal of Behavioural Sciences*, **6**, 385–396.

Ruggeri, M. (1994) Patient's and relatives' satisfaction with psychiatric services: the state of the art of its measurement. *Social Psychiatry and Psychiatric Epidemiology*, **29**, 212–227.

—— (1996) Satisfaction with psychiatric services. In *Mental Health Outcomes Measures* (eds G. Thornicroft & M. Tansella), pp. 27–51. Heidelberg: Springer-Verlag.

—— & Dall'Agnola, R. (1993) The development and use of the Verona Expectations for Care Scale (VECS) and the Verona Service Satisfaction Scale (VSSS) for measuring expectations and satisfaction with community-based psychiatric services in patients, relatives and professionals. *Psychological Medicine*, **23**, 511–523.

——, ——, Agostini, C., *et al* (1994) Acceptability, sensitivity and content validity of VECS and VSSS in measuring expectations and satisfaction in psychiatric patients and their relatives. *Social Psychiatry and Psychiatric Epidemiology*, **29**, 265–276.

—— & Greenfield, T. (1995) The Italian version of the Service Satisfaction Scale (SSS–30) adapted for community-based psychiatric services: development, factor analysis and application. *Evaluation and Program Planning*, **18**, 191–202.

—— & Tansella, M. (1995) Evaluating outcome in mental health care. *Current Opinion in Psychiatry*, **8**, 116–121.

——, Dall'Agnola, R., Greenfield, T., *et al* (1996) Factor analysis of the Verona Service Satisfaction Scale–82 and development of reduced versions. *International Journal of Methods in Psychiatric Research*, **6**, 23–38.

—— & TANSELLA, M. (1996) Individual patient outcomes. In *Mental Health Service Evaluation* (eds H. C. Knudsen & G. Thornicroft), pp. 281–295. Cambridge: Cambridge University Press.

——, BIGGERI, A., RUCCI, P., *et al* (1998*a*) Multivariate analysis of outcome of mental health care using graphical chain models. The South-Verona Outcome Project 1. *Psychological Medicine*, **28**, 1421–1431.

——, RIANI, M., RUCCI, P., *et al* (1998*b*) Multidimensional assessment of outcome in psychiatry: the use of graphical displays. The South-Verona Outcome Project 2. *International Journal of Methods in Psychiatric Research*, **7**, 186–198.

SABOURIN, S., GENDREAU, P. & FRENETTE, L. (1987) Le neveau de satisfaction des cas d'abandon dans un service universitaire de psychologie. *Canadian Journal of Behavioral Sciences*, **19**, 314–323.

SALMON, P., SHARMA, N., VALORI, R., *et al* (1994) Patients' intentions in primary care: relationship to physical and psychological symptoms, and their perception by general practitioners. *Social Science and Medicine*, **38**, 585–592.

SHEPPARD, M. (1993) Client satisfaction, extended intervention and interpersonal skills in community mental health. *Journal of Advanced Nursing*, **18**, 246–259.

SISHTA, S. K., RINCO, S. & SULLIVAN, J. C. F. (1986) Clients' satisfaction survey in a psychiatric inpatient population attached to a general hospital. *Canadian Journal of Psychiatry*, **31**, 123–128.

SLATER, V., LINN, M. W. & HARRIS, R. (1981) Outpatient evaluation of mental health care. *Southern Medical Journal*, **74**, 1217–1219.

SMITH, G. R., MANDERSCHEID, R. W., FLYNN, L. M., *et al* (1997) Principles for assessment of patient outcomes in mental health care. *Psychiatric Services*, **48**, 1033–1036.

STEINWACHS, D. M., CULLUM, H., DORWART, R. A., *et al* (1992). Service systems research. *Schizophrenia Bulletin*, **18**, 627–668.

TANSELLA, M. (1989) Evaluating community psychiatric services. In *The Scope of Epidemiological Psychiatry* (eds P. Williams, C. Wilkinson & K. Rawnsley), pp. 386–403. London: Routledge.

—— (ed.) (1991) *Community-Based Psychiatry: Long Term Patterns of Care in South-Verona.* Psychological Medicine Monograph Supplement 19. Cambridge: Cambridge University Press.

THORNICROFT, G. & TANSELLA, M. (1999) *The Mental Health Matrix. A Manual to Improve Services.* Cambridge: Cambridge University Press.

TONELLI, G. & MERINI, A. (1995) La valutazione del Servizio di Salute mentale della I Clinica Psichiatrica dell'Università di Bologna tramite la Verona Service Satisfaction Scale (VSSS). *Rivista Sperimentale di Frenatria*, **119**, 825–842.

WARE, J. E. & DAVIES, A. R. (1983) Behavioral consequences of consumer dissatisfaction with medical care. *Evaluation and Program Planning*, **6**, 291–298.

—— & SNYDER, M. K. (1976) Dimensions of patients' attitudes regarding doctors and medical care services. *Medical Care*, **13**, 669–683.

——, ——, WRIGHT, W. R., *et al* (1983) Defining and measuring patient satisfaction with medical care. *Evaluation and Program Planning*, **6**, 247–263.

5 Measuring family or care-giver burden in severe mental illness: the instruments

AART H. SCHENE, RICHARD C. TESSLER, GAIL M. GAMACHE and BOB VAN WIJNGAARDEN

Until the middle of the twentieth century, neither society nor psychiatry as the principal responsible discipline could offer people with severe mental illness much more than hospital care for periods ranging from months to years. The recognition of the detrimental effects of hospitalisation, and developments in psychopharmaceutical, psychotherapeutic and social treatments, gave impetus to deinstitutionalisation and opened doors to new approaches now associated with community psychiatry and community care.

Over the past four decades this movement away from hospital care resulted in a great interest in the community adjustment of psychiatric patients (Weissman, 1975, 1981). Treating patients in the least restrictive environment and consumer empowerment made social functioning and social performance important concepts, not only for patients, practitioners and researchers, but certainly also for patients' relatives (Fisher *et al*, 1990). Confronted with care-giving tasks taken away from them since the start of institutionalism in the early nineteenth century, family members had to learn to cope again with the dysfunctional behaviour inherent in most of the severe mental illnesses.

Family or care-giver burden

Care-giving refers to the relationship between two adult individuals who are typically related through kinship. One, the care-giver,

48

assumes an unpaid and unanticipated responsibility for another, the care recipient, whose mental health problems are disabling, long term in nature, and essentially incurable. The care recipient is unable to fulfil the reciprocal obligations associated with normative adult relationships and the mental health problems are serious enough to require substantial amounts of care. What makes the situation particularly burdensome is the addition of the care-giving role to the already existing family role (Gubman & Tessler, 1987; Gubman *et al*, 1987; Tessler *et al*, 1989; Gallop *et al*, 1991).

Although the concept is referred to as 'family' burden, most studies have sampled primary 'care-givers'. Care-giver burden has a narrower perspective than family burden, as the latter includes the consequences for family members other than the main care-giver, such as the interpersonal relations within the family, the consequences for children of patients and the social network of the whole family.

Measuring burden

The adverse consequences of psychiatric disorders for relatives have been studied since the early 1950s, for different reasons: at first, to determine the feasibility of discharging patients into the community; later, to refine the concept of care-giving, its content and its underlying structure; and, most recently, to measure burden as an outcome variable in programme evaluations and controlled clinical trials (Schene *et al*, 1996). Although a number of instruments or scales have been developed to measure care-giver burden, there is still no standard instrument generally accepted within the scientific community. The application of burden measures in routine clinical settings – to screen for burden, to identify individual family members at risk, and to monitor changes in burden over time – is certainly in its infancy.

The present paper updates earlier reviews of family burden instruments (e.g., Platt, 1985; Schene, 1990; Schene *et al*, 1996). We identify relevant instruments and discuss their suitability for both routine clinical and research use. The protocols are described in terms of their method and comprehensiveness, precursors and theoretical foundations, and types of psychometric information available. The instruments in the following references are not included in the review because to our knowledge they have not been used in the last 10 years, or because they have been superseded by other instruments that have built upon them and that are included in the current review: Grad & Sainsbury (1963, 1968), Hoenig & Hamilton (1966*a*,*b*) and Hoenig (1968), Pasamanick *et al* (1967), Spitzer *et al* (1971), Test & Stein (1980) and Creer *et al* (1982).

Method

For the initial review, conducted in 1994, we contacted researchers to identify instruments available in English. We used our own personal knowledge of researchers in the field and identified others from the literature on family burden. A letter describing our purpose asked researchers whether they were adaptors or developers of family burden instrumentation, and also to name other persons who might be working in the area of family burden.

An 80-item Family Burden Researchers' Questionnaire was sent to 52 of the original 128 researchers that the authors believed had

TABLE 5.1
Family or care-giver burden instruments and main references

No.	Instrument	References
1	Social Behaviour Assessment Schedule	Platt *et al* (1980, 1983)
2	Burden on Family Interview Schedule	Pai & Kapur (1981, 1982)
3	Family Distress Scale for Depression	Jacob *et al* (1987)
4	Scale for Assessment of Family Distress	Gopinath & Chaturvedi (1986, 1992)
5	Family Burden Scale	Madianos *et al* (1987), Madianos & Madianou (1992)
6	Family Distress Scale	Birchwood & Smith (1992)
7	Thresholds Parental Burden Scale	Cook & Pickett (1987)
8	Texas Inventory of Grief – Mental Illness Version	Miller *et al* (1990)
9	Family Burden Questionnaire	Fadden (1984), Fadden *et al* (1987*a,b*)
10	Significant Other Scale	Herz *et al* (1991)
11	Family Problems Questionnaire	Morosini *et al* (1991), Magliano *et al* (1998)
12	Involvement Evaluation Questionnaire	Schene (1990), Schene & Van Wijngaarden (1992)
13	Family Burden Interview Schedule	Tessler *et al* (1992)
14	Family Caregiving of Persons with Mental Illness Survey	Biegel *et al* (1994)
15	Family Burden and Services Questionnaire	Greenberg *et al* (1993)
16	Burden Assessment Scale	Reinhard *et al* (in press)
17	Family Economic Burden Interview	Clark & Drake (1994)
18	Experience of Caregiving Inventory	Szmukler *et al* (1996*a,b*)
19	Perceived Family Burden Scale	Levene *et al* (1996)
20	Victorian Carers Program Questionnaire	Schofield *et al* (1997)

developed or adapted measures that could be shared with other researchers. When possible, the original author was contacted. Researchers were *not* sent a questionnaire if they failed to respond to the first letter, if they replied that they were not developers or adaptors, or if they were using an instrument developed by someone already represented in the sample. Instruments developed primarily for use with care-givers other than those of the severely mentally ill (e.g. geriatric patients) were also excluded.

To update the initial review, in 1999 we screened the 1994–1999 literature with regard to the instruments included in the 1994 review. Also, the Family Burden Researchers' Questionnaire was sent to another three researchers who had published new scales between 1994 and 1999. With this method we found a final sample of 20 family burden instruments.

Results

Table 5.1 shows the names of the 20 instruments, as well as their developers and the year of the main reference(s). The instruments are listed according to the year in which they were first printed or included in a published report (see Table 5.4 for these years). The difference between the year the instrument was introduced and the year of the main reference exists because of the lag between instrument development and publication in scientific journals.

To the best of our knowledge, the list in Table 5.1 represents the state of the art of burden measures that are currently in use or in advanced stages of development. For brevity of presentation, the numbers shown in Table 5.1 are used to identify specific instruments throughout the text and in the other tables.

Conceptual issues and content

Researchers were asked to describe the theoretical foundations underlying their measures and to check from a list of 20 the dimensions included in their instruments. All researchers but one considered burden to be a multi-dimensional concept (see Table 5.2). Some researchers consider patient symptoms and behaviours to be the origin of burden. Dysfunctional behaviour disrupts the household routine as well as the care-giving tasks for close relatives. Others suggest that care-giving may result in role strain because it is added to the culturally defined relationships between family members. Some researchers also referred to the stress research literature. They

TABLE 5.2
Dimensions assessed by family or caregiver burden instruments

Dimension	1	2	3	4	5	6	7	8	9	10	11	12	13	14	15	16	17	18	19	20
Effect on:																				
family interaction		+	+	+	+	+	+		+	+	+	+	+	+		+		+		+
family routine		+	+	+	+	+	+		+	+	+	+	+	+	+	+	+	+		
leisure	+	+	+	+	+	+	+		+	+	+	+	+	+	+	+	+	+		+
work/employment	+	+		+	+	+			+	+	+	+	+	+	+	+	+			+
mental health	+	+	+	+	+		+	+	+	+	+	+	+	+				+		+
physical health	+	+	+				+			+	+	+	+	+						+
use of psychotropics					+					+		+								
social network	+	+		+	+	+	+		+	+	+	+	+	+	+	+		+		+
others outside household	+			+	+	+	+		+	+	+	+	+	+	+	+	+	+		
children	+				+	+	+		+	+	+	+		+			+			
Financial consequences	+	+		+	+	+	+		+			+	+	+	+	+	+			+
Helping the patient with:																				
activities of daily living	+			+	+	+	+		+	+	+	+	+	+	+	+		+		+
Supervising the patient				+	+	+	+		+	+	+	+	+	+		+	+	+		+
Encouraging the patient						+	+					+	+	+	+	+	+	+		
Distress	+	+	+	+	+	+	+	+	+	+	+	+	+	+	+	+		+		+
Stigma		+	+	+	+				+	+	+	+	+	+	+	+		+		+
Worrying	+	+	+	+	+	+	+		+	+		+	+	+	+	+	+	+	+	+
Shame						+			+				+	+		+	+	+	+	+
Guilt				+		+					+			+	+		+	+	+	+
Global burden		+		+	+		+		+	+		+	+	+	+			+		
Total no. of dimensions	10	11	7	12	16	17	18	2	15	14	13	16	14	16	11	12	6	15		14

[1] Instrument number refers to Table 5.1

consider patients' dysfunctioning and its different consequences as chronic stressors with which family members must learn to cope. Standard neoclassical economic theory was the basis for a specialized instrument (no. 17).

A major theoretical distinction made by many researchers is that between objective and subjective burden. However, definitions of objective and subjective burden are implicit rather than explicit and operationalisations differ. The following approaches can be distinguished. Platt (no. 1) considers symptoms and dysfunctioning as objective and assesses the informant's distress (subjective burden) in relation to each particular problem or difficulty associated with the patient's illness. Gopinath (no. 4) and Tessler (no. 13) also use this approach. However, the latter also includes measures of subjective burden such as anger, depression, and embarrassment that are separate from measures of objective care-giving.

Schene (no. 12) argues that burden should be measured in terms of behaviour that can be measured objectively, which involves determining how often relatives have to perform specific care-giving tasks. Like Tessler, he also measures distress, tension and worrying, but not directly related to patient behaviour. Pai (no. 2) measures subjective burden with one question: "How much would you say you have suffered owing to the patient's illness?" Reinhard (no. 16) considers subjective burden to be affective dimensions subjectively felt, such as shame, stigma, guilt, resentment, grief and worry. The instrument developed by Szmukler (no. 18) concentrates on the cognitive and emotional experience of care-giving.

Table 5.2 shows that some dimensions are included in almost all instruments. Worrying ($n = 16$), distress ($n = 16$), the effect of the patient's disorder on the family routine ($n = 16$), leisure ($n = 16$) and family interaction ($n = 15$), and financial consequences ($n = 15$) are most frequently included. Among the less frequently measured dimensions are use of psychotropics ($n = 3$), having to encourage the patient ($n = 7$), effects on the physical health of the care-giver ($n = 8$), and care-givers' feelings of guilt ($n = 8$) and shame ($n = 9$).

More than half the researchers mentioned additional burden dimensions, including: cognitive preoccupation (no. 7), feelings of loss and grief (no. 8), positive aspects of care-giving and knowledge about the illness (no. 9), problems with patients using alcohol or drugs, feeling threatened (no. 12), having to change personal plans for the future, and being upset about the change in the patient from his or her former self (no. 16).

The average number of dimensions is 12.5. These may be represented by a single item or by a fully developed scale. A measure of global burden is included in 55% of the instruments. It may comprise a single general item, summary scales or cumulative indexes constructed from items or interviewer assessments.

Another way to examine the structure underlying the burden concept is to use results from factor analyses (see Table 5.4). These results show some empirical basis for the dimensions of worrying, effect on family routine/interaction (tension, familial discord, disruption), care and control (supervision, urging, ongoing responsibility), behavioural problems, economic hardship, preoccupation (also emotional over-involvement), distress and stigma.

Specialised instruments

Some instruments have been developed for specific purposes. Those of Jacob (no. 3) and Fadden (no. 9) have been designed in particular for family members of patients with depression. Cook's instrument (no. 7) has been developed for parents residing with chronically mentally ill offspring. Coverage includes parental feelings of connection to the ill child, preoccupation, and feelings of ongoing responsibility, among others. Miller (no. 8) adapted an instrument used to measure both initial and present symptoms of grief. In his view, families of the severely mentally ill undergo a syndrome of grief and mourning akin to that experienced by individuals suffering other forms of real or psychic loss. Finally, Clark (no. 17) developed an instrument especially to measure economic burden. Costs are defined as direct dollar expenditures, time expended and opportunities forgone.

Precursors and influences

Table 5.3 summarises the influence of older instruments on the development of newer ones. The vast majority of burden instruments in current use are adapted or influenced at least in part by the work of earlier researchers. The instruments of Platt *et al* (1980) (no. 1), Grad & Sainsbury (1963), Creer *et al* (1982), Pasamanick *et al* (1967), and Tessler *et al* (1987) appear to have had the most influence. While some instruments were influenced by one or two precursors, others acknowledge multiple influences. The instruments developed by Schene (no. 12), Greenberg (no. 15) and Reinhard (no. 16) give credit to a variety of sources.

How did researchers collect their items if not by using pre-existing instruments? Gopinath (no. 4) held open interviews with a number of relatives and chose the most frequent and important distressing

TABLE 5.3
Instruments based on or influenced by other (earlier) instruments

Based on/influenced by:	Instrument[1]																			
	1	2	3	4	5	6	7	8	9	10	11	12	13	14	15	16	17	18	19	20
Freeman & Simmons (1958)															+	+				
Grad & Sainsbury (1963)	+	+													+	+				
Hoenig & Hamilton (1966a,b)	+										+	+								
Pasamanick et al (1967)			+			+								+						
Spitzer et al (1971)										+						+				
Test & Stein (1978)												+	+		+	+				
Platt et al (1980)									+		+		+			+				
Pai & Kapur (1982)					+							+								
Thompson & Doll (1982)									+						+					
Creer et al (1982)									+			+	+		+					
Fadden et al (1987a,b)											+	+								
Coyne et al (1987)												+								
Jacob et al (1987)												+								
Tessler et al (1987)												+			+	+	+			

[1] Instrument number refers to Table 5.1

behaviours. Cook (no. 7) used the work of Hatfield (1978, 1981; Hatfield & Lefley, 1987) and Falloon *et al* (1984). Szmukler (no. 18) organised focus groups with relatives, Schofield (no. 20) held in-depth interviews with care-givers, and Miller (no. 8), as noted above, modified a pre-existing grief instrument. Morosini (no. 11) used the literature on expressed emotion.

Structure and psychometrics

Table 5.4 contains an overview of the instruments, country of origin, and most important psychometric characteristics. Nine instruments are from the USA, four from the UK, two from India, and one each from Greece, Italy, The Netherlands, Canada and Australia.

Nine instruments are self-administered questionnaires, of which three can also be used as personal interviews, two also as postal questionnaires, and one also as a telephone interview. Twelve instruments can be used as personal interviews, of which seven can be used only as such, two can also be used as telephone interviews, and two also as self-administered questionnaires. Two instruments can be used only as telephone interviews.

The instruments that use an interview format all require an interviewing background on the part of the interviewer, while seven also require knowledge of severe mental illness, and seven require a clinical background. For eight of the instruments the interviewers require special training, for four instruments a training guide is currently available (others are being developed) and for six instruments interviewer judgements or ratings are required.

The number of questions ranges from 19 to 437, with a mean of 96. One-third of the instruments have fewer than 30 questions. If we do not include the lengthiest interviews (nos 14, 15 and 20) the mean number of questions is 54. Most of the briefer instruments contain care-giving burden questions only. The instruments with more than 70 questions also incorporate non-burden items, such as asking about the patient, the family, the care-giver, social support, use of mental health services, opinions about mental health services, coping, and patients' contributions to the household.

Of the nine self-administered questionnaires, more than half have fewer than 30 questions, and take 5–45 minutes to complete (the average is 18 minutes). The self-administered questionnaires of Morosini (no. 11) and Schene (no. 12) take the most time because they also gather information about the patient, the family, the household, contact with the patient, and so on. Of the personal and telephone interviews, five have over 100 questions, and take between one and two hours to complete. Nine interviews take half an hour or less, with a mean of 37 questions.

For the majority of instruments the time frame is the past four weeks or 30 days, and for one it is six months. Approximately a quarter use no time frame. For one it is the "current time". In longitudinal studies, the time frames may vary from baseline to follow-up.

Table 5.4 also shows whether information is available about construct validity, internal consistency, interrater reliability (if applicable), test–retest reliability and sensitivity for change. Slightly more than half of the researchers have information on construct validity and internal consistency. Of the 20 instruments, seven have information about test–retest reliability, and seven have information about sensitivity for change. Twelve instruments produce subscale scores as well as a summary score, five produce only subscale scores, one produces only summary scores, and two produce neither. For nine instruments subscale scores are probably associated with factor analyses.

Regarding the type of patient populations in relation to which burden was measured, researchers' descriptions in the questionnaire were used. Most studied family members of severely mentally ill patients. Neurotic patients were studied by only two researchers. Another two studied only relatives of patients with affective disorders. Parents have been most often studied ($n = 13$), followed by siblings ($n = 11$), indicating a tendency to focus on the family of origin. Significant others, partners and offspring have been studied less often.

We know of two instruments that have been translated into different European languages and that have been used in BIOMED-funded research projects: Magliano (no. 11) and Schene (no. 12).

Individual instruments

In the following sections, a summary description of each instrument is given. Instruments are divided into two categories: suitable for research use only and suitable for clinical use too, according to the authors of the instruments. All 20 instruments are considered suitable for research use, while 14 are also considered suitable for clinical use.

Scales suitable for research use only

1. Social Behaviour Assessment Schedule

This interview, developed in the UK, is still used, although the author himself is no longer active in the field (personal communication to the senior author of this chapter). This instrument is administered

Table 5.4
Psychometric characteristics of family or care-giver burden instruments

Instrument (year of publication)	Main author (country)	Number of questions / Completion time / Time frame / Type of instrument[1]	Information available on[2]					Subscale scores	Summary score	Factor analyses
			CV	IC	IR	TRR	SFC			
1. Social Behaviour Assessment Schedule (1980)	Platt (UK)	186 questions / 90 minutes / 4 weeks / SPI	–	–	+	–	–	+	–	–
2. Burden on Family Interview Schedule (1981)	Pai (India)	28 questions / 25 minutes / no time frame / SSPI	+	+	+	–	+	+	+	–
3. Family Distress Scale for Depression (1983)	Jacob (USA)	25 questions / 10 minutes / several weeks / SSPI	–	–	–	–	–	–	+	–
4. Scale for Assessment of Family Distress (1986)	Gopinath (India)	26 questions / 20 minutes / 4 weeks / SAQ, SSPI	+	+	+	+	–	+	+	six factors (data not yet reported)
5. Family Burden Scale (1987)	Madianos (Greece)	34 questions / 30 minutes / ? / SPI	–	–	+	+	–	+	+	–
6. Family Distress Scale (1987)	Birchwood (UK)	46 questions / 10 minutes / 4 weeks / SAQ	–	+	na	+	+	+	+	–

TABLE 5.4 (contd...)

Instrument (year of publication)	Main author (country)	Number of questions / Completion time / Time frame / Type of instrument[1]	Information available on[2]					Subscale scores	Summary score	Factor analyses
			CV	IC	IR	TRR	SFC			
7. Thresholds Parental Burden Scale (1988)	Cook (USA)	29 questions / 10 minutes / current time / SAQ, SPI, SSPI	+	+	+	+	–	+	+	feelings of connection, preoccupation, ongoing responsibility, behavioural problems, familial discord, worries
8. Texas Inventory of Grief – Mental Illness Version (1990)	Miller (USA)	24 questions / 10 minutes / ? / SAQ	+	+	na	–	–	+	–	–
9. Family Burden Questionnaire (1990)	Fadden (UK)	95 questions / 90 minutes / not specified / SSPI	–	–	–	+	–	–	–	–
10. Significant Other Scale (1991)	Herz (USA)	50 questions / 15 minutes / last month	–	–	+	–	–	+	+	–
11. Family Problems Questionnaire (1991)	Morosini (Italy)	29 questions / 15 minutes / 8 weeks / SAQ	+	+	na	+	–	+	+	objective burden, subjective burden, support, positive attitude, criticism of patient

TABLE 5.4 (contd...)

Instrument (year of publication)	Main author (country)	Number of questions / Completion time / Time frame / Type of instrument[1]	Information available on[2]					Subscale scores	Summary score	Factor analyses
			CV	IC	IR	TRR	SFC			
12. Involvement Evaluation Questionnaire (1992)	Schene (The Netherlands)	77 questions 30 minutes 4 weeks SAQ, MQ	+	+	na	+	+	+	+	tension, worrying, supervision, urging
13. Family Burden Interview Schedule (1992)	Tessler (USA)	100 questions 60 minutes 4 weeks TIS, SPI	+	+	–	–	+	+	+	care, control, disruption
14. Family Caregiving of Persons with Mental Illness Survey (1992)	Biegel (USA)	437 questions 70 minutes no time frame SPI	+	+	–	–	–	+	+	overall burden, family disruption, client dependency, stigma, strain
15. Family Burden and Services Questionnaire (1992)	Greenberg (USA)	300 questions 90 minutes 4 weeks TIS	+	+	–	–	–	+	–	subjective burden, worry, patient harming self, patient harming others, stigma, positive/ negative feelings about involvement
16. Burden Assessment Scale (1992)	Reinhard (USA)	19 questions 5 minutes 6 months SAQ, TIS, SPI	+	+	–	–	+	+	+	disrupted activities, personal distress, time perspective, guilt, basic social functioning

TABLE 5.4 (contd...)

Instrument (year of publication)	Main author (country)	Number of questions / Completion time / Time frame / Type of instrument[1]	Information available on[2]					Subscale scores	Summary score	Factor analyses
			CV	IC	IR	TRR	SFC			
17. Family Economic Burden Interview (1993/94)	Clark (USA)	70 questions 30 minutes 2 and 4 weeks TIS, SPI	–	–	–	–	–	+	–	–
18. Experience of Caregiving Inventory (1996)	Szmukler (UK)	66 questions 15 minutes 4 weeks SAQ, MQ	+	+	na	–	+	+	+	difficult behaviour, negative symptoms, stigma, problems with services, effects on family, need to back-up, dependency, loss
19. The Perceived Family Burden Scale (1996)	Levene (Canada)	24 questions – – SAQ	+	+	na	+	+	–	–	–
20. Victorian Carers Program Questionnaire (1996)	Schofield (Australia)	249 questions 50 minutes No time frame TIS	–	+	–	–	–	+	–	–

[1] SAQ, self-administered questionnaire; MQ, mail questionnaire; TIS, telephone interview (structured); TISS, telephone interview (semistructured); SPI, structured personal interview; SSPI, semistructured personal interview.
[2] CV, construct validity; IC, internal consistency; IR, interrater reliability; TRR, test–retest reliability; SFC, sensitivity for change; na, not applicable.

by trained interviewers, for whom a training guide is available, and information on interrater reliability is available. The instrument is comprehensive, and measures social behaviour as well as burden. For routine clinical use this interview may be too lengthy.

6. Family Distress Scale

This self-administered questionnaire, developed in the UK, is an expanded version of Pasamanick's scale. It especially measures subjective burden (Smith *et al*, 1993), and was designed for use with first-degree relatives of schizophrenic patients. It takes 10 minutes and covers a large number of burden dimensions. The psychometric properties are well established.

9. Family Burden Questionnaire

This 95-item interview, developed in the UK, is one of two that concentrates especially on family members of patients with depression. It has been used effectively in descriptive studies. Psychometrics are not well established. According to the author, the interview would probably be perceived as too long for routine clinical work.

13. Family Burden Interview Schedule

This 100-item structured personal interview was developed in the USA. It takes about 60 minutes to administer in person and can also be used as a briefer telephone interview, as has been done in two follow-up assessments. Interviewers do not need a special background, and a manual is available describing the modular structure of the instrument. Psychometric information is available (Tessler & Gamache, 1994)

15. Family Burden and Services Questionnaire

This telephone interview was developed in the USA. Interviewers do not need a special background, but have to be trained. It contains approximately 300 questions, of which some 57 are about burden. The other items measure attributions of the cause of the illness, coping, opinions about mental health services, patient behaviour and clients' contributions to the family. The entire instrument takes 90 minutes to administer, of which about 45 minutes are devoted to burden. Factor analysis resulted in a six-factor structure, and information is available pertaining to reliability and validity.

17. Family Economic Burden Interview

This personal or telephone interview was developed in the USA. It contains 70 questions, and is the only instrument that is devoted mainly to economic burden. It has been used for relatives of people with severe mental disorder who also suffer from substance misuse. Its primary focus is on objective burden. Psychometric information has not been published.

Scales suitable for both clinical and research use

2. Burden on Family Interview Schedule

This interview, developed in India, takes 25 minutes to administer, its psychometric properties are well established, and information about sensitivity for change is available. Interviewer ratings and special training are required. Developed in the early 1980s, this instrument has since been used by a number of other researchers (e.g., Raj *et al*, 1991; Chakrabarti *et al*, 1992).

3. Family Distress Scale for Depression

This interview is based on Pasamanick's instrument, but was greatly modified to assess the distress associated with depressive symptoms and behaviour. It takes 10 minutes to complete. Its brevity and ease of administration are advantages for use in routine clinical practice. However, its comprehensiveness of coverage is low, and the psychometric properties are not well established.

4. Scale for Assessment of Family Distress

This self-administered questionnaire, a second Indian contribution to burden measurement, takes 20 minutes to complete. The scale focuses on the distress that psychotic symptoms and behaviour produce in family members, rather than on the measurement of care-giving *per se*. It can also be used as an interview, for which interviewers require a clinical background, but not special training. This scale has been used mainly in association with psychiatric patients, but a variant scale is available for patients with substance misuse. Extensive psychometric analyses have been done.

5. Family Burden Scale

This instrument, developed in Greece, is a structured personal interview requiring 30 minutes to administer. It is designed for use with first-degree relatives of schizophrenic patients. Interviewers require a clinical background but no special training. Some psycho-metric information is currently available, and the authors report that the scale is undergoing standardisation. The authors also developed the Family Atmosphere Scale, which is a supplementary instrument.

7. Thresholds Parental Burden Scale

This 29-item self-administered questionnaire, developed in the USA, was designed to be used for parents of offspring with severe mental illness. Recently it has been used in analyses of the relationship of parental burden to race, age, residence, and stage in the life course. The psychometric properties are well established (Cook *et al*, 1994). The scale has also been administered to the parents of a sample of non-disabled, same-aged offspring.

8. Texas Inventory of Grief – Mental Illness Version

This 24-item self-administered questionnaire can be completed in 10 minutes. It concentrates on grief reactions of family members of persons with severe mental disorder. Although this is one of the least comprehensive burden instruments, it provides the most extensive measures of grief that are available. Separate subscale scores are produced for initial and present feelings about the relative's loss of mental health. Psychometric information is available pertaining to internal consistency and construct validity.

10. Significant Other Scale

This personal interview with family members whose relative is a patient with schizophrenia takes 15 minutes to administer. It is comprehensive and designed to generate separate scores for subjective and objective burden. The instrument has been used in a randomised trial, comparing intermittent and maintenance medication. Psychometric information is only available pertaining to interrater reliability.

11. Family Problems Questionnaire (FPQ)

This was developed in Italy for use in routine clinical practice. Its first version (Questionnaire for Family Problems; Morosini *et al*, 1991), a comprehensive self-administered questionnaire, was admin-istered to a variety of relatives of recently admitted psychiatric patients at two points in time. An international version of the questionnaire, the FPQ, has been developed and validated in five European languages (English, German, Greek, Italian and Portuguese). It was used in a BIOMED study on family burden and coping in schizophrenia (Magliano *et al*, 1998, 1999). It contains 29 items grouped in five factors. Three of these have to do with burden: objective burden, subjective burden and criticism. The other two factors concern support and positive attitudes towards the patient. The psychometric properties are well established.

12. Involvement Evaluation Questionnaire (IEQ)

This instrument was initially developed in The Netherlands to compare the family impact of day hospitalisation against in-patient hospitalisation (Schene, 1987). It was subsequently revised to render it suitable for a survey of a large organisation of relatives of patients with psychotic disorders (Schene *et al*, 1998). The core IEQ is a 31-item questionnaire and may be used as a self-administered or mail questionnaire. It is extended with six extra modules, containing the 12-item General Health Questionnaire, sociodemographic variables, and items on extra financial expenses, care-giver's use of professional help, and consequences for the patient's children. The whole 77-item instrument takes about 30 minutes to administer. Psychometric properties are well established. Factor analysis identified four factors, which can be added into a total score (see Table 5.4). The IEQ is available in nine languages. The English, Danish, Italian and Spanish translations have been developed, validated and used in the BIOMED-financed Epsilon study of schizophrenia in five European countries (van Wijngaarden *et al*, 2000). The Finnish, German, French and Portuguese versions have not been validated yet.

14. Family Caregiving of Persons with Mental Illness Survey

This structured personal interview was developed in the USA. It includes 53 burden items contained within a broader instrument that also measures client and care-giver demographic characteristics, client illness characteristics and behavioural problems, social network and social support, and health status. The burden items take 10 minutes to administer, while the larger instrument requires 70 minutes. It has been administered to a heterogeneous population of relatives of persons with mental illness. Extensive psychometric information is available, including results from factor analysis (see Table 5.4).

16. Burden Assessment Scale

This instrument, developed in the USA, can be administered as a personal interview, a telephone interview and as a self-administered questionnaire. The 19 questions can be answered in five minutes. A six-month time frame is recommended, which contrasts with the four weeks used in most other instruments. The instrument is appropriate for use with a variety of family members of the severely mentally ill, including (but not limited to) the primary care-giver. Psychometric information is available. Factor analysis identified five factors (see Table 5.4).

18. Experience of Caregiving Inventory (ECI)

This questionnaire was developed in the UK by collecting items from in-depth interviews and focus groups with 120 care-givers. It takes about 15 minutes to complete and has two main sections. The first section contains 52 statements and care-givers are asked how often during the last month they have thought about the issue outlined in the statement. The second section contains 14 questions about symptoms, in the format "During the past month how often have you thought about her being ... [symptom]". The questionnaire has been used in descriptive, epidemiological and programme-evaluation studies, as well as in randomised clinical trials. The psychometric properties are well established (Szmukler *et al*, 1996*a*,*b*).

19. Perceived Family Burden Scale

This 24-item questionnaire was developed in Canada for the measurement of burden experienced by relatives of patients with schizophrenia. Items were generated from a literature review and consultation of relatives' groups. Psychometrics were tested in a small sample ($n = 52$) and further replication in a larger sample is needed according to the authors (Levene *et al*, 1996). So far, the scale has been used only in descriptive studies.

20. Victorian Carers Program Questionnaire

This 249-item interview was developed in Australia to study a random sample of carers of the population of Victoria. It measures attitudes and feelings about care-giving and the amount of help needed and given in various activities of daily living. It takes 50 minutes to administer and has been used in epidemiological studies.

Discussion

Family or care-giver burden research has a history that begins after the Second World War. During the last decade, however, the field has undergone rapid growth. At the end of the 1980s we were able to identify 12 burden instruments (Schene, 1990). The current review identifies 20. The emergence of new family burden instruments indicates the growing importance accorded to burden within the mental health field. This scientific tradition continues in the USA and, to a lesser extent, in the UK. Not only were the 'classic' scales developed in those two countries, but also most of the recent ones. However, we were able to identify three instruments from other European countries, and two from India.

Researchers thus have 20 scales from which to make a selection. Since the authors of this review are each identified with their own burden instruments, we do not feel it is appropriate to recommend one instrument over another. In any case, the final choice of instrument depends on a variety of considerations, including the purpose(s) for which the study is being conducted. Depending on the research aims, the following should be considered as guidelines in making a selection.

If the purpose is to conduct a theoretical study linking burden with other constructs, then the following instruments may be relevant: nos 1, 9, 13, 14 and 15. If the purpose is to study the family burden associated with caring for a person with depression, then the following instruments should be considered: nos 1, 3, 9, 12 and 18. For those whose research interest is relatives of persons with schizophrenia, the following instruments are appropriate: nos 1, 4, 5, 6, 8, 10, 11, 12, 18 and 19. For more general use with heterogeneous patient populations, researchers may find the following instruments useful: nos 1, 2, 4, 8, 12, 13, 14, 15, 16, 18 and 20. For specialised economic studies, no. 17 should be used. For studying grief reactions, no. 8 is appropriate. For measuring change in longitudinal studies, the following instruments should be considered, as they have previously been used for this purpose: nos 2, 6, 11, 12, 13, 15, 17 and 18. However, one has to check whether sensitivity for change has been studied (see Table 5.4).

The section on individual instruments and Table 5.4 may also be useful in helping researchers to select an instrument that meets other specific requirements, such as time to administer, interviewer background and method of administration. For example, if one knows in advance that a brief, self-administered questionnaire is to be used, then this narrows down the range of options. However, we recommend that researchers do not make final choices based on this review alone, but contact the authors of the instruments directly and obtain copies of their instruments before making a final choice. A list of addresses is available from the first author of this chapter upon request.

Morosini *et al* (1991) suggest that "family evaluation should not be performed only at specific requests for help, but offered routinely to families at the first contact with the patient". If we take this as a *modus operandi*, then the following criteria may be applied in choosing an instrument for clinical use: brevity and ease of administration, comprehensiveness of coverage, appropriateness for different types of patients and family members, and adequate psychometric properties. While a number of the instruments reviewed appear to meet these criteria and thus have potential use in routine clinical settings, it should be noted that the measurement of burden in routine clinical practice is relatively new. No authors have reported clinical norms or cut-off points that can be used to detect individual family members at risk from over-burden, or to serve as a basis for clinical intervention for the family member.

Conclusions

Researchers more or less agree about the dimensions that comprise the concept of family burden. There is less agreement with regard to the definition of burden and how best to measure objective and subjective burden. These disagreements influence how specific dimensions are operationalised. Some burden researchers use single items denoting different aspects of burden as part of a summary scale, while others have turned to a modular approach, with multi-item scales devoted to separate dimensions.

It is encouraging that some theoretical models describing the structure of burden or care-giving have been published (Tessler *et al*, 1989, 1991; Schene, 1990; Biegel *et al*, 1991; Schene *et al*, 1998). This is significant, because the measurement of burden hinges largely on how it is conceptualised. Further research is needed to elaborate these models, so that the theory and measurement of family burden are better integrated. The relationship between patient and care-giver characteristics, care-giving tasks and the role of social and professional support need further empirical and theoretical work.

In conclusion, although it is encouraging to see that the field is growing, we believe that some standardisation is needed and therefore recommend that burden researchers join and develop a few standard instruments, with acceptable psychometric properties, for both research and routine clinical use.

References

Biegel, D. E., Sales, E. & Schulz, R. (1991) *Family Caregiving in Chronic Illness*. London: Sage.

——, Song, L. Y. & Chakravarthy, V. (1994) Predictors of caregiver burden among support group members of persons with chronic mental illness. In: *Family Caregiving Across the Lifespan* (eds E. Kahana, D. E. Biegel & M. L. Wykle), pp. 178–215. Family Caregiver Applications Series, **4**. Newbury Park, California: Sage.

Birchwood, M. & Smith, J. (1992) Specific and non-specific effects of educational intervention for families living with schizophrenia. *British Journal of Psychiatry*, **160**, 645–652.

Chakrabarti, S., Kulhara, P. & Verma, S. K. (1992) Extent and determinants of burden among families of patients with affective disorders. *Acta Psychiatrica Scandinavica*, **86**, 247–252.

Clark, R. E. & Drake, R. E. (1994) Expenditures of time and money by families of people with severe mental illness and substance use disorders. *Community Mental Health Journal*, **30**, 145–163.

Cook, J. A. & Pickett, S. A. (1987) Feelings of burden and criticalness among parents residing with chronically mentally ill offspring. *Journal of Applied Social Sciences*, **12**, 79–107.

——, Lefley, H. P., Pickett, S., *et al* (1994) Age and family burden among parents of offspring with severe mental illness. *American Journal of Orthopsychiatry*, **64**, 435–447.

Coyne, J. C., Kessler, R. C., Tal, M., *et al* (1987) Living with a depressed person. *Journal of Consulting and Clinical Psychology*, **55**, 347–352.

Creer, C., Sturt, E. & Wykes, T. (1982) The role of relatives. In *Long Term Community Care Experience in a London Borough* (ed. J. K. Wing), pp. 29–39. Psychological Medicine, Monograph Supplement 2.

Fadden, G. B. (1984) *The Relatives of Patients with Depressive Disorders: A Typology of Burden and Strategies of Coping*. MPhil thesis, Institute of Psychiatry, University of London.

——, Bebbington, P. & Kuipers, L. (1987*a*) The burden of care: the impact of functional psychiatric illness on the patient's family. *British Journal of Psychiatry*, **150**, 285–292.

——, —— & —— (1987*b*) Caring and its burdens. A study of the spouses of depressed patients. *British Journal of Psychiatry*, **151**, 660–667.

Falloon, I. R. H., Boyd, J. L. & McGill, C. W. (1984) *Family Care of Schizophrenia*. New York: Guilford Press.

Fisher, G. A., Benson, P. R. & Tessler, R. C. (1990) Family response to mental illness: developments since deinstitutionalization. *Research in Community and Mental Health*, **6**, 203–236.

Freeman, H. E. & Simmons, O. G. (1958) Mental patients in the community. Family settings and performance level. *American Sociological Review*, **22**, 147–154.

Gallop, R., McKeever, P., Mohide, E. A., *et al* (1991) *Family Care and Chronic Illness: The Caregiving Experience. A Review of the Literature*. Toronto: Faculty of Nursing, University of Toronto.

Gopinath, P. S. & Chaturvedi, S. K. (1986) Measurement of distressful psychotic symptoms perceived by the family: preliminary findings. *Indian Journal of Psychiatry*, **28**, 343–345.

—— & —— (1992) Distressing behaviour of schizophrenics at home. *Acta Psychiatrica Scandinavica*, **86**, 185–188.

Grad, J. & Sainsbury, P. (1963) Mental illness and the family. *Lancet*, **8**, 544–547.

—— & —— (1968) The effects that patients have on their families in a community care and a control psychiatric service. *British Journal of Psychiatry*, **114**, 265–278.

Greenberg, J. S., Greenley, J. R., McKee, D., *et al* (1993) Mothers caring for an adult child with schizophrenia: the effects of subjective burden on maternal health. *Family Relations*, April, **442**, 205–211.

Gubman, G. D. & Tessler, R. C. (1987) The impact of mental illness on families. *Journal of Family Issues*, **8**, 226–245.

——, —— & Willis, G. (1987) Living with the mentally ill: factors affecting household complaints. *Schizophrenia Bulletin*, **13**, 727–736.

Hatfield, A. (1978) Psychological costs of schizophrenia to the family. *Social Work*, **23**, 355–359.

—— (1981) Coping effectiveness in families of the mentally ill: an exploratory study. *Journal of Psychiatric Treatment and Evaluation*, **3**, 11–19.

—— & LEFLEY, H. P. (1987) *Families of the Mentally Ill. Coping and Adaptation*. London: Cassell Educational.

HERZ, M. I., GLAZER, W. & MOSTERT, M. (1991) Intermittent vs maintenance medication in schizophrenia. *Archives of General Psychiatry*, **48**, 333–339.

HOENIG, J. (1968) The de-segregation of the psychiatric patient. *Proceedings of the Royal Society of Medicine*, **61**, 115–120.

—— & HAMILTON, M. W. (1966*a*) The schizophrenic patient in the community and the effect on the household. *International Journal of Social Psychiatry*, **26**, 165–176.

—— & —— (1966*b*) The burden on the household in an extramural psychiatric service. In *New Aspects of the Mental Health Services* (eds H. L. Freeman & W. A. J. Farndale), pp. 612–635. Oxford: Pergamon Press.

JACOB, M., FRANK, E., KUPFER, D. J., *et al* (1987) Recurrent depression: an assessment of family burden and family attitudes. *Journal of Clinical Psychiatry*, **48**, 395–400.

LEVENE, J. E,. LANCEE, W. J. & SEEMAN, M. V. (1996) The perceived family burden scale: measurement and validation. *Schizophrenia Research*, **22**, 151–157.

MADIANOS, M., GOURNAS, G., TOMARAS, V., *et al* (1987) Family atmosphere on the course of chronic schizophrenia treated in a community mental health center: a prospective longitudinal study. In *Schizophrenia: Recent Biosocial Developments* (eds C. Stefanis & A. Rabavilas), pp. 246–256. New York: Human Sciences Press.

—— & MADIANOU, D. (1992) The effects of long-term community care on relapse and adjustment of persons with chronic schizophrenia. *International Journal of Mental Health*, **21**, 37–49.

MAGLIANO, L., FADDEN, G., MADIANOS, M., *et al* (1998) Burden on the families of patients with schizophrenia: results of the BIOMED I study. *Social Psychiatry and Psychiatric Epidemiology*, **33**, 405–412.

——, ——, FIORILLO, A., *et al* (1999) Family burden and coping strategies in schizophrenia: are key relatives really different to other relatives? *Acta Psychiatrica Scandinavica*, **99**, 10–15.

MILLER, F., DWORKIN, J., WARD, M., *et al* (1990) A preliminary study of unresolved grief in families of seriously mentally ill patients. *Hospital and Community Psychiatry*, **41**, 1321–1325.

MOROSINI, P., RONCONE, R., VELTRO, F., *et al* (1991) Routine assessment tool in psychiatry: a case of questionnaire of family attitudes and burden. *Italian Journal of Psychiatry and Behavioural Sciences*, **1**, 95–101.

PAI, S. & KAPUR, R. L. (1981) The burden on the family of a psychiatric patient: development of an interview schedule. *British Journal of Psychiatry*, **138**, 332–335.

—— & —— (1982) Impact of treatment intervention on the relationship between dimensions of clinical psychopathology, social dysfunction and burden on the family. *Psychological Medicine*, **12**, 651–658.

PASAMANICK, B., SCARPITTI, F. R. & DINITZ, S. (1967) *Schizophrenics in the Community: An Experimental Study in the Prevention of Hospitalization*. New York: Appleton-Century-Crofts.

PLATT, S. (1985) Measuring the burden of psychiatric illness on the family: an evaluation of some rating scales. *Psychological Medicine*, **15**, 383–393.

——, WEYMAN, A., HIRSCH, S., *et al* (1980) The Social Behaviour Assessment Schedule (SBAS): rationale, contents, scoring and reliability of a new interview schedule. *Social Psychiatry*, **15**, 43–55.

——, —— & —— (1983) *Social Behaviour Assessment Schedule* (SBAS, 3rd edn). Windsor: NFER-Nelson.

RAJ, L., KULHARA, P. & AVASTHI, A. (1991) Social burden of positive and negative schizophrenia. *International Journal of Social Psychiatry*, **37**, 242–250.

REINHARD, S., GUBMAN, G., HORWITZ, A., *et al* (in press) Burden assessment scale for families of the seriously mentally ill. *Evaluation and Program Planning* (in press).

Schene, A. H. (1987) *The Burden on the Family Scale.* Utrecht: Department of Ambulatory and Social Psychiatry, University of Utrecht, The Netherlands.

—— (1990) Objective and subjective dimensions of family burden. Toward an integrative framework for research. *Social Psychiatry and Psychiatric Epidemiology*, **25**, 289–297.

—— & van Wijngaarden, B. (1992) *The Involvement Evaluation Questionnaire.* Amsterdam: Department of Psychiatry, University of Amsterdam, The Netherlands.

——, Tessler, R. C. & Gamache, G. M. (1996) Caregiving in severe mental illness; conceptualization and measurement. In *Mental Health Service Evaluation* (eds H. C. Knudsen & G. Thornicroft), pp. 296–316. Cambridge: Cambridge University Press.

——, van Wijngaarden, B. & Koeter, M. W. J. (1998) Family caregiving in schizophrenia: domains and distress. *Schizophrenia Bulletin*, **24**, 609–618.

Schofield, H., Murphy, B., Herrman, H., *et al* (1997) Family caregiving: measurement of emotional well being and various aspects of the caregiving role. *Psychological Medicine*, **27**, 647–657.

Smith, J., Birchwood, M., Cochrane, R., *et al* (1993) The needs of high and low expressed emotion families: a normative approach. *Social Psychiatry and Psychiatric Epidemiology*, **28**, 11–16.

Spitzer, R. L., Giboon, M. & Endicott, J. (1971) *Family Evaluation Form.* New York: New York State Department of Mental Hygiene.

Szmukler, G. I., Burgess, P., Herrman, H., *et al* (1996*a*) Caring for relatives with serious mental illness: the development of the Experience of Caregiving Inventory. *Social Psychiatry and Psychiatric Epidemiology*, **31**, 137–148

——, Herrman, H., Colusa, S., *et al* (1996*b*) A controlled trial of a counselling intervention for caregivers of relatives with schizophrenia. *Social Psychiatry and Psychiatric Epidemiology*, **31**, 149–155.

Tessler, R. C., Killian, L. M. & Gubman, G. D. (1987) Stages in family response to mental illness: an ideal type. *Psychosocial Rehabilitation Journal*, **10**, 3–16.

——, Fisher, G. & Gamache, G. (1989) A role strain approach to the measurement of family burden: the properties and utilities of a new scale. Paper presented at the Annual Meetings of the Eastern Sociological Society, Baltimore.

——, —— & —— (1991) *Conceptualizing and Measuring the Burden of Caregiving on Families of the Severely Mentally Ill.* Amherst, MA: Social and Demographic Research Institute, University of Massachusetts.

——, —— & —— (1992) *The Family Burden Interview Schedule Manual.* Amherst MA: Social and Demographic Research Institute, University of Massachusetts.

—— & Gamache, G. (1994) Continuity of care, residence, and family burden in Ohio. *Milbank Memorial Fund Quarterly*, **72**, 149–169.

Test, M. A. & Stein, L. I. (1978) *Alternatives to Mental Hospital Treatment.* New York: Plenum Press.

—— & —— (1980) Alternative to mental hospital treatment: III Social cost. *Archives of General Psychiatry*, **37**, 409–412.

Thompson, E. H. & Doll, W. (1982) The burden of families coping with the mentally ill: an invisible crisis. *Family Relations*, **31**, 379–388.

Weissman, M. M. (1975) The assessment of social adjustment. A review of techniques. *Archives of General Psychiatry*, **32**, 357–365.

—— (1981) The assessment of social adjustment. An update. *Archives of General Psychiatry*, **38**, 1250–1258.

van Wijngaarden, B., Schene, A. H., Koeter, M., *et al* (2000) Caregiving in schizophrenia: development, internal consistency and reliability of the Involvement Evaluation Questionnaire – European version. *British Journal of Psychiatry*, **177** (suppl. 39), s21–s27.

6 Measures of quality of life for people with severe mental disorders

ANTHONY F. LEHMAN

This chapter provides clinicians, researchers, programme evaluators and administrators with current information on the assessment of quality-of-life (QOL) outcomes for people with severe mental disorders. Measures are summarised according to purpose, content, psychometric properties, patient subgroups with whom used and key references. Fifteen QOL measures are summarised and reflect considerable variability in the parameters examined. Comprehensive, reliable and valid measures of QOL are available, although further development of QOL assessment methodologies is needed. More importantly, we must strive for a better understanding of how to interpret and use QOL outcome information.

The broad impact that severe mental illnesses have on people's lives and the resulting complexity of the needs generated by such illnesses pose a particular challenge in the assessment of the outcomes of services for these persons (Schulberg & Bromet, 1981; Lehman *et al*, 1982). Relevant outcome domains include psychiatric symptoms, functional status, access to resources and opportunities, subjective well-being, family burden and community safety. Because of this broad array of relevant outcomes and because of a prevailing concern that outcome assessments should include the patient's perspective, there has been increased attention paid over the past decade to the development of measures of patients' QOL.

Before describing the measures that are reviewed, it is important to acknowledge those that are not. 'Quality of life' is a broad term and conceptually could cover all outcome measures, including measures of clinical symptoms and functional status. However, many of these measures are reviewed elsewhere in this volume or have been reviewed previously. Therefore, they are not included in this chapter. Also excluded are measures of such concepts as 'family burden' and client satisfaction with services, because these are considered not to be patient outcomes *per se* (but see Chapters 4 and 5).

Rather, the measures reviewed here are those that emphasise the patient's QOL, that is, measures covering patients' perspectives on what they have, how they are doing and how they feel about their life circumstances. At a minimum, QOL covers people's sense of well-being; often it also includes how they are doing (functional status) and what they have (access to resources and opportunities). In order to be selected for this review, a measure had at least to assess the domain of subjective well-being; as will be seen, most of these measures also cover the broad areas of functioning and resources.

Specific measures

The vast majority of QOL measures identified were designed for mixed diagnostic groups of persons with mental illnesses, primarily schizophrenia, but also including affective disorders and a variety of other chronic axis I disorders. This section is organised according to the mental illnesses targeted by the various measures: severe and persistent mental illnesses, schizophrenia, depression and anxiety disorders. Each measure is summarised in terms of its name, key reference(s), original purpose, types of patient studied, type of instrument, number of items, length of administration, summary content and psychometric properties.

Severe and persistent mental illnesses

Community Adjustment Form (CAF)

This semistructured self-report interview (Stein & Test, 1980) was developed to assess life satisfaction and other QOL outcomes in a randomised study of an experimental system of community-based care for the severely mentally ill versus standard care in Dane County, Wisconsin. It consists of 140 items and requires approximately 45 minutes to complete. The areas assessed include: leisure activities; quality of living situation; employment history and status; income sources and amounts; free lodging and/or meals; contact with friends; family contact; legal problems; life satisfaction (21 items); self-esteem; medical care; and agency utilisation. No psychometric properties have been reported. The original patient sample studied included 130 patients seeking admission to a state hospital. Over half (55%) were men and their mean age was 31 years. Half carried a diagnosis of schizophrenia. They were treated both in the state hospital and in an 'assertive community treatment programme'. The results of the original Wisconsin study were replicated in Australia using the same measures (Hoult & Reynolds, 1984).

Quality of Life Checklist (QLC)

This instrument (Malm *et al*, 1981) was developed to provide information about which aspects of QOL are particularly important to patients and clinician raters to assist in therapeutic planning. The 93-item rating scale is completed by a trained interviewer after conducting a one-hour semistructured interview. Scoring for all areas assessed is dichotomised as 'satisfactory' or 'unsatisfactory'. The areas assessed include: leisure activities, work, vocational rehabilitation, economic dependency, social relationships, knowledge and education, psychological dependency, inner experience, housing standard, medical care (psychiatric and general), and religion. No psychometric properties are reported. Data analyses report simple frequencies of 'satisfactory' or 'unsatisfactory' by item. The patients studied included 40 persons with chronic schizophrenia in a Swedish out-patient clinic. They ranged in age from 18 to 50 years and the sample was 68% male.

Satisfaction with Life Domains Scale (SLDS)

This instrument (Baker & Intagliata, 1982; Johnson, 1991) was developed to evaluate the impact of the Community Support Program (CSP) in New York state on the quality of life of chronically mentally ill patients. It is a self-report scale administered by a trained interviewer, consists of 15 items, and requires approximately 10 minutes. Its individual items cover: satisfaction with housing, neighbourhood, food to eat, clothing, health, people lived with, friends, family, relations with other people, work/day programming, spare time, fun, services and facilities in area, economic situation, place lived in now compared with state hospital. These can be summed into a total life satisfaction score. The total life satisfaction score correlates with scores on both the Bradburn Affect Balance Scale (Bradburn, 1969) ($r = 0.64$) and the Global Assessment Scale (Endicott *et al*, 1976) ($r = 0.29$). No other psychometric data are provided. The frequencies and means on the individual items can be compared with item scores in a national QOL survey of the general population (Andrews & Withey, 1976). The patients studied included 118 chronically mentally ill out-patients, aged 18–86 years, in two community support programmes. They had a mean age of 53.3 years; 61% were women, and 84% lived in supervised residential settings. Diagnoses included 56% schizophrenia, 14% affective disorders, 5% substance misuse and 3% organic mental syndromes.

Oregon Quality of Life Questionnaire (OQLQ)

The OQLQ (Bigelow *et al* 1982*a,b*, 1991*a,b*; Bigelow & Young, 1991) was originally based upon the Denver Community Mental Health Scale, but has undergone a series of developments since 1981. Its original purpose was to assess QOL outcomes among clients served by community mental health programmes, especially those developed under the CSP initiative of the National Institute of Mental Health (NIMH). Originally published in 1982, the OQLQ has been updated by its developer with more recent psychometric data, alternative versions, and further programme applications.

The OQLQ exists in two versions: a structured self-report interview (263 items) and a semistructured interviewer-rated interview (146 items). Both are administered by a trained (not necessarily clinical) interviewer. The theory underlying the OQLQ states that QOL derives from the social contract between an individual and society. Individuals' *needs* are met to the extent that they fulfil the *demands* placed upon them by society.

Most of the items use fixed, ordinal response categories, and the interview requires approximately 45 minutes to administer. The OQLQ yields 14 scale scores: psychological distress, psychological well-being, tolerance of stress, total basic need satisfaction, independence, interpersonal interactions, spouse role, social support, work at home, employability, work on the job, meaningful use of time, negative consequences of alcohol use, negative consequences of drug use.

The psychometric properties of the OQLQ have been evaluated extensively. Cronbach's alpha for the 14 scales on the self-report interview version range from 0.05 to 0.98, with a median of 0.84. Eight of the scales have excellent reliability (alpha > 0.8), two have intermediate reliability (alpha between 0.8 and 0.4) and four have poor reliability (< 0.4). Test–retest reliabilities (interval not specified) ranged from 0.37 to 0.64, with a median of 0.50. The interrater reliability for the interviewer-rated version has been assessed in a small sample study (*n* = 6) and produced interrater agreement levels of between 58% and 100% on the interviewer judgements. More than half the items showed greater than 90% agreement, and Cronbach's alpha ranged from 0.32 to over 0.80 (more than half over 0.80). The predictive validity of the OQLQ has been evaluated by comparing:

clients in different types of community mental health programmes (CSP, drug, alcohol and general psychiatric clinics); general community respondents from economically distressed and non-distressed communities; and changes in community mental health clients over time. Results of these analyses support the overall predictive validity of the OQLQ.

The OQLQ has been applied to out-patients of mental health programmes as well as to samples of the general population. The out-patient samples included patients at intake to community mental health programmes in Oregon (including chronically mentally ill, drug misusing, alcoholic and general psychiatric patients). Their mean age was 33.8 years (range 18–85); the sample was included 60% male and 96% 'non-Hispanic'. The community sample had a mean age of 36.8 years and was 43% male and was 92% non-Hispanic.

Lehman Quality of Life Interview (QOLI)

The QOLI (Lehman *et al*, 1982, 1986, 1991, 1992, 1995; Lehman, 1983*a,b*, 1988; Franklin *et al*, 1987; Simpson *et al*, 1989; Levitt *et al*, 1990; Sullivan *et al*, 1992; Huxley & Warner, 1992; Rosenfield, 1992; Rosenfield & Neese-Todd, 1993; Mechanic *et al*, 1994) assesses the life circumstances of people with severe mental disorders in terms of both what they actually do and experience ('objective' QOL) and how they feel about these experiences ('subjective' QOL). It provides a broad assessment of the recent and current life experiences of the respondent in a wide variety of life areas of potential interest.

The QOLI is a structured self-report interview administered by trained lay interviewers. Its original, core version consists of 143 items and requires approximately 45 minutes to administer. It has undergone a variety of revisions over the past 10 years, primarily to improve its psychometric properties and to shorten it. The core version contains a global measure of life satisfaction as well as measures of objective and subjective QOL in eight life domains: living situation, daily activities and functioning, family relations, social relations, finances, work and school, legal and safety issues, and health. The sections on each life domain are organised such that information is first obtained about objective QOL and then about level of life satisfaction in that life area. This pairing of objective and subjective QOL indicators by domain is essential to the QOL assessment model (Lehman, 1988).

All of the life satisfaction items in the interview utilise a fixed interval scale, which originally was developed in a national survey of the quality of American life (Andrews & Withey, 1976). The types of objective QOL indicators used vary considerably across the domains.

In general, they can be viewed as of two types: measures of functioning (e.g. frequency of social contacts or daily activities) and measures of access to resources and opportunities (e.g. income support or housing type). The QOL indicators include both individual items (e.g. monthly income support) and scales (e.g. frequency of social contacts).

The variables generated by the QOLI are the objective and subjective QOL indicators. The objective indicators are: residential stability, homelessness, daily activities, frequency of family contacts, frequency of social contacts, total monthly spending money, adequacy of financial supports, current employment status, number of arrests during the past year, victim of violent crime during the past year, victim of non-violent crime during the past year, and general health status. The subjective QOL indicators are reflect satisfaction with: living situation, leisure activities, family relations, social relations, finances, work and school, legal and safety issues, and health.

The psychometric properties of the QOLI have been extensively assessed. Internal consistency ranges from 0.79 to 0.88 (median 0.85) for the life satisfaction scales, and from 0.44 to 0.82 (median 0.68) for the objective QOL scales. These reliabilities have been replicated in two separate studies of persons with severe mental illnesses. Test–retest reliabilities (one week) have also been assessed for the QOLI: life satisfaction scales, 0.41–0.95 (median 0.72); and objective QOL scales, 0.29–0.98 (median 0.65). Construct and predictive validity have been assessed as good by confirmatory factor analyses and multivariate predictive models. The QOLI also differentiates between patients living in hospitals and supervised community residential programmes in the USA and Britain (Lehman *et al*, 1986; Simpson *et al*, 1989). Individual life satisfaction items clearly discriminate between persons with severe mental illness and the general population (Lehman *et al*, 1982). Further construct validation has been assessed in studies of the predictors of QOL among day treatment patients in Britain (Levitt *et al*, 1990) and the relationship between QOL and feelings of empowerment among persons with severe mental illnesses in the USA (Rosenfield & Neese-Todd, 1993). A variety of methodological papers have explored such other issues as the relationship between QOL and clinical symptoms (Lehman, 1983*b*); gender, race and age (Lehman *et al*, 1992, 1995), and housing type (Lehman *et al*, 1991; Slaughter & Lehman, 1991).

The QOLI has been used almost exclusively with people with severe mental disorders. The samples in published studies have included approximately equal numbers of men and women, about 75% of whom were white, ranging in age from 18 to 65 years. The predominant diagnosis in these studies has been schizophrenia (57–76% of patients). General population norms for individual life satisfaction items are available (Andrews & Withey, 1976).

A brief version of the QOLI is now available (Health Services Research Institute, 1995). As with the core version, this brief version provides a broad-based QOL assessment. It consists of 78 questions from the full version and is again a self-report interview administered by trained lay interviewers. It requires on average 16 minutes and measures the same life domains as the core version, including the global measure of life satisfaction as well as measures of objective and subjective QOL in the eight life domains.

This brief QOLI has been tested in a pilot study on a sample of 50 individuals with severe mental illness from a local psychosocial rehabilitation programme. Diagnoses included schizophrenia ($n =$ 17) and major depression ($n = 17$). Internal consistency was comparable to that for the full version, ranging from 0.70 to 0.87 (median 0.83). Internal consistency for the objective brief QOLI scales ranged from 0.56 to 0.82 (median 0.65).

Client Quality of Life Interview (CQLI)

The CQLI (Goldstrom & Manderscheid, 1986; Mulkern *et al*, 1986) was developed as part of a battery of instruments to assess outcomes among persons with severe mental disorders who were served by the NIMH CSP. These instruments include the Uniform Client Data Instrument (UCDI), the UCDI–Short Form and the CSP Participant Follow-Up Form, as well as the CQLI. The content of these instruments overlap to a considerable extent. All but the CQLI are completed by case managers or other professionals serving the clients and generally focus on functioning, services and clinical outcomes. Only the CQLI asks clients directly about the quality of their lives and therefore only it is reviewed here. The conceptual model underlying the CQLI assumes that certain life essentials are necessary precursors to a good QOL. One major purpose of the CSP was to provide these essentials and thus to enhance QOL.

The CQLI is a structured self-report interview administered by a trained lay interviewer. It consists of 46 items rated by the respondent as well as 19 interviewer ratings. Ratings are done on fixed, ordinal scales. The content areas covered include: essentials of life (food, clothing, shelter, health and hygiene, money and safety), job training and education, daily activities and recreation, privacy, social supports, social time, self-reliance, and peace of mind. In each area questions generally cover both the quantity of resources or activity as well as the respondent's subjective feelings about these resources and activities. Many of the item sets lend themselves readily to composite scales, although the development or scoring of these scales is not available for the CQLI. Some of the scales parallel those of the UCDI, for which computation guidelines as well as psychometric properties are available.

No formal psychometric analyses of the CQLI are available. Correlations of CQLI items rated by clients with comparable items from the UCDI rated by the case manager were quite low. The CQLI ratings remained stable over a 14-month follow-up. The subsample in the CSP study who completed the CQLI were 109 severely mentally ill clients from six exemplary CSP projects. The sample was 51% male, 82% white, 11% black, 6% Hispanic and 1% other, and had a mean age of 41.5 years. No diagnoses are indicated, but all were severely mentally ill.

California Well-Being Project Client Interview (CWBPCI)

The California Well-Being Project was a three-year initiative funded by the California Department of Mental Health to develop a better understanding of the health and well-being concerns of people who have been treated for mental illness, the so-called 'psychiatrically labelled'. The most unique aspect of this initiative is that it was designed and conducted entirely by mental health care consumers. The Project consisted of three components: research and analysis of well-being factors for individuals, assessed through a structured survey of consumers, family members and professionals; the production of educational materials based upon this survey; and the dissemination of these educational materials to consumers, family members and mental health providers.

Three versions of the CWBPCI (Campbell *et al*, 1989) were developed for consumers (151 items), family members (76 items) and mental health professionals (77 items). The time required for administration is not indicated. The questionnaires consist predominantly of Likert-scaled questions, but with some open-ended questions interspersed. The questionnaires are designed to be administered in face-to-face interviews (conducted by trained consumers), self-administered by mail, or self-administered in a group with an interviewer available to answer questions. The instrument is thus designed for flexibility in administration to provide the multiple perspectives of consumers, family members and professionals.

In the California Project, the CWBPCI was administered to 331 persons who were 'psychiatrically labelled' and living in various settings, including psychiatric hospitals (non-state), skilled nursing facilities, board-and-care homes, satellite houses, community residential treatment centres, drop-in centres, client self-help groups, organisations serving people identified as 'homeless mentally ill' and on the streets. The final sample consisted of 61 randomly selected members of the California Network of Mental Health Consumers (surveyed by mail), 249 volunteer respondents from various facilities in California (who were given face-to-face interviews and who were not randomly selected) and 21 randomly selected Project return clients. The sample was 52% male, 67.5% white, 14.7% black and 4.6% Hispanic. They were predominantly young, with 41% below the age of 35 and 75% below 45 years, and the authors describe them as predominantly chronically mentally ill, but no further clinical details are given.

No information is provided on the instrument's psychometric properties, and for the most part data from individual items are reported as frequencies (or percentages) in a narrative section that discusses the many concerns of the respondents. Topics covered in this narrative include: illness factors, family and social supports, activities, sense of well-being and stigma, among others.

A key measure derived from the interview is the 'well-being quotient'. This measure is derived from two questions providing information about the relative importance assigned to various factors that may affect well-being and whether the respondent currently lacks these factors. The questions read: "Below is a list of things that some people have said are essential for their well-being. Please mark all of those things that you believe are *essential* for your well-being" and "Of the things that people have mentioned that are essential for well-being, which of the following, if any, do you lack in your everyday life?" The response factors include happiness, health, adequate income, meaningful work or achievement, comfort, satisfying social life, satisfying spiritual life, adequate resources, good food and a decent place to live, satisfying sexual life, creativity, basic human freedoms, warmth and intimacy, safety, and other. Besides simply rank ordering these factors according to the percentages of respondents who identify each factor in each of the questions, four well-being profiles are computed: (1) for each factor, the proportion of respondents who indicate that they lack a well-being factor that they consider essential; (2) the proportion of respondents who do not lack a factor they consider essential; (3) the proportion of clients who consider a factor essential regardless of whether they have it; and (4) the proportion of respondents who lack a given factor regardless of whether or not it is deemed essential.

The most noteworthy aspect of this instrument is that it was entirely consumer-generated. This enhances its face validity even though no formal psychometric analyses have been conducted. The researchers consider this instrument is in a developmental stage.

Lancashire Quality of Life Profile (LQOLP)

The LQOLP was developed in the UK during the late 1980s by Oliver and colleagues (Oliver, 1991–92; Oliver & Mohamad, 1992) in response to a mandate by the British government that all community-care programmes serving persons with severe mental disorders assess the impact of their services on patients' QOL. The LQOLP is based upon the Lehman QOLI, but modified to reflect cultural variations and the broader survey intent of the government mandate for service-based evaluation of QOL. The theory underlying the LQOLP is essentially the same as that described under the Lehman QOLI above.

The LQOLP is a structured self-report patient interview designed for administration by clinical staff in community settings. It consists of 100 items and requires approximately one hour to administer. It assesses objective QOL and life satisfaction in nine life domains: work/education, leisure/participation, religion, finances, living situation, legal and safety, family relations, social relations, and health. In addition, it includes a measure of general well-being and self-concept. Objective QOL information is collected by means of categorical or continuous measures, depending upon the content area. Life satisfaction ratings are on a seven-point Likert scale.

Psychometric properties of the LQOLP have been evaluated in a series of pilot studies (Oliver, 1991–92). Test–retest reliabilities for life satisfaction scores range from 0.49 to 0.78, depending upon the patient sample. The internal consistency (Cronbach's alpha) of these scales ranges from 0.84 to 0.86. Content, construct and criterion validities were also assessed using a variety of techniques and judged to be adequate.

The LQOLP has been used with chronically mentally ill patients in a variety of community-care settings in both the UK and Colorado. Details of sample characteristics are not available. A briefer version of the LQOLP has been developed.

Quality of Life Self-Assessment Inventory (QLSAI)

The QLSAI (Skantze, 1993) provides information about which aspects of QOL are particularly important to patients and natural raters (care providers) to assist in therapeutic planning. It is an updated version of the QLC (see above) and has been used with out-patients with chronic schizophrenia ($n = 66$). The QLSAI is a 100-item self-report inventory completed by patient, followed by a semistructured interview with a clinician to confirm the patient's ratings of satisfaction and dissatisfaction and to discuss implications for treatment planning. It takes approximately 10 minutes for the patient to complete the self-rated inventory, and another 40–50 minutes for the semistructured clinical interview.

The domains assessed include physical health, finances, household and self-care, contacts, dependence, work and leisure, knowledge and education, inner experiences, mental health, housing, housing environment, community services, and religion. For all areas, ratings are 'satisfactory' or 'unsatisfactory'. The test–retest (7–10 days) correlation for the overall scale is 0.88. Comparative data are available from healthy university students.

Quality of Life Index for Mental Health (QLI-MH)

The QLI-MH (Becker *et al*, 1993) provides a patient-focused assessment of QOL that is intended to be responsive to the needs and constraints of clinical practice and research and which incorporates the multiple perspectives of patients, families and clinicians. It is designed as a self-administered questionnaire, but assistance may be given to more severely impaired patients. Versions exist for patients, families and clinicians. It consists of 113 items; the patient version requires about 20–30 minutes and the provider version about 10–20 minutes. It has been field tested with a convenience sample of 40 out-patients meeting DSM–III–R criteria for schizophrenia.

The QLI-MH produces eight scaled scores in the following domains: life satisfaction, using 15 items from Andrews & Withey (1976); occupational activities; psychological well-being, using the Bradburn Affect Balance Scale (Bradburn, 1969); physical health; activities of daily living, using the Life Skills Profile (Rosen *et al*, 1989) and the QL Index (Spitzer *et al*, 1981); social relationships, using items from the International Pilot Study of Schizophrenia (Strauss & Carpenter, 1974); economics; (adequacy and satisfaction with finances); and symptoms, using the Brief Psychiatric Rating Scale (Overall & Gorham, 1962). The QLI-MH also includes some open-ended questions to generate individual goals for improvement with treatment. Finally, the instrument includes ratings of the importance of each domain to assess the salience of the scales to patients' overall QOL.

Test–retest reliabilities have been assessed on a subsample of 10 patients with schizophrenia over 3–10 days. The 'percentage match' for the various domains ranged from 0.82 to 0.87. Content validity is supported by the use of some previously developed scales and a scale development process that used key informants, including patients, family members and providers. Criterion validity has been assessed through correlations between patient QLI-MH scores and provider ratings on the Spitzer QL Index (0.58).

Quality of Life Interview Scale (QOLIS)

The QOLIS (Holcomb *et al*, 1993) is a semistructured interview administered by trained clinical interviewers and consists of 87 items. Length of time to administer is not reported. The QOLIS was used with 201 severely mentally ill patients, including 100 long-term in-patients and 101 patients in surrounding community residences. Diagnoses included schizophrenia (45%), organic mental disorders (16%) and major affective disorders (11%). QOLIS items are rated on a Likert scale from 'strongly agree' to 'strongly disagree' and generate seven factors: autonomy, self-esteem, social support, physical health, anger/hostility, emotional autonomy, and personal fulfilment.

Factor analysis of an initial pool of 148 items yielded the eight factors with 87 items. Alpha coefficients for these factors range from 0.72 to 0.93 (median 0.77). Step-wise multiple regression analyses were used to predict self-reported life satisfaction using the SLDS (see above) and Global Assessment of Functioning scale (Endicott *et al*, 1976) ($P < 0.0001$ for both analyses). All of the QOLIS subscales significantly discriminated between the in-patient and the community-based samples. Canonical analysis of the QOLIS subscales and the scales from the Heinrichs–Carpenter Quality of Life Scale (Heinrichs *et al*, 1984) showed substantial redundancy.

Schizophrenia

Although all of the QOL measures reviewed above have been used with patient samples with a predominance of schizophrenia, none was specifically developed as a disease-specific QOL measure. Only one schizophrenia-specific QOL measures exists.

Quality of Life Scale (QLS)

The QLS (Heinrichs *et al*, 1984) was developed to assess the deficit syndrome in patients with schizophrenia. It is a semi-structured interview rated by trained clinicians. Its 21 items are rated on fixed interval scales based upon the interviewer's judgement of the patient's functioning in each of the 21 areas. The interview takes approximately 45 minutes. The 21 items of the QLS cover: commonplace activities, occupational role, work functioning, work level, possession of com-monplace objects, interpersonal relations (household, friends, acquaintances, social activity, social network, social initiative, social withdrawal, sociosexual functioning), sense of purpose, motivation, curiosity, anhedonia, aimless inactivity, empathy, emotional inter-action, and work satisfaction. These items reduce to four scales:

intrapsychic foundations, interpersonal relations, instrumental role, and total score.

The interrater reliabilities on conjointly conducted interviews range from 0.84 to 0.97 on summary scales. Individual item intraclass correlations range from 0.5 to 0.9. Confirmatory factor analysis has been conducted. This scale is widely used in the evaluation of psychopharmacological treatments for schizophrenia, predominantly with out-patients (e.g. Meltzer *et al*, 1990).

Depression and anxiety disorders

Quality of Life Enjoyment and Satisfaction Questionnaire (Q-LES-Q)

The intent of the Q-LES-Q (Endicott *et al*, 1993) is to provide an easy-to-use assessment of patients' enjoyment and satisfaction with their lives. It is a self-administered, 93-item questionnaire. The time required to complete it has not been reported.

The Q-LES-Q has been used with 95 out-patients meeting DSM–III–R criteria for major depression. It yields eight summary scale scores. Five of these are relevant to all subjects: physical health, subjective feelings, leisure time activities, social relationships, and general activities. Three can be scored for appropriate subgroups: work, household duties, and school/course work. Items are posed as questions and respondents rate their degree of enjoyment or satisfaction on a five-point scale. The Q-LES-Q also includes single items assessing satisfaction with medication and overall life satisfaction.

Test–retest reliabilities (interval not specified) were assessed on 54 stable out-patients; these intra-class correlations ranged from 0.63 to 0.89 (median 0.74) on the various scales. The internal consistency of each scale is over 0.90 (median 0.92). Validity has been assessed by correlating Q-LES-Q scores with illness severity and depression measures. The correlations of the Q-LES-Q scales ranged from –0.34 to –0.68 (median –0.54) with the Clinical Global Impressions scale (CGI; National Institute of Mental Health, 1985) and showed comparable correlations with the Hamilton Rating Scale for Depression (HRSD; Hamilton, 1960), the Beck Depression Inventory (BDI; Beck & Beamesderfer, 1974), and the Symptom Checklist–90 (Derogatis *et al*, 1973). Changes in the Q-LES-Q correlated with changes in the CGI and the HRSD (correlations of change scores ranged from –0.30 to –0.54; median –0.46).

SmithKline Beecham Quality of Life Scale (SBQOL)

The SBQOL (Stoker *et al*, 1992) was specifically designed to provide a method for assessing QOL in patients with affective disorders. It is a 28-item self-report questionnaire (time to complete not specified). It was developed with 129 out-patients presenting in general practice and meeting the DSM–III–R criteria for either major depression or generalised anxiety disorder. The items in the SBQOL are rated on a 10-point scale anchored by positive and negative extremes of the various constructs. Domains covered include psychic well-being, physical well-being, social relationships, activities/interests/hobbies, mood, locus of control, sexual function, work/employment, religion, and finances. To provide an idiographic component, respondents are asked to rate themselves on these constructs from three perspectives: self now, ideal self, and sick self. A summary score is then generated across the domains for the differences between self now and either ideal self or sick self.

Changes in the self now/sick self and self now/ideal self difference scores paralleled improvements in clinical depression (measured by the HRSD) over a 12-week therapeutic period. The self now/sick self and self now/ideal self 'distances' correlated with ratings on the Sickness Impact Profile (Bergner *et al*, 1981) and the General Health Questionnaire (Goldberg, 1979), two generic health-related QOL measures. One-day test–retest reliabilities for the self now, sick self, ideal self, self now/sick self and self now/ideal self scores ranged from 0.66 to 0.83 (median 0.70). Internal consistency for these scores ranged from 0.85 to 0.95 (median = 0.90).

Quality of Life in Depression Scale (QLDS)

The QLDS (Hunt & McKenna, 1992*a,b*) was designed to assess the impact of depression on the QOL of patients. It is a 34-item, self-report questionnaire (time to complete not specified). It has been used in a study of 74 patients with depression in the UK. The QLDS generates a summary score encompassing six dimensions: domestic activities, interpersonal relationships, social life, cognition, personal hygiene, and leisure activities and relaxation. The two-week test–retest reliability coefficient was 0.81 and the internal consistency was 0.93. The QLDS score had a correlation coefficient of 0.79 with the General Well-Being Index (DuPuy, 1984). These results have been replicated on samples of non-elderly and elderly Dutch patients with major depression (Greoire *et al*, 1994).

Discussion

Selecting a QOL measure

Given that none of these QOL measures has been widely used or accepted as a standard, the choice of a measure must rest with the investigator's particular purpose and needs. Some general comments and caveats are warranted for the investigator or programme evaluator seeking a QOL measure for the severely mentally ill, whether one of those described above or some other. First, a major concern with using normative QOL measures in this population is that floor effects are frequently encountered, especially in role-functioning domains (e.g. spouse, parent, employment roles). Therefore, special attention must be paid to instrument sensitivity. Such floor effects are typically not a problem in the domains of life satisfaction and resources. Second, many of these patients have problems with task perseverance and comprehension. Therefore, pencil-and-paper questionnaires are ill-advised. Note that nearly all of the instruments discussed here are interviews. Finally, psychopathology affects patients' ratings of their QOL. Therefore, QOL assessments of these patients should be accompanied by a concomitant assessment of psychopathological symptoms, to reduce the confounding effects of psychiatric syndromes on QOL assessments.

Interpreting QOL information

A gnawing issue is whether persons with mental illness can provide truly valid assessments of their QOL. On a general level, it can be argued that psychometric studies of the validity of QOL measures for persons with mental illness have produced positive results (Lehman, 1996). That is, these have tended to support the construct, predictive and criterion validity of QOL measures. Nonetheless, it has been repeatedly shown that the so-called objective and subjective aspects of QOL are not highly correlated. For example, income typically does not predict life satisfaction (Andrews & Withey, 1976). Patients with schizophrenia, although functionally more impaired, express somewhat greater life satisfaction than do depressed patients (Lehman, 1983*b*; Oliver *et al*, 1996; Atkinson *et al*, 1997). Similarly, African-American patients report lower incomes and rates of employment but somewhat greater life satisfaction than do white patients (Lehman *et al*, 1995). The maxim 'You can't buy happiness' seems to hold.

   Still, the issue of validity of patient self-reports frequently arises when QOL findings do not coincide with clinical, research or societal expectations. We must assume that this concern is valid. As mentioned earlier, we do know that disorders of mood substantially affect the level of life satisfaction. Mood may also affect self-assessments of functional status. For example, a depressed patient may report low life satisfaction and cognitively distort and underestimate prior work achievements. Conversely, psychosis on average is only modestly related to level of life satisfaction (Lehman, 1983*b*; Oliver *et al*, 1996;

Atkinson *et al*, 1997), probably because the effects of psychosis on life satisfaction depend upon the nature of the psychosis. Grandiose delusions may raise life satisfaction, while persecutory delusions will lower it. By definition, psychotic people may distort the reality of their level of functioning.

To some extent, the issue reduces to our willingness to accept inconsistencies in outcomes as rated by patients versus others (clinicians, family members) and to incorporate such differences of perception into treatment planning and research. A recent example illustrates this point. In a randomised trial of clozapine in patients with treatment-refractory schizophrenia, Cramer *et al* (2000) found that clozapine was associated with a significant improvement in clinical symptoms and clinicians' ratings of patients' QOL (using the Heinrichs–Carpenter QLS), but there was no significant change in patients' self-rated QOL (using the Lehman QOLI). They concluded that patient self-reports of QOL are not as sensitive as clinician ratings of QOL to the types of clinical change observed in clinical trials. At the very least we are left with the ambiguous finding that clozapine was associated with improved clinical symptoms and a perception by clinicians that patients were doing better, but the perception by patients that things had not changed significantly in their lives. This can be taken either as a plausible set of circumstances to inform future efforts to improve care or as evidence that patients misperceive their circumstances. If we are to adhere to the philosophy underlying QOL assessment – that the goal is to address the patients' well-being as judged by the patient – then dismissing patient self-reports as invalid is not productive.

Rather than reflecting measurement limitations, such inconsistent QOL findings may offer valuable information for clinical interventions and service planning. Contradictory QOL results may reflect idiosyncratic views and values of persons afflicted by severe mental illness and should affect the clinician's approach to service planning. Patients are unlikely to be motivated to change circumstances with which they are content, even if the clinician and family feel otherwise. Conversely, failure to address an area of life with which a patient is dissatisfied, even though the clinician and family view the patient's circumstances as satisfactory, can adversely affect the treatment alliance with the patient. Such disagreements about QOL may signal the need for a period of negotiation regarding treatment and service goals.

Counterintuitive QOL findings also may represent patients' accommodation to adversity. Patients who have lived with social isolation, unemployment, poverty and other adverse living circumstances for extended periods may nonetheless report being satisfied with life. Their satisfaction reflects an accommodation to adversity and does not necessarily mean that they would not desire an improvement in life circumstances if the hope and opportunity for such changes were offered. Conversely, interventions that promote positive change, such as vocational rehabilitation or a novel anti-psychotic medication (e.g. clozapine), may produce transient decreases in life satisfaction because of patients' renewed awareness of how their lives could be better. Such possibilities form the basis for caution and more thoughtful consideration about how we expect interventions to affect QOL.

Research needs

Studies are needed to examine in more detail the relationships between QOL judgements and psychopathology. A variety of research questions can be raised. How do people's ratings of their QOL vary when they are and are not experiencing major symptoms? That is, holding objective life circumstances constant, how does life satisfaction vary with symptoms? If it does vary, how should this affect the timing of collection of life satisfaction assessments? Holding symptoms constant, how does life satisfaction vary across time as changes occur in objective life circumstances? Does psychopathology override the effects of changes in life circumstance on life satisfaction? Does depression dampen the effects of improvements in objective life circumstances? Does psychosis distort changes in life satisfaction due to changes in life circumstances? For example, do we see expected changes in housing satisfaction among the homeless who are psychotic when they achieve decent housing? Many of these questions could be answered from reanalyses of existing data-sets or from longitudinal studies that concurrently assess psycho-pathology, life satisfaction and objective life changes.

An additional issue that must be addressed in QOL research is whether perceptions of QOL are primarily 'state' or 'trait'. Lykken & Tellegen (1996) suggested that there may be a strong hereditary component to 'happiness'. These investigators found intra-class correlations on a measure of subjective well-being in the range 0.44–0.52 among monozygotic twins, whether reared together or apart, contrasting with correlations of −0.02 to 0.08 among dizygotic twins. Hence we must ask whether QOL is a state or a trait. In contrast to the question raised above about the effects of current mental status (a state) on subjective well-being, this question asks whether life satisfaction is primarily a function of enduring personality character-istics. In essence, are people inherently optimistic or pessimistic and is this the main determinant of life satisfaction? Again, this question should be examined through longitudinal studies to determine whether and how life satisfaction changes as circumstances change.

Do people have an internal set for life satisfaction to which they tend to return despite changes in life circumstances? How should this be incorporated into QOL research? Some data suggest that such enduring temperament characteristics may affect measures of general life satisfaction more than measures of domain-specific life satisfaction, such as housing or job satisfaction (Lehman *et al*, 1991; Slaughter & Lehman, 1991; Lykken & Tellegen, 1996).

Finally, we need a better understanding of how QOL varies naturally over time in psychiatric populations, the predictive validity of QOL measures as regards illness course and outcome, and the sensitivity of QOL measures for detecting treatment effects among these patients, who may at best experience very modest improvements. There is a need for basic conceptual work to develop better models for integrating QOL data into a general model of outcome for people with severe mental disorders.

References

ANDREWS, F. M. & WITHEY, S. B. (1976) *Social Indicators of Well-Being.* New York: Plenum Press.

ATKINSON, M., ZIBIN, S. & CHUANG, H. (1997) Characterizing quality of life among patients with chronic mental illness: a critical examination of the self-report methodology. *American Journal of Psychiatry*, **154**, 99–105.

BAKER, F. & INTAGLIATA, J. (1982) Quality of life in the evaluation of community support systems. *Evaluation and Program Planning*, **5**, 69–79.

BECK, A. T. & BEAMESDERFER, A. (1974) Assessment of depression: the depression inventory. In *Modern Problems in Pharmacopsychiatry* (ed. P. Pichot), pp. 151–169. Basel: S. Karger.

BECKER, M., DIAMOND, R. & SAINFORT, F. (1993) A new patient focused index for measuring quality of life in persons with severe and persistent mental illness. *Quality of Life Research*, **2**, 239–251.

BERGNER, M., BOBBIT, R. A., CANTER, W. B., *et al* (1981) The Sickness Impact Profile: development and final revision of a health status measure. *Medical Care*, **19**, 787–805.

BIGELOW, D. A., BRODSKY, G., STEWARD, L., *et al* (1982*a*) The concept and measurement of quality of life as a dependent variable in evaluation of mental health services. In *Innovative Approaches to Mental Health Evaluation* (eds G. Stahler & W. Tash), pp. 345–366. New York: Academic Press.

—, GAREAU, M. J. & YOUNG, D.J. (1982*b*) A quality of life interview. *Psychosocial Rehabilitation Journal*, **14**, 94–98.

—, McFARLAND, B. H., GAREAU, M. J., *et al* (1991*a*) Implementation and effectiveness of a bed reduction project. *Community Mental Health Journal*, **27**, 125–133.

—, — & OLSON, M. M. (1991*b*) Quality of life of community mental health program clients: validating a measure. *Community Mental Health Journal*, **27**, 43–55.

— & YOUNG, D. J. (1991) Effectiveness of a case management program. *Community Mental Health Journal*, **27**, 115–123.

BRADBURN, N. M. (1969) *The Structure of Psychological Well-Being.* Chicago: Aldine.

CAMPBELL, J., SCHRAIBER, R., TEMKIN, T., *et al* (1989) *The Well-Being Project: Mental Health Clients Speak for Themselves.* Report to the California Department of Mental Health.

CRAMER, J. A., ROSENHECK, R. & CHARNEY, D. S. (2000) Quality of life in schizophrenia: a comparison of instruments. *Schizophrenia Bulletin*, in press.

DEROGATIS, D. A., LIPMAN, R. S. & COVI, L. (1973) SCL–90: an outpatient psychiatric rating scale: preliminary report. *Psychopharmacology Bulletin*, **9**, 13–28.

DRAKE, R. E., McHUGO, G. J., BECKER, D. R., *et al* (1996) The New Hampshire study of supported employment for people with severe mental illness. *Journal of Consulting and Clinical Psychology*, **64**, 391–399.

DUPUY, H. (1984) The Psychological General Well-Being Index. In *Assessment of Quality of Life in Clinical Trials of Cardiovascular Therapies* (ed. N. Wenger), pp. 170–183. New York: Le Jacq.

ENDICOTT, J., SPITZER, R., FLEISS, J., *et al* (1976) The Global Assessment Scale: a procedure for measuring overall severity of psychiatric disturbance. *Archives of General Psychiatry*, **33**, 766–771.

——, NEE, J., HARRISON, W., *et al* (1993) Quality of life enjoyment and satisfaction questionnaire: a new measure. *Psychopharmacology Bulletin*, **29**, 321–326.

FRANKLIN, J. L., SOLOVITZ, B., MASON, M., *et al* (1987) An evaluation of case management. *American Journal of Psychiatry*, **77**, 674–678.

GOLDBERG, D. (1979) *Manual of the General Health Questionnaire.* Windsor: NFER Publishing.

GOLDSTROM, I. D. & MANDERSCHEID, R. W. (1986) The chronically mentally ill: a descriptive analysis from the Uniform Client Data Instrument. *Community Support Services Journal*, **2**, 4–9.

GREGOIRE, J., DE LEVAL, N., MESTERS, P., *et al* (1994) Validation of the Quality of Life in Depression Scale in a population of adult depressive patients aged 60 and above. *Quality of Life Research*, **3**, 13–19.

HAMILTON, M. (1960) A rating scale for depression. *Journal of Neurology, Neurosurgery and Psychiatry*, **23**, 56–62.

HEALTH SERVICES RESEARCH INSTITUTE (1995) *Quality of Life Toolkit.* Boston, MA: HSRI.

HEINRICHS, D. W., HANLON, T. E. & CARPENTER, W. T. (1984) The Quality of Life Scale: an instrument for rating the schizophrenic deficit syndrome. *Schizophrenia Bulletin*, **10**, 388–398.

HOLCOMB, W. R., MORGAN, P., ADAMS, N. A., *et al* (1993) Development of a structured interview scale for measuring quality of life of the severely mentally ill. *Journal of Clinical Psychology*, **49**, 830–840.

HOULT, J. & REYNOLDS, J. (1984) Schizophrenia: a comparative trial of community oriented and hospital oriented psychiatric care. *Acta Psychiatrica Scandinavica*, **69**, 359–372.

HUNT, S. M. & McKENNA, S. P. (1992a) A new measure of quality of life in depression: testing the reliability and construct validity of the QLDS. *Health Policy*, **22**, 321–330.

—— & —— (1992b) The QLDS: a scale for measurement of quality of life in depression. *Health Policy*, **22**, 307–319.

HUXLEY, P. & WARNER, R. (1992) Case management, quality of life, and satisfaction with services of long-term psychiatric patients. *Hospital and Community Psychiatry*, **43**, 799–802.

JOHNSON, P. J. (1991) Emphasis on quality of life of people with severe mental illness in community-based care in Sweden. *Psychosocial Rehabilitation Journal*, **14**, 23–37.

LEHMAN, A. F. (1983a) The effects of psychiatric symptoms on quality of life assessments among the chronic mentally ill. *Evalation and Program Planning*, **6**, 143–151.

—— (1983b) The well-being of chronic mental patients: assessing their quality of life. *Archives of General Psychiatry*, **40**, 369–373.

—— (1988) A quality of life interview for the chronically mentally ill. *Evaluation and Program Planning*, **11**, 51–62.

—— (1996) Measures of quality of life among persons with severe and persistent mental disorders. *Social Psychiatry and Psychiatric Epidemiology*, **31**, 78–88.

——, WARD, N. & LINN, L. (1982) Chronic mental patients: the quality of life issue. *American Journal of Psychiatry*, **10**, 1271–1276.

——, POSSIDENTE, S. & HAWKER, F. (1986) The quality of life of chronic mental patients in a state hospital and community residences. *Hospital and Community Psychiatry*, **37**, 901–907.

——, SLAUGHTER, J. C. & MYERS, C. P. (1991) The quality of life of chronically mentally ill persons in alternative residential settings. *Psychiatric Quarterly*, **62**, 35–49.

——, —— & —— (1992) Quality of life of the chronically mentally ill: gender and decade of life effects. *Evaluation and Program Planning*, **15**, 7–12.

——, RACHUBA, L. T. & POSTRADO, L. T. (1995) Demographic influences on quality of life among persons with chronic mental illnesses. *Evaluation and Program Planning*, **18**, 155–164.

LEVITT, A. J., HOGAN, T. P. & BUCOSKY, C. M. (1990) Quality of life in chronically mentally ill patients in day treatment. *Psychological Medicine*, **20**, 703–710.

LYKKEN, D. & TELLEGEN, A. (1996) Happiness is a stochastic phenomenon. *Psychological Science*, **7**, 186–189.

MALM, U., MAY, P. R. A. & DENCKER, S. J. (1981) Evaluation of the quality of life of the schizophrenic outpatient: a checklist. *Schizophrenia Bulletin*, **7**, 477–487.

MECHANIC, D., MCALPINE, D., ROSENFIELD, S., *et al* (1994) Effects of illness attribution and depression on the quality of life among persons with serious mental illness. *Social Science and Medicine*, **39**, 155–164.

MELTZER, H. Y., BURNETT, S., BASTANI, B., *et al* (1990) Effects of six months of clozapine treatment on the quality of life of chronic schizophrenic patients. *Hospital and Community Psychiatry*, **41**, 892–897.

MULKERN, V., AGOSTA, J. M., ASHBAUGH, J. W., *et al* (1986) *Community Support Program Client Follow-Up Study*. Report to the NIMH, Bethesda, MA.

NATIONAL INSTITUTE OF MENTAL HEALTH (1985) Special feature: rating scales and assessment instruments for use in pediatric psychopharmacology research. *Psychopharmacology Bulletin*, **21**, 839–843.

OLIVER, J., HUXLEY, P., BRIDGES, K., *et al* (1996) *Quality of Life and Mental Health Services*. London: Routledge.

OLIVER, J. P. J. (1991–92) The social care directive: development of a quality of life profile for use in community services for the mentally ill. *Social Work and Social Science Review*, **3**, 5–45.

—— & MOHAMAD, H. (1992) The quality of life of the chronically mentally ill: a comparison of public, private, and voluntary residential provisions. *British Journal of Social Work*, **22**, 391–404.

OVERALL, J. E. & GORHAM, D. R. (1962) The Brief Psychiatric Rating Scale. *Psychological Reports*, **10**, 799–812.

ROSEN, A., HADZI-PAVLOVIC, D. & PARKER, G. (1989) The Life Skills Profile: a measure assessing function and disability in schizophrenia. *Schizophrenia Bulletin*, **15**, 325–337.

ROSENFIELD, S. (1992) Factors contributing to the subjective quality of life of the chronically mentally ill. *Journal of Health and Social Behavior*, **33**, 299–315.

—— & NEESE-TODD, S. (1993) Elements of a psychosocial clubhouse program associated with a satisfying quality of life. *Hospital and Community Psychiatry*, **44**, 76–78

SCHULBERG, H. & BROMET, E. (1981) Strategies for evaluating the outcome of community services for the chronically mentally ill. *American Journal of Psychiatry*, **138**, 930–935.

SIMPSON, C. J., HYDE, C. E. & FARAGHER, E. B. (1989) The chronically mentally ill in community facilities: a study of quality of life. *British Journal of Psychiatry*, **154**, 77–82.

SKANTZE, K. (1993) *Defining Subjective Quality of Life Goals in Schizophrenia: The Quality of Life Self-Assessment Inventory, QLS–100, A New Approach to Successful Alliance and Service Development*. Gothenburg: Department of Psychiatry, Sahlgrenska Hospital, University of Gothenburg, Sweden.

SLAUGHTER, J. C. & LEHMAN, A. F. (1991) Quality of life of severely mentally ill adults in residential care facilities. *Adult Residential Care Journal*, **5**, 97–111.

SPITZER, W. O., DOBSON, A., HALL, J., *et al* (1981) Measuring the quality of life in cancer patients: a concise Q/L index for use by physicians. *Journal of Chronic Disease*, **34**, 585–597.

STEIN, L. I. & TEST, M. A. (1980) Alternative to mental hospital treatment: I. Conceptual model, treatment program and clinical evaluation. *Archives of General Psychiatry*, **37**, 392–397.

STOKER, M. J., DUNBAR, G. C. & BEAUMONT, G. (1992) The SmithKline Beecham 'quality of life' scale: a validation and reliability study in patients with affective disorder. *Quality of Life Research*, **1**, 385–395.

STRAUSS, J. S. & CARPENTER, W. T. (1974) The prediction of outcome in schizophrenia: II. Relationships between predictor and outcome variables: a report from the WHO international pilot study of schizophrenia. *Archives of General Psychiatry*, **31**, 37–42.

SULLIVAN, G. S., WELLS, K. B. & LEAKE, B. (1992) Clinical factors associated with better quality of life in a seriously mentally ill population. *Hospital and Community Psychiatry*, **43**, 794–798.

7   Quality of mental health care: from process to attributable outcomes

TRAOLACH S. BRUGHA and FIONA LINDSAY

Health care outcomes reflect the quality of care at its most fundamental level. There should be no need to justify a chapter on quality
in a book on mental health outcome measures. However, the topic
subsumes wider considerations than the specific concern with
process–outcome relationships considered here. Broader issues will
be influenced by non-clinical perspectives, including managerial
concerns with the values of a wider range of stakeholders (Coleman
& Hunter, 1995; Chowanec, 1996), the full range of goals of the
organisation (Lavender *et al*, 1995) and the special requirements and
information limitations of the service context, as in the contrasting
examples of primary care in the community (Chisholm *et al*, 1997)
and prison health care (Reed & Lyne, 1997).

What does outcomes research have to offer? The title of this chapter
reflects two questions about psychiatric care:

1   Is care being implemented according to good practice criteria?
2   Does it work?

The first of these two questions takes account of relational aspects
(especially doctor–patient communication), environmental aspects
(e.g. accessibility) and the technical aspects of the process (provision
of care that is most likely to lead to a better health outcome)
(Donabedian, 1989). Leading on from these two questions, we may
ask:

> Does properly implemented *care* lead to better subsequent
> health *status* (and functioning, satisfaction)? If not, what
> should we measure and rely upon – the *process* of care, or health

93

> status *subsequent* to care provision, or a *combination* of process
> and health status, even when they appear to be unrelated?

The question of whether to monitor process or outcome is a major problem in quality assurance (Fauman, 1990). The term health *status* is emphasised at this point rather than health *outcome*. Donabedian (1992) defined outcomes as the states or conditions attributable to antecedent health care. If we accept this definition of outcome, then it follows logically that we can use this term only when we are able to show that status is significantly associated with and therefore *attributable* to antecedent care.

In the early 1990s it was argued that outcomes had been generally ignored, largely because the structural indicators of input and process were more easily accessed (Jenkins, 1990). When an earlier version of this chapter appeared (Brugha & Lindsay, 1996), more explicit outcome measures were already in vogue and, as we shall see below, there has been no diminution in interest since. Measures of the process of care have received less attention, but this has not been an obstacle to achieving further refinements. The most difficult aspect – the judgement of whether outcomes can be judged to be attributable to care – has also been advanced, most notably by the evaluations referred to below (see also Britton *et al*, 1998).

Review methodology

In preparing this chapter we have updated an earlier review (Brugha & Lindsay, 1996) of the literature on quality of care in medicine and psychiatry and the published literature on audit in psychiatry. We conducted searches (in PSYCHLIT, MEDLINE, SSCI and HMIC) for journal articles, textbooks, chapters and cross-references covering historical and definitional aspects, methods of assessment and examples of their use in the field of psychiatry. A selection of relevant articles from the appropriate areas of medical statistics and epidemiology was included also.

Our first aim was to try to reach a conclusion concerning the relative benefits and feasibility of quality assessments that rely upon aspects of process assessment and those that are based on outcomes. Our second aim, also difficult to achieve, was to try to structure the evidence in the literature in a cyclical fashion, as recommended in quality assurance and audit programmes. The chapter covers: definitional issues; the establishment of quality standards; guidelines and policies; measurement and assessment issues; interpretation and appraisal as in peer group audit activities; and finishes with implementation strategies, including the final stage of the audit cycle, the experimental evaluation of clinical guidelines in routine practice and a brief mention of commissioning.

Definitions and history

In 1910, Codman proposed the "end result idea", according to which "every hospital should follow *every* patient it treats, long enough to determine whether or not the treatment has been successful, and then to inquire 'if not, why not?' with a view to preventing a similar failure in the future"; in essence it was equivalent to monitoring outcomes (Donabedian, 1989). Codman suggested concurrent assessment of care and its consequences, with the occurrence of adverse outcomes being the only occasion for process assessment. In order to establish the relation between care and its results, observations were needed on the causes for not attaining perfection. Codman believed that the end result was the only true product of health care and the main purpose of the end result system was to bring improvements in health care (Donabedian, 1989).

Quality of care is defined as the level of performance or accomplishment that characterises the health care provided (Last, 1988). Structure refers to manpower, facilities, resources, numbers and qualifications of professionals, characteristics of administrative organisations and physical facilities (Tugwell, 1979). Process refers to technical styles (investigations, physiological monitoring and treatment prescribed; diagnostic and therapeutic procedures) or interpersonal (patient education) styles (Tugwell, 1979). Donabedian's (1992) definition of outcomes as the states or conditions attributable to antecedent health care is not uncontroversial. Outcome can refer to death or disability rate, disease (cure or not), effect on patient health and satisfaction (Ruggeri *et al*, 1994) and discomfort, or social and psychological well-being (Tugwell, 1979).

Quality assurance and audit

Medical audit has been defined as "the systematic, critical analysis of the quality of medical care, including the procedures used for diagnosis and treatment, the use of resources and the resulting outcome and quality of life for the patient" (Department of Health, 1989). In what way does audit relate to our basic question about the relationship between process and outcome? Audit is inclined to be insensitive to outcome, but sensitive to structure and process (Holman, 1989).

The aim of audit is to produce change, but it does this only if it extends to health care workers and managers (Moss & Smith, 1991). Quality assessment refers to the determination of the degree of quality of care, and quality assurance refers to all measures used to protect, maintain and improve the quality of care (Donabedian, 1992). Quality assurance implies a good-quality service achieved at minimum expenditure, but in health care this means any procedure(s) improving quality of care (Jacyna, 1992). Audit is about continuing improvement. Construction of an audit involves adopting a standard, defining an indicator, setting a target and defining the monitoring method (DeLacey, 1992). The sequence of separate activities linked to and from the 'audit cycle' should include stages of observation, comparison and taking action (Robinson, 1991). The audit cycle must be completed if it is to be beneficial, that is to improve patient care (Hatton & Renvoize, 1991; Moss & Smith, 1991; McClelland, 1992). The indicated practice change may be the most difficult and challenging step in the process. Steps must be charted and measured. Identification of what improvements can be made should be followed by further assessment once improvements are instituted (Feldman, 1992). The operational definitions of quality assurance all have the feedback cycle in common (McClelland, 1992).

Quality standards and practice guidelines

Standards in psychiatry

Standards of care will depend increasingly on regularly updated overviews, systematic reviews and meta-analyses of evidence of the effectiveness of psychiatric treatments and related interventions (Wing, 1992; Depression Guideline Panel, 1993). The diversity of professional providers in psychiatry has complicated the development of standards, classifications of intervention problem groupings, and thus methods for monitoring the quality of care (Wells & Brook, 1988). Both national governments and agencies and the World Health Organization have promoted standards.

The Health Advisory Service (HAS), the Mental Health Act Commission – particularly in its biennial reports (e.g. 1993) and its second-opinion system – the mental health review tribunals and the approval exercise of the Royal College of Psychiatrists are all examples of formal institutional audit (Garden *et al*, 1989). The introduction throughout the National Health Service (NHS) of the Care Programme Approach (Burns, 1997) has been initiated through similar statutory procedures.

The Royal Australian and New Zealand College of Psychiatrists set up the Quality Assurance in Aspects of Psychiatric Practice Project (Holman, 1989), which resulted in the development of possibly the first ever treatment recommendations for depressive disorders (Quality Assurance Project, 1983). It was concerned with more than just audit; a series of treatment outlines for major conditions was developed as a basis for peer review and research. Holman (1989) suggested that a clinical focus should be maintained in audit, especially by the use of care plans and established guidelines similar to those established by the Australian Quality Assurance Project. More precise treatment guidelines have also been developed elsewhere (Depression Guideline Panel, 1993), and these make use of diagnostic and treatment decision trees and algorithms.

Policy aspects

The role of central government in establishing standards and in monitoring their quality includes a range of activities, such as central monitoring, survey programmes (Jenkins *et al*, 1997) and audits. In the UK, the Audit Commission (1992) has a statutory duty to promote economy, efficiency and effectiveness in the bodies that it audits, which since 1990 has included the NHS. Its role is to prioritise the patient perspective, community care and joint audits; and develop tools for direct use, quality exchange, accreditation and league tables.

In England, the Department of Health introduced the requirement that every consultant be involved in a form of medical audit agreed between management and the profession locally, making this a contractual obligation. Similar steps were followed in other parts of the UK. Audit became a condition for the training of junior staff, without which hospitals could not be accredited for higher specialist training (Department of Health, 1989). Well-publicised negative outcomes in NHS surgical practice heightened public concerns over the following decade. Regardless of earlier warnings (*Lancet*, 1993), newly elected health ministers responded quickly. A health policy White Paper introduced the new rubric 'clinical governance' (Department of Health, 1998), promising to tie together standards of care and outcome indicators at an organisational level, as well as at the level of the individual clinical practitioner and team. At a public level, survival following surgery can now be tracked like school test results (Oakley Davies & Marshall, 1999). A key part of this strategy is the National Institute for Clinical Excellence (NICE), which took up responsibility early in 1999 for the appraisal of new and existing health technologies, the development of clinical guidelines and the promotion of clinical audit and confidential enquiries (Rawlins,

1999). The old HAS (referred to above) was also relaunched as HAS2000, building on the earlier work of the Clinical Standards Advisory Group project on schizophrenia (College Research Unit & Department of Health, 1995). HAS2000 is setting standards for the major psychiatric service speciality groupings used in periodic service evaluations within the NHS throughout the UK. Whether these policy-strategy driven (and principally centrally funded) developments, including ever-growing investments into inputs of care and service frameworks (Department of Health, 1999), will produce more tangible dividends will depend on our ability to assess and interpret high-quality information on inputs, processes and outcomes.

Quality measurement

Quality is judged by individual professionals comparing with a standard; but it may be perceived differently by users. Donabedian (1966) considered the sources and methods of obtaining information: sampling and selection; clinical research, and the limitations of direct observation especially in general practice; measurement standards (empirical and normative), measurement scales and reliability, bias and validity.

The classic work of Donabedian is fraught with the problems of using each dimension (e.g. structure) in isolation (Turner, 1989). Turner (1989) suggests other quality-of-care perspectives: first, patient perceptions, that is patients may judge quality more by how they are treated than by the health outcome; and second, adherence to standards. Despite being a multi-dimensional approach, the focus is still on outcome. Monitoring quality in medical practice has come to be synonymous with the growing practice of audit.

There has been a long debate on the right way to measure the quality of care: whether to use process or outcome criteria. Ierodiakonou & Vandenbroucke (1993) have argued that the ultimate judgement of quality rests on the evaluation of process (as suggested by both the ancient Greek philosophers and modern theoreticians of quality assurance). Some administrators are convinced that quality of performance should be measured according to what they assert to be outcome criteria, principally mortality rates, but there are dangers involved in ranking the appropriate criteria (Ierodiakonou & Vandenbroucke, 1993). To use outcome as a quality measure, continuous evaluation of all individual patient characteristics is needed, which is a gigantic and perhaps unrealistic research effort (Ierodiakonou & Vandenbroucke, 1993).

Tugwell (1979) clearly advocated process-based approaches in a quote from Cochrane: "the core of quality of medical care is the extent to which scientifically proven effective methods of treatment are properly applied to patients who can benefit from them". A strong case for a process-driven quality-of-care strategy has been made by Micossi *et al* (1993).

Evaluation of structure and input

The emphasis on structure, particularly in governmental policies – for example on deinstitutionalisation and the division between health and social care – has hardly been accompanied by a commensurate emphasis on definitions and measures of structure.

The World Health Organization (Janca & Chandrashekar, 1993) published details of six instruments designed to be used in quality assurance assessments: these consist of national assessments of mental health policy, mental health programmes, out-patient mental health facilities; and, within a given setting, assessments of primary health care facilities and residential facilities for the elderly mentally ill. The former cover such matters as decentralisation, equity and community participation; the latter cover such matters as cleanliness, privacy, water and food. Both types of measure cover such matters as staffing, physical environment, interaction with families and the community. Within the NHS there have also been attempts systematically to describe the profile of community-based service provision (Griffiths *et al*, 1992).

Measurement of process

Micossi *et al* (1993) have argued that since an outcomes-based approach is generally impracticable (randomisation is rarely feasible) and usually unreliable (due to unknown imbalances in treatment allocations), a 'profiles-of-care' approach is preferable, centred on the symptoms presented by patients when first seen by a doctor, which determine the resources utilised and the costs incurred. Profiles of care represent blocks of symptoms or intermediate diagnoses that are associated with corresponding objectives and procedures. Quality control can therefore be based on the comparison between observed and expected actions.

Within psychiatry, process-based approaches to quality-of-care assessment have grown rapidly in number, if not in use. Shepherd (1988) argued that the most systematic approximation to a process method of quality assessment in the field of psychiatry was the Needs for Care Assessment, first described by Brewin *et al* (1987). This is based on an individualised assessment of clinical and social problems, or deficits in functioning, linked with a schedule that prescribes appropriate actions, or 'forms of care' for the defined problems; its widespread use has been discussed since (Brewin & Wing, 1993).

Researchers have reported achieving acceptable levels of reliability in the use of this method, although it does depend on the use of judgements, both of what constitutes potentially worthwhile care and of whether realistic attempts have been made to provide it. Notable achievements have been a general population version (Bebbington *et al*, 1996), a similarly structured short assessment form, designed to systematise community social and health care assessments (Slade *et al*, 1996; Bonsack & Lesage, 1998), and a fascinating prospective case series demonstrating the usefulness of the original method in clinical practice within a rehousing programme (Higgins *et al*, 1997; O'Leary & Webb, 1999).

Process measures must be considered in the context of agreed standards of treatment, despite suggestions of a problem with the sheer variety of approaches and modalities (Turner, 1989). These standards have been much expanded in recent times under the banner of evidence-based medicine and psychiatry (Lewis, 1997).

Tugwell (1979) proposed methodological criteria to assist process measurement:

1   *Validity.* A statistical association is needed between process and outcome measures. Tugwell's review of the literature showed few correlations in process–outcome studies. Methodological reasons were suggested, for example sample size, inappropriate sampling and inappropriate measures. These same criticisms have recently been applied to the evidence base in relation to case management for the severely mentally ill (Brugha & Glover, 1998).

2   *Clinical credibility of the process criteria with health professionals.* Credibility will decrease if items are unlikely to influence management.

3   *Accuracy.* A measure must reflect the actual clinical process, despite the fact that even simply giving doctors questionnaires to complete may alter their usual clinical behaviour.

4   *Comprehensiveness.* Items must include all the important aspects of the process of care. For example, patient education is often omitted.

5   *Sensitivity.* This relates both to differences between practices and to improvements or deteriorations over time.
6   *Amenability to index construction.* The results should enable statistical analysis.
7   *Feasibility and cost.* Measurement must be simple and acceptable. This could be achieved in a number of different ways, including record review, direct observation and the use of doctor and patient questionnaires.

Williamson (1971) developed a strategy for process and outcome assessment. The strategy was based on factors likely to have the greatest probability of effecting significant improvement in the health status of a target population. The four elements of the strategy were diagnostic, therapeutic, process and outcome. The strategy involved the development of outcome criteria. To determine whether a study of processes was required, they compared outcomes achieved. Thus, a process study would clarify the direction and priorities for action to improve outcomes. This strategy could be seen to enhance educational effectiveness.

Brook (1977) questioned the validity of process criteria on the grounds that only 'technical' not 'humanitarian' aspects of care were being measured. He cited a study that reported no relation between a process and an outcome assessment of quality of care, and claimed that this invalidated process audit unless, perhaps, one focused on very simple process criteria. Alternatively, efforts to bypass measuring the process of care and to concentrate on outcome could be considered, possibly by using short-term 'proximate' outcomes (Brook, 1977).

Measurement of outcomes

A broad range of purposes for assessing a variety of different kinds of outcomes at the individual and structural level can be considered (Lyons *et al*, 1997; Srebnik *et al*, 1997). Donabedian (1992) has argued that outcomes are the paramount criterion of good quality; that is, they remain the ultimate validators of effectiveness and quality of medical care (Fessel & Van Brunt, 1972). Donabedian (1992) has drawn up a classification of outcomes of health care and has discussed the uses of outcomes in quality assessment. For example, they permit only inference (not direct assessment) about process (and structure); with the role of intercurrent factors, outcomes may be misleading indicators. Outcomes are 'integrative' also; that is, they are of value but need process analysis.

Outcome indicators

An indicator is a measurable variable related to facilities, or treatment, or outcome of care (Fauman, 1990). The identification of indicators and the definition of clinical criteria are specialised tasks and need extra training. Measurements of process and structure are acceptable as quality indicators only if they predict outcome, generally in terms of functional status or patient survival (Tugwell, 1979).

Jenkins (1990) proposed a system of outcome indicators for mental health care for monitoring and evaluation by clinicians, health authorities and directors of public health. She considered the indicators of input, process and outcome for schizophrenia, affective psychosis, neurosis, dementia, child psychiatry, forensic psychiatry, mental handicap, disability and mortality. Process indicators for all illness types could be regarded simply as "activity on [input indicators]". Jenkins (1990) concluded that it is more useful to measure inputs and outcomes and to use process measures only when necessary to investigate shortfalls in achieving objectives. This key paper presaged the centrally driven development of outcome scales for use in secondary care, as part of the evaluation of *Health of the Nation* health targets set by central government for England (Department of Health, 1991). Outcomes were also to be assessed, by means of trends in suicide rates and by means of a programme of national surveys of psychiatric morbidity (Jenkins *et al*, 1997). It will be some time yet before this long-term strategy (Charlwood *et al*, 1999) can be evaluated. Nevertheless, real difficulties with the assessment of national outcomes remain to be resolved both at the level of national survey measures (Bartlett & Coles, 1998; Brugha *et al*, 1999) and within health services, possibly because of variations in the quality of training (Bebbington *et al*, 1999).

There are problems with the use of outcome measures; many variables in addition to the process of care itself may contribute to the final outcome (Tugwell, 1979). Thus poor outcome does not necessarily imply poor quality of care (Fauman, 1989) and, arguably, good outcome does not mean that credit can be apportioned to the health care system. Therefore, risk factors or covariates must be controlled for in any analysis. Confounding is defined as the failure of a crude association to reflect properly the magnitude and direction of an exposure effect because of a different distribution of extraneous risk factors among exposed and unexposed individuals (Datta, 1993). A confounder is associated with disease (outcome) and exposure (process) factors; and is extraneous to these two main variables but can distort their relation (Datta, 1993). Once a strong cause–effect relationship has been established, process can be monitored as a surrogate for outcome of care (Fauman, 1989).

Methods of audit

Robinson (1991) outlines the various methods of audit; some involve process measures and others outcome. Case-note review has been used by the Royal College of Physicians' audit in the reaccreditation of training posts. Criterion-based audit is used in peer review. Outcome audit is the most sophisticated and valid, but has difficulties. Information-based audit involves a review of aggregated activity and financial data. Topic-based audit and intermediate outcomes are two other forms of audit. Hatton & Renvoize (1991) also considered the use of a random case-note sample, criterion-based and covering adverse occurrences.

In the USA, local professional standards review organisations and the Joint Commission on Accreditation of Hospitals (JCAH) have performed audit. Both were found to be costly and without obvious benefit (Garden *et al*, 1989). The JCAH focused on diagnosis-related groups. In Canada and The Netherlands, a legal requirement to perform quality-of-care or quality-assurance programmes was introduced.

The JCAH, later known as the Joint Commission on Accreditation of Healthcare Organizations (JCAHO), became involved in monitoring, owing to public demands for accountability and the requirement for institutional accreditation (Fauman, 1989; Elliott, 1994). This approach involved an emphasis on clinical outcome rather than on delivery of care. Criteria could be: classified in relation to structure, process or outcome; implicit or explicit (specified in advance); referents (the problem or diagnosis to which criteria apply); or normative or empirical source (derived by consensus or by empirical investigation). Indicators, tracers (broadly defined health problems) and thresholds triggering more intensive evaluation could be used in monitoring (Fauman, 1989). The JCAHO planned to identify indicators (of outcome) in psychiatry. It became the main driving force in the development and application of standards of quality of medical care (Fauman, 1990; Elliott, 1994). The JCAHO developed an audit system, termed the Performance Evaluation Procedure, but it was later discontinued.

There is a conflict between ensuring quality of treatment and controlling expenditure; therefore attempts are required to link quality assurance with 'cost-effectiveness analysis' (Cahn & Richman, 1985). There is a distinction between quality assessment and quality assurance; quality assurance means measuring both the level of care and when necessary improving it (Cahn & Richman, 1985). The processes of quality assurance include medical audit as well as, for example, the Performance Evaluation Procedure.

Because audit is to a substantial degree part of routine service work in the NHS, annually reported by providers to commissioning health authorities, little information on this area of activity appears in the medical literature. However, attention has been devoted to obstacles to routine outcome data collection by computer-based systems (Marks, 1998) and the development of multi-disciplinary approaches (Riordan & Mockler, 1997).

Illustrative quality-of-care studies in psychiatry

The influence of health care on suicide is uncertain; nonetheless, it has been considered by a number of writers to be an important mental health service outcome indicator (Hawton, 1987; Jenkins, 1990) and recent work does confirm the importance of maintaining levels of care of persons at high risk of suicide (Appleby *et al*, 1999). Morgan & Priest (1991) carried out a study following on from an initiative by the Royal College of Psychiatrists; in essence it was an audit of unexpected deaths. Demographic and clinical data, including diagnosis and treatment, were collected by means of a questionnaire completed by the responsible consultant. The results pointed to a number of possible risk factors for suicide and other unexpected deaths; they included misleading clinical improvement in the absence of a corresponding alleviation of situational problems, and social alienation of the patient. The study was felt to have implications for service development, with major reductions in bed numbers planned; and this method of audit would need to be evaluated. The Confidential Inquiry into Suicides and Homicides by Mentally Ill People continues and further reports will be published periodically (Steering Committee of the Confidential Inquiry into Homicides and Suicides by Mentally Ill People, 1996).

Structure, process and outcome quality evaluations in psychiatry

Structure

Education can be considered to be a structural influence on the process of care. Rutz *et al* (1992) carried out a much-discussed study in which they followed up the long-term development of an educational programme for general practitioners (GPs) on the prevention and treatment of depression. All GPs on a Swedish island completed the programme. Process and outcome measures of the quality of care, including the number of referrals, the number of emergencies, sick leave, prescription of psychotropics, in-patient care and suicide frequency, were made before and after the programme. The results of the study indicated that the effects, strictly related in time to the educational programmes, which included a lowered suicide rate, were real and not only a coincident local trend. This open study still represents one of the most compelling pieces of evidence that suicide can be an outcome of antecedent care. Similar work evaluated by means of a random-allocation design in a representative setting seems unlikely because of the substantial sample size required in such a study (Appleby *et al*, 1999).

Process

Previous reviewers have noted the small number of studies that have focused on the process of psychiatric care and particularly on aspects of drug treatment (Wells & Brook, 1988). The Needs for Care Assessment system referred to above has been used in a number of studies evaluating the process of care, particularly for long-term patients (Brewin & Wing, 1993). The first such study, carried out on 145 long-term users of psychiatric day care, showed that benzo-diazepine tranquillisers and anticholinergic preparations were frequently being used without the need for them being reviewed by the responsible clinician. Episodes of depression and anxiety disorder were sometimes untreated and psychotic symptoms were often under-treated. Deficits in role skills that were being particularly neglected included self-care and literacy skills, for which remedial training or shelter was unlikely to have been offered (Brewin *et al*, 1988). When a similar methodology was applied to physical health problems in the same population (Brugha *et al*, 1989) almost half (44%) of those with such problems had not received appropriate assessment or treatment.

Met and unmet needs for care have also been evaluated in the community (Bebbington *et al*, 1997) and these principles have been used to quantify treatment receipt nationally (Meltzer *et al*, 1995). Elsewhere, one of us has discussed the particular problem of the under-treatment of depression in both primary and secondary care (Brugha, 1995), referring to longitudinal studies revealing surprising failures in the provision of effective care and some suggestions that this is reflected in poor outcomes (Brugha *et al*, 1992; Wells *et al*, 1992).

Outcome

Recently the use of high-quality, clinical databases and well-designed and executed analyses of treatment outcome information has been advocated (Black, 1999). Although there have been observational outcome studies of community mental health care initiatives and psychotherapy services (i.e. structural inputs), in general there is very little outcomes research in relation to detailed information on the process of psychiatric care. In an overview of the strength and quality of evidence for the effectiveness of treatments for neurotic, affective and functional psychotic disorders (Wing, 1992), no citations were based on well-designed cohort or case-controlled analytic studies (from more than one research group). In one open study evaluating a deinstitutionalisation programme, better clinical status appeared to be associated with higher costs (Beecham & Knapp, 1992). Schuster (1991) reported that outcome studies will be critical in preventing further limitations in psychiatric care and its funding; this promise has not yet been clearly fulfilled. He suggested that quality and cost containment should be improved by concentrating on treatment settings and who gives the treatment (i.e. process).

The structure–process–outcome paradigm

The structure–process–outcome paradigm provides information from which inferences about quality of care may be made; that is, they are not attributes of quality unless they are causally related. It has been argued that process and outcome should be measured together (Williamson, 1971; Fessel & Van Brunt, 1972; Wells & Brook, 1988). Only one of the published studies in which the Needs for Care Assessment system referred to above, or similar systems, was used has examined the relationship between these very detailed indices of quality of care process and later health status, as an outcome validator (O'Leary & Webb, 1999). Even in the field of depression treatment, where there is a substantial evidence base to inform practice, there is a surprising lack of such prospective research (Brugha, 1995). Concerns about the validity of data analyses in studies in which treatments are not subject to random allocation may partly underlie this information deficit, a point we shall turn to shortly. However, the position may be beginning to improve (Ruggeri *et al*, 1994).

Implementing change

Glick *et al* (1989) discuss the reasons for disparity between the quality of the scientific base and quality of care, and outline the obstacles to improving quality of care. A central failing of quality assessment is that it is rarely used to change behaviour (Brook, 1977). However, the principal shortcoming of intervention studies is the lack of internal and external validity of the 'outcome' measures (Moskowitz, 1993).

Commissioning for quality

There is evidence elsewhere in medicine that some patients receive care they do not need while others are denied care they could benefit from and that these discrepancies occur not only in well- but also in poorly resourced and funded settings (Gill, 1993). A criticism of attempts to reform the management of the NHS early in the 1990s was that *activity* was the principal measure of performance: the more health care provided, the better (Sheldon & Borowitz, 1993). Improvement in quality would thus depend on a shift from commissioning activity to the commissioning of effective techniques. It was suggested that commissioners should contract for evidence-based protocols (Sheldon & Borowitz, 1993), a process that NICE may yet help to encourage in the first decade of the new millennium. The way that providers organise and monitor their own activity and thus quality is therefore an important topic.

Responsibility for commissioning in the NHS has undergone a series of changes over this period and at the time of writing is increasingly favouring the influence of primary-care professionals, who also retain provider roles. Whether a more localised focus for planning and commissioning will resolve the issues discussed here remains to be seen. In reality, both commissioners and providers can and should influence quality cooperatively and with greater sophistication. For example, an interesting and analytically advanced use of quality indicators based on inputs (such as bed numbers), process of care (including the use of more expensive medications) and of user perspectives has recently been reported from a public mental health setting in Maine (Davis *et al*, 1997, 1998).

Experimental and independent evaluation

Work has been carried out on the effects of different payment methods on later mental health outcomes (Rogers *et al*, 1993). Not surprisingly, perhaps, we have been unable to find any comparable evaluative evidence of the effectiveness of such organisational and management strategies in relation to psychiatric services and outcome within the NHS. Clearly, if there is any prospect of their widespread acceptance, they should be the subject of experimental evaluation.

There is encouraging evidence, already, of the beneficial effects of locally, experimentally introduced clinical guidelines into medical practice. Grimshaw *et al* (1997) found a number of factors that influenced whether guidelines were accepted and implemented. In a few experimentally evaluated studies, evidence in most cases pointed to an association between increased adherence to guidelines and subsequent enhanced health status. The durability of such changes in practice is not known.

None of the experimental studies cited (Grimshaw *et al*, 1997) focused on structural or process aspects of psychiatric care. Of possible relevance is separate research showing that when different methods of fee payment were randomised, clinical outcomes did not differ (Rogers *et al*, 1993). One study experimentally evaluating the effects of clinical guidelines and protocols on the process and outcome of care for depression has been conducted (Katon *et al*, 1996). This follows on the development of suitable assessment and treatment protocols (Depression Guideline Panel, 1993). One hundred and fifty-three primary-care patients with current depression were entered into this randomised controlled trial (Katon *et al*, 1996). Intervention patients received a structured depression treatment programme within primary care in Seattle, USA, that included both behavioural treatment to increase use of adaptive coping strategies and counselling to improve medication adherence. Control patients received the 'usual' care by their general practitioner. Outcome measures included adherence to antidepressant medication, satisfaction with care of depression and with antidepressant treatment, and reduction of depressive symptoms over time. At four-month follow-up, significantly more intervention patients with major and minor depression than usual-care patients adhered to antidepressant medication and rated the quality of care they received for depression as good to excellent. The severity of major depression among the intervention patients decreased significantly more over time compared with usual-care patients on all four outcome analyses. The positive outcome of this Seattle study may lie in the use of a specifically trained team of providers. Other studies currently in progress have been designed to evaluate methods for increasing the effectiveness of depression treatment by existing primary-care providers in the UK and The Netherlands. Therefore, we would urge caution about the premature introduction of guidelines in commissioning agreements involving local practitioners until the benefits have been empirically tested.

From process to attributable outcomes

Clearly, the difficulties that we have encountered in attributing health outcomes to care processes do not apply to interventions with dramatic effects, such as inhumane, degrading or punishing environments. Our difficulties have been to do with less substantial and obvious effects of routine care, some of them delayed over time, such as the effect of a course of antidepressants, or a series of cognitive–behavioural therapy sessions on depressive or anxiety symptoms, weeks and months later. It is clearly recognised that it is only for these less substantial effects, which can be difficult to detect in an unbiased way, that sophisticated instruments and research designs are required (NHS Management Executive, 1992). Randomised designs are a fundamental part of any such strategy. What can be said concerning observational methods, given that most quality assurance activity will be based in some way on these?

Arguably, later health status cannot be reliably interpreted because we cannot be certain that, when care is not randomly assigned, later status is not due to antecedent factors that have not been considered or measured (Datta, 1993). Arguably, therefore, "outcome measurements cannot be adopted as standard tools to assess the performance of healthcare facilities" (Micossi *et al*, 1993). For example, having identified post-treatment health status indicators (perhaps erroneously assumed to be outcomes) that are less than optimal, attention may focus logically on the supposedly antecedent factors of structure and process, in that order. Whether this is a good or a bad thing depends also on the appropriateness of the targets and the effects on the health care system of any change in focus: "setting inappropriate targets often has the effect of diverting effort from the legitimate activity of the organisation" (*Lancet*, 1993).

In effect, in real-world practice settings, if outcome cannot be relied upon, then quality can be judged only by assessing the extent to which care that service users are capable of benefiting from is provided according to criterion standards, in other words, 'the evidence base'.

According to this argument, measurement of quality should be based on the size of the gap between observed and expected (ideal) care actions. This brings the focus back to the process and structural factors (service resources, training and organisation) that underpin care activity, in which case, should these criterion standards be determined from scientifically verified evaluations of the effectiveness of care actions, which in conventional practice means the results of randomised controlled trials (RCTs)? But RCTs may not be the perfect 'yardstick' for setting down such standards because "the way that patients are recruited for a randomised study can seriously impair the generalisability of results" (see US Government Accounting Office, 1992).

Clearly, we face a dilemma, which in orthodox academic circles leads to a call for more research. Fortunately, the efforts of the NHS research and development programme (Peckham, 1991) are beginning to bear fruit. A recent health technology assessment systematic review bears on many of these issues, including, in particular, the internal and external validity of randomised and non-randomised treatment evaluations and comparisons of these two approaches where both have been used with the same medical condition (Britton *et al*, 1998). It suggests that the results of non-randomised studies may be more reliable than was previously supposed, but this will depend on adherence to clear standards of design, data collection and *planned* data analysis.

Unfortunately, no suitable examples in the mental disorder field were available to these reviewers (apart from evaluations of interventions for drug misuse). The reviewers may not have had access to two recently published studies of note. The results of a recent non-randomised comparison of different community models of care for adults with psychosis (Thornicroft *et al*, 1998) showed similar results to those found in earlier randomised comparisons. In the field of depression, a Medicaid database has been used recently to examine treatment prospectively over two years in over 4000 patients with depression, and the findings do confirm predictions from randomised studies; for example, those who discontinued medication early were more likely to relapse (Melfi *et al*, 1999). Both clinical and activity indicators have been studied prospectively in community mental health service data of good quality using graphical chain models (Ruggeri *et al*, 1998).

Before considering more seriously the proposition that intervention evaluations based on non-randomised designs can be relied upon, several caveats must be underlined. First, it may well be that the mental health field poses additional challenges, particularly at the level of objective outcomes assessment, which cautions us not to rush to the same conclusion as that reached in areas such as the treatment of heart disease. Second, we have emphasised in particular the need for rigorously *planned* and executed methods of data analysis, of the kind that methodologists have increasingly been discussing (US Government Accounting Office, 1992). Unfortunately, with a few exceptions, we have found that the data available from routine practice are either non-existent or strikingly inadequate and, in particular, incomplete. The now much quoted Depression in Primary Care guideline (Depression Guideline Panel, 1993), recently updated (Schulberg *et al*, 1999), refers only to randomised studies. Our hope is that the inevitable universal adoption of computer-supported monitoring of the care process and of outcomes will bring the facility of high-quality databases and their analysis into the mental health field (Marks, 1998).

The particular example of depression

In discussions of quality of psychiatric care, in what way does the process–outcome debate apply to the major and the commoner psychiatric disorders? The topic of depression has been given particular attention and we have referred to it several times here. First, evidence for potential effectiveness, for the most part, has been found from randomised designs in which clinical outcome tends to be assessed over a single or brief period of time (Depression Guideline Panel, 1993). But it is increasingly being recognised that recurrence and chronicity rather than prolonged remission characterise the more severe of these disorders (Lee & Murray, 1988). How should clinical management protocols for depression increasingly define as targets of intervention remission mainten-ance and relapse prevention (Depression Guideline Panel, 1993) and altered management for non-responders (Brugha, 1995)? If commissioners (purchasers and payers) are to contract for quality based on demonstrable effectiveness, and therefore outcomes, confirming that they are getting what they are paying for, how should this be effected? Will the call for commissioning agreements based on treatment protocols (Sheldon & Borowitz, 1993) be applicable to this aspect of quality of care in the field of psychiatry? Should an outcomes strategy be chosen, as in the assessment of the quality of surgical services, based on the implementation of high-quality clinical databases that are rigorously and independently analysed?

Conclusions

We have seen that there are at least two ways in which outcomes data could be used. First, outcomes data may be used to assess effectiveness: there is encouraging evidence that this may become more possible in the future. Carefully analysed process and outcome practice data could furnish thus an 'effectiveness lead' approach. Second, we could make use of Codman's nineteenth-century lesson (Donabedian, 1989) that when the end results of health care are less than expected, then it is time to go back and ask why. This model has been followed in the case of inquiries into deaths, whether by homicide or suicide, although with questionable usefulness in terms of change that yields tangible benefits.

How should the case for an outcomes-managed health service be achieved at a local level? When deficiencies in care are identified locally, clinical supervision based on direct observation and feedback by a locally recognised expert is known to be effective (Wells & Brook, 1988). The educational effectiveness of such direct feedback teaching methods in achieving measurable enhancements in skills has been clearly shown in the area of doctor–patient communication and clinical assessment (Maguire *et al*, 1978); many recent medical graduates are already accustomed to this style of learning and would find it acceptable. Effective health care team models (Pritchard, 1996) will need to replace existing, outmoded, hierarchical managerial models. Overcoming deficiencies and maintaining improvements may be crucially dependent on sharing of information between different professional groups and agencies, and greater sophistication in the use of clinical information systems (Harris & Conner, 1994; Rigby *et al*, 1998).

So where does this leave commissioners and providers with responsibility now for assuring quality? Major changes in the structure, including the management, of health services (and we can be assured that periods of such change will continue to be the norm) provide an opportunity for developing and evaluating outcomes-focused models of the kind argued for in this chapter. Until a sound, research-informed, case for introducing such procedures can be made, changes in practice should follow the systematic route of adopting process protocols that reflect best clinical practice. In certain limited areas, such as suicide audits, outcomes may direct useful attention to process deficiencies. Changes of the kind discussed here may be brought to bear upon the medical profession by commissioners and payers, unless the profession itself guides its introduction (Horton, 1993). The endorsement by the medical profession of NICE suggests that the profession in the UK will be increasingly involved, if not actually in charge.

References

APPLEBY, L., DENNEHY, J. A., THOMAS, C. S., *et al* (1999) Aftercare and clinical characteristics of people with mental illness who commit suicide. *Lancet*, **353**, 1397–1400.

AUDIT COMMISSION (1992) *Minding the Quality*. London: Audit Commission.

BARTLETT, C. J. & COLES, E. C. (1998) Psychological health and well-being: why and how should public health specialists measure it? Part 1: rationale and methods of the investigation, and review of psychiatric epidemiology. *Journal of Public Health Medicine*, **20**, 281–287.

BEBBINGTON, P., BREWIN, C. R., MARSDEN, L., *et al* (1996) Measuring the need for psychiatric treatment in the general population: the community version of the MRC Needs for Care Assessment. *Psychological Medicine*, **26**, 229–236.

——, MARSDEN, L. & BREWIN, C. R. (1997) The need for psychiatric treatment in the general population: the Camberwell Needs for Care Survey. *Psychological Medicine*, **27**, 821–834.

——, BRUGHA, T., HILL, T., *et al* (1999) Validation of the Health of the Nation Outcome Scales. *British Journal of Psychiatry*, **174**, 389–394.

BEECHAM, J. & KNAPP, M. (1992) Costing psychiatric interventions. In *Measuring Mental Health Needs* (eds G. Thornicroft, C. R. Brewin & J. Wing), pp. 163–183. London: Gaskell.

BLACK, N. (1999) High-quality clinical databases: breaking down barriers. *Lancet*, **353**, 1205–1206.

BONSACK, C. & LESAGE, A. (1998) Two instruments to evaluate mental health care needs: a comparative study in highly institutionalized persons. *Annales Medico-Psychologiques*, **156**, 244–257.

BREWIN, C. R., WING, J. K., MANGEN, S. P., *et al* (1987) Principles and practice of measuring needs in the long-term mentally ill: the MRC Needs for Care Assessment. *Psychological Medicine*, **17**, 971–981.

——, ——, ——, *et al* (1988) Needs for care among the long-term mentally ill: a report from the Camberwell High Contact Survey. *Psychological Medicine*, **18**, 457–468.

—— & —— (1993) The MRC Needs for Care Assessment: progress and controversies. *Psychological Medicine*, **23**, 837–841.

BRITTON, A., MCKEE, M., BLACK, N., *et al* (1998) Choosing between randomised and non-randomised studies: a systematic review. *Health Technology Assessment*, **2**, 1–124.

BROOK, R. H. (1977) Quality – can we measure it? *New England Journal of Medicine*, **296**, 170–171.

BRUGHA, T. S. (1995) Depression undertreatment – lost cohorts, lost opportunities. *Psychological Medicine*, **25**, 3–6.

——, WING, J. K. & SMITH, B. (1989) Physical health of the long-term mentally ill in the community: is there unmet need? *British Journal of Psychiatry*, **155**, 777–781.

—— & BEBBINGTON, P. E. (1992) The undertreatment of depression. *European Archives of Psychiatry and Clinical Neuroscience*, **242**, 103–108.

——, ——, MACCARTHY, B., *et al* (1992) Antidepressives may not work in practice: a naturalistic prospective survey. *Acta Psychiatrica Scandinavica*, **86**, 5–11.

—— & LINDSAY, F. (1996) Quality of mental health service care: the forgotten pathway from process to outcome. *Social Psychiatry and Psychiatric Epidemiology*, **31**, 89–98.

—— & GLOVER, G. (1998) Process and health outcomes: need for clarity in systematic reviews of case management for severe mental disorders. *Health Trends*, **30**, 76–79.

114　Brugha & Lindsay

——, BEBBINGTON, P. E., JENKINS, R., *et al* (1999) Cross validation of a household population survey diagnostic interview: a comparison of CIS–R with SCAN ICD–10 diagnostic categories. *Psychological Medicine,* **29,** 1029–1042.

BURNS, T. (1997) Case management, care management and care programming. *British Journal of Psychiatry,* **170,** 393–395.

CAHN, C. & RICHMAN, A. (1985) Quality assurance in psychiatry. *Canadian Journal of Psychiatry,* **30,** 148–152.

CHARLWOOD, D., MASON, A, GOLDACRE, M., *et al* (1999) *Health Outcome Indicators: Severe Mental Illness.* Report of a working group to the Departmnet of Health. Oxford: National Centre for Health Outcomes Development.

CHISHOLM, M., HOWARD, P. B., BOYD, M. A., *et al* (1997) Quality indicators for primary mental health within managed care: a public health focus. *Archives of Psychiatric Nursing,* **11,** 167–181.

CHOWANEC, G. D. (1996) The fall and rise of TQM at a public mental health hospital. *Joint Commission Journal on Quality Improvement,* **22,** 19–26.

COLEMAN, R. L. & HUNTER, D. E. (1995) Contemporary quality management in mental health. *American Journal of Medical Quality,* **10,** 120–126.

COLLEGE RESEARCH UNIT & DEPARTMENT OF HEALTH (1995) *Schizophrenia. Volume 2: Protocol for Assessing Services for People with Severe Mental Illness.* Report of a CSAG Committee on Schizophrenia. London: Department of Health.

DALY, O. E. (1991) Reading about ... medical audit. *Psychiatric Bulletin,* **15,** 209–210.

DATTA, M. (1993) You cannot exclude the explanation you have not considered. *Lancet,* **342,** 345–347.

DAVIS, G. E., LOWELL, W. E. & DAVIS, G. L. (1997) Measuring quality of care in a psychiatric hospital using artificial neural networks. *American Journal of Medical Quality,* **12,** 33–43.

——, —— & —— (1998) Determining the number of state psychiatric hospital beds by measuring quality of care with artificial neural networks. *American Journal of Medical Quality,* **13,** 13–24.

DELACEY, G. (1992) What is audit? Why should we be doing it? *Hospital Update,* **18,** 458–466.

DEPARTMENT OF HEALTH (1989) *Working for Patients. Medical Audit.* London: HMSO.

—— (1991) *Health of the Nation: A Strategy for England* (Cm. 1986). London: HMSO.

—— (1998) *The New NHS: Modern, Dependable* (Cm 3807). London: The Stationary Office.

—— (1999) National Service Frameworks for Mental Health. London: Department of Health.

DEPRESSION GUIDELINE PANEL (1993) *Depression in Primary Care: Volume 2. Treatment of Major Depression.* AHCPR Publication No. 93–0551. Clinical Practice Guideline No. 5. Rockville, MD: US Department of Health and Human Services, Public Health Service, Agency for Health Care Policy and Research.

DONABEDIAN, A. (1966) Evaluating the quality of medical care. *Milbank Memorial Fund Quarterly,* **44** (suppl. 206).

—— (1989) The end results of health care: Ernest Codman's contribution to quality assessment and beyond. *Milbank Memorial Fund Quarterly,* **67,** 233–256.

—— (1992) The role of outcomes in quality assessment and assurance. *Quality Review Bulletin,* **18,** 356–360.

ELLIOTT, R. L. (1994) Applying quality improvement principles and techniques in public mental-health systems. *Hospital and Community Psychiatry,* **45,** 439–444.

FAUMAN, M. A. (1989) Quality assurance monitoring in psychiatry. *American Journal of Psychiatry,* **146,** 1121–1130.

—— (1990) Monitoring the quality of psychiatric care. *Psychiatric Clinics of North America,* **13,** pp. 73–88.

FELDMAN, M. M. (1992) Audit in psychotherapy: the concept of Kaizen. *Psychiatric Bulletin,* **16,** 334–336.

FESSEL, W. J. & VAN BRUNT, E. E. (1972) Assessing quality of care from the medical record. *New England Journal of Medicine,* **286,** 134–138.

GARDEN, G., OYEBODE, F. & CUMELLA, S. (1989) Audit in psychiatry. *Psychiatric Bulletin*, **13**, 278–281.

GILL, M. (1993) Purchasing for quality: still in the starting blocks? *Quality in Health Care*, **2**, 179–182.

GLICK, I. D., SHOWSTACK, J. A., COHEN, C., *et al* (1989) Between patient and doctor. Improving the quality of care for serious mental illness. *Bulletin of the Menninger Clinic*, **53**, 193–202.

GRIFFITHS, S., WYLIE I. & JENKINS, R. (1992). *Creating a Common Profile for Mental Health*. London: HMSO.

GRIMSHAW, J., FREEMANTLE, N., WALLACE, S., *et al* (1997) Developing and implementing clinical practice guidelines. *Quality in Health Care*, **4**, 55–64.

HARRIS, C. S. & CONNER, C. B. (1994) Building a computer-supported quality improvement system in one year: the experience of a large state psychiatric hospital. *Joint Commission Journal on Quality Improvement*, **20**, 330–342.

HATTON, P. & RENVOIZE, E. B. (1991) Psychiatric audit. *Psychiatric Bulletin*, **15**, 550–551.

HAWTON, K. (1987) Assessment of suicide risk. *British Journal of Psychiatry*, **150**, 145–153.

HIGGINS, A., WEBB, M., O'NEILL, G., *et al* (1997) The needs for care of the chronic mentally ill relocating from psychiatric hospital to the community: a pilot study. *Irish Journal of Psychology*, **18**, 307–320.

HOLMAN, C. (1989) Medical audit in psychiatry. *Psychiatric Bulletin*, **13**, 281–284.

HORTON, R. (1993) Data-proof practice. *Lancet*, **342**, 1499–1500.

IERODIAKONOU, K. & VANDENBROUCKE, J. P. (1993) Medicine as a stochastic art. *Lancet*, **347**, 542–548.

JACYNA, M. R. (1992) Audit assesses quality: but what is quality? A clinician's view. *Hospital Update*, **18**, 822–824.

JANCA, A. & CHANDRASHEKAR, C. R. (1993) *Catalogue of Assessment Instruments Used in the Studies Co-ordinated by the WHO Mental Health Programme*. WHO/MNH/92.5. Geneva: WHO

JENKINS, R. (1990) Towards a system of outcome indicators for mental-health-care. *British Journal of Psychiatry*, **157**, 500–514.

——, BEBBINGTON, P., BRUGHA, T., *et al* (1997) The national psychiatric morbidity surveys of Great Britain – strategy and methods. *Psychological Medicine*, **27**, 765–774.

KATON, W., ROBINSON, P., VON KORFF, M., *et al* (1996) A multifaceted intervention to improve treatment of depression in primary care. *Archives of General Psychiatry*, **53**, 924–932.

LANCET (1993) Dicing with death rates. *Lancet*, **341**, 1183–1184.

LAST, J. M. (1988) *A Dictionary of Epidemiology*. New York: Oxford University Press.

LAVENDER, A., LEIPER, R., PILLING, S., *et al* (1995) Quality assurance in mental health: the QUARTZ system. *British Journal of Clinical Psychology*, **33**, 451–467.

LEE, A. S. & MURRAY, R. M. (1988) The long-term outcome of Maudsley depressives. *British Journal of Psychiatry*, **153**, 741–751.

LEWIS, G. (1997) New evidence is required. *British Journal of Psychiatry*, **171**, 227.

LYONS, J. S., HOWARD, K. I., O'MAHONEY, M. T., *et al* (1997) *The Measurement and Management of Clinical Outcomes in Mental Health*. Chichester: Wiley.

MAGUIRE, P., ROE, P., GOLDBERG, D., *et al* (1978) The value of feedback in teaching interviewing skills to medical students. *Psychological Medicine*, **8**, 695–704.

MARKS, I. (1998) Overcoming obstacles to routine outcome measurement: the nuts and bolts of implementing clinical audit. *British Journal of Psychiatry*, **173**, 281–286.

McCLELLAND, R. (1992) The quality issue. *Psychiatric Bulletin*, **16**, 411–413.

MELFI, C. A., CHAWLA, A. J., CROGHAN, T. W., *et al* (1999) The effects of adherence to antidepressant treatment guidelines on relapse and recurrence of depression. *Archives of General Psychiatry*, **55**, 1128–1132.

MELTZER, H., GILL, B., PETTICREW, M., *et al* (1995) *OPCS Surveys of Psychiatric Morbidity in Great Britain. Report 2: Physical Complaints, Service Use and Treatment of Adults with Psychiatric Disorder*. London: HMSO.

MENTAL HEALTH ACT COMMISSION (1993) *Fifth Biennial Report 1991–1993*. London: HMSO.

MICOSSI, P., CARBONE, M., STANCANELLI, G., *et al* (1993) Measuring products of health care systems. *Lancet*, **341**, 1566–1567.

MORGAN, H. G. & PRIEST, P. (1991) Suicide and other unexpected deaths among psychiatric in-patients. *British Jouranl of Psychiatry*, **158**, 368–374.

MOSKOWITZ, J. M. (1993) Why reports of outcome evaluations are often biased or uninterpretable. *Evaluation and Program Planning*, **16**, 1–9.

MOSS, F. & SMITH, R. (1991) From audit to quality and beyond. *British Medical Journal*, **303**, 199–200.

NHS MANAGEMENT EXECUTIVE (1992) *Assessing the Effects of Health Technologies*. London: Department of Health.

OAKLEY DAVIES, H. T. & MARSHALL, M. N. (1999) Public disclosure of performance data: does the public get what the public wants? *Lancet*, **353**, 1639–1640.

O'LEARY, D. & WEBB, M. (1999) The needs for care assessment – a longitudinal approach. *Psychiatric Bulletin*, **20**, 134–136.

PECKHAM, M. (1991) Research and development for the National Health Service. *Lancet*, **338**, 367–371.

PRITCHARD, R. D. (1996) *Measuring and Improving Organizational Productivity: The Productivity Measurement and Enhancement System (ProMES)*. Unpublished mimeo, Department of Psychology, Texas A&M University, USA.

QUALITY ASSURANCE PROJECT (1983) A treatment outline for depressive disorders. *Australian and New Zealand Journal of Psychiatry*, **17**, 129–146.

RAWLINS, M. (1999) In pursuit of quality: the National Institute for Clinical Excellence. *Lancet*, **353**, 1079–1082.

REED, J. & LYNE, M. (1997) The quality of health care in prison: results of a year's programme of semistructured inspections. *British Medical Journal*, **315**, 1420–1424.

RIGBY, M. L., LINDMARK, J. & FURLAN, P. M. (1998) The importance of developing an informatics framework for mental health. *Health Policy*, **45**, 57–67.

RIORDAN, J. & MOCKLER, D. (1997) *Clinical Audit in Mental Health: Towards a Multidisciplinary Approach*. Chichester: Wiley.

ROBINSON, M. (1991) Medical audit: basic principles and current methods. *Psychiatric Bulletin*, **15**, 21–23.

ROGERS, W. H., WELLS, K. B., MEREDITH, K. B., *et al* (1993) Outcomes for adult outpatients with depression under prepaid or fee-for-service financing. *Archives of General Psychiatry*, **50**, 517–525.

RUGGERI, M., DALL'AGNOLA, R., AGOSTINI, C., *et al* (1994) Acceptability, sensitivity and content validity of the VECS and VSSS in measuring expectations and satisfaction in psychiatric patients and their relatives. *Social Psychiatry and Psychiatric Epidemiology*, **29**, 265–276.

——, BIGGERI, A., RUCCI, P., *et al* (1998) Multivariate analysis of outcome of mental health care using graphical chain models – the South-Verona outcome project 1. *Psychological Medicine*, **28**, 1421–1431.

RUTZ, W., VON KNORRING, L. & WALINDER, J. (1992) Long-term effects of an educational program for general practitioners given by the Swedish Committee for the Prevention and Treatment of Depression. *Acta Psychiatrica Scandinavica*, **85**, 83–88.

SCHULBERG, H. C., KATON, W., SIMON, G. E., *et al* (1999) Treating major depression in primary care practice. An update of the Agency for Health Care Policy and Research practice guidelines. *Archives of General Psychiatry*, **55**, 1121–1127.

SCHUSTER, J. (1991) Ensuring highest quality care for the cost: coping strategies for mental health providers. *Hospital and Community Psychiatry*, **42**, 774–776.

SHEA, M. T., ELKIN, I., IMBER, S. D., *et al* (1992) Course of depressive symptoms over follow up: findings from the National Institute of Mental Health Treatment of Depression Collaborative Research Program. *Archives of General Psychiatry*, **49**, 782–787.

SHELDON, T. & BOROWITZ, M. (1993) Changing the measure of quality in the NHS: from purchasing activity to purchasing protocols. *Quality of Health Care*, **2**, 149–150.

SHEPHERD, G. (1988) Evaluation and service planning. In *Community Care in Practice* (eds A. Lavender & F. Holloway), pp. 91–114. Chichester: Wiley.

SLADE, M., PHELAN, M., THORNICROFT, G., *et al* (1996) The Camberwell Assessment of Need (CAN): comparison of assessments by staff and patients of the needs of the severely mentally ill. *Social Psychiatry and Psychiatric Epidemiology*, **31**, 109–113.

SREBNIK, D., HENDRYX, M., STEVENSON, J., *et al* (1997) Development of outcome indicators for monitoring the quality of public mental health care. *Psychiatric Services*, **48**, 903–909.

STEERING COMMITTEE OF THE CONFIDENTIAL INQUIRY INTO HOMICIDES AND SUICIDES BY MENTALLY ILL PEOPLE (1996) *Report of the Confidential Inquiry into Homicides and Suicides by Mentally Ill People.* London: Royal College of Psychiatrists.

THORNICROFT, G., WYKES, T., HOLLOWAY, F., *et al* (1998) From efficacy to effectiveness in community mental health services. PRiSM Psychosis Study. 10. *British Journal of Psychiatry*, **173**, 423–427.

TUGWELL, P. (1979) A methodological perspective on process measures of the quality of medical care. *Clinical and Investigative Medicine*, **2**, 113–121.

TURNER, W. E. (1989) Quality care comparisons in medical/surgical and psychiatric services. *Administration and Policy in Mental Health*, **17**, 79–90.

US Government Accounting Office (1992) *Cross Design Synthesis: A New Strategy for Medical Effectiveness Research.* Report No. B244808. Washington, DC: US GAO.

WELLS, K. B. & BROOK, R. H. (1988) *The Quality of Mental Health Services: Past Present and Future.* New York: Plenum.

——, BURNAM, M. A., ROGERS, W., *et al* (1992) The course of depression in adult outpatients. Results from the medical outcomes study. *American Journal of Psychiatry*, **49**, 788–794.

WILLIAMSON, J. W. (1971) Evaluating quality of patient care. *Journal of the American Medical Association*, **218**, 564–569.

WING, J. K. (1992) Mental illness. In *Health Care Needs Assessment: The Epidemiologically Based Needs Assessment Reviews* (eds A. Stevens & J. Raftery), pp. 202–304. London: Radcliffe Medical Press.

8 Measuring social disabilities in mental health

DURK WIERSMA

Mental disorders are in general strongly associated with social dysfunction, particularly schizophrenia and the major affective disorders. For a long time, social dysfunctioning was considered an epiphenomenon of the disease process. Nonetheless, criteria for the diagnosis of a mental disorder were and still often are derived from the domains of work and social relationships. There are at least two related reasons why social functioning deserves a closer look:

1   There is an increasing trend to treat patients in the community instead of in the hospital. The changing orientation towards community care needs careful evaluation with respect to its consequences. To what extent is survival in the community possible and what is the quality of life like there? Are community programmes better than hospital treatment, and for whom? The answer to these questions requires the separate measurement of social functioning in analyses of the outcome, costs and benefits of these programmes.

2   There is growing evidence that the courses of symptoms and social dysfunctioning may vary relatively independently: the social disablement of a patient may be characterised much more by social disabilities than by persistent psychiatric symptoms; the former may call for interventions different in kind from those usually available. For example, psychosocial rehabilitation focuses on those cognitive and social abilities of the patient that are crucial for a more or less independent life. Therefore, separate measurement of social functioning is again justified for the sake of the right choice of treatment.

The usual diagnostic systems such as the World Health Organization's (1992) *International Classification of Mental and Behavioural Disorders* and the American Psychiatric Association's (1987) *Diagnostic*

118

and Statistical Manual offer no adequate solution to the problem of the classification and assessment of social dysfunctioning as a consequence of mental disorder. We have to look to other classification systems, such as *The International Classification of Impairments, Disabilities and Handicaps* (ICIDH) of the World Health Organization (1980), which offers a conceptual model to study the long-term consequences of functional disabilities and social handicaps, and the effectiveness of health care to handle these kinds of problem (Badley, 1993).

Some conceptual models of disability

The ICIDH has been developed in order to improve the quantity and quality of information on what health care systems do to individuals, and in particular to evaluate the outcome of treatment. This classification distinguishes three levels of experience and consequences for the individual (Fig. 8.1).

Disease or disorder refers to an intrinsic situation within the individual and to pathological changes in the structure or functioning of the body.

Impairments (I) are considered as "any loss or abnormality of psychological, physiological or anatomical structure or function"; "I" represents the exteriorisation of the pathological state and reflects disturbances at the level of the organ.

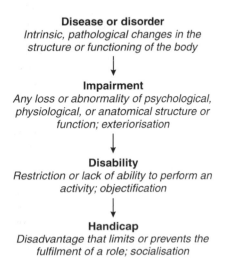

Disease or disorder
Intrinsic, pathological changes in the structure or functioning of the body

↓

Impairment
Any loss or abnormality of psychological, physiological, or anatomical structure or function; exteriorisation

↓

Disability
Restriction or lack of ability to perform an activity; objectification

↓

Handicap
Disadvantage that limits or prevents the fulfilment of a role; socialisation

Fig. 8.1. The ICIDH classification of the consequences of disease

Disabilities (D) are defined as "any restriction or lack of ability to perform an activity in the manner or in the range considered normal for a human being"; "D" represents objectification of "I" and reflects disturbances at the level of the person; "I" and "D" categories are supposed to be value free.

Handicaps (H) represent the disadvantages experienced by the individual as a result of the impairments and disabilities and reflect the interaction with the social environment that limit or prevent the fulfilment of social roles. It is supposed to be a classification of circumstances in which disabled people find themselves.

The conceptual model of this classification is rather simple and linear. It is assumed that I may cause D, which in their turn may give rise to H; sometimes I may directly cause H without the intermediate steps of D, for example in the case of a social stigma. Although it has, to a certain extent, been recognised as a valuable tool for assessment and research, it has already been criticised because of many conceptual problems with respect to the distinction between concepts. There is a lack of internal coherence within the framework with respect to how concepts are defined and used, and how categories are drawn up. There is much overlap between the three classifications.

This is even more so in its application to mental health. In general, mental disorders are complex, are somewhat imprecisely defined and may cause disturbances at all three levels, I, D and H. It is therefore difficult to take properly into account factors such as lack of motivation, the psychological reaction of the individual to the disorder, the impact on social functioning and the reaction of others in the community (stigma).

Some further problems have to be mentioned. The problem that bothers us most is the distinction between role disability and handicap. Both classifications deal with social functioning (at work or in the household, with a partner or children) and use the concept of role with regard to disabilities in relationships and handicaps in occupational and social integration. For example, social integration with respect to family, work colleagues, spouse, peers and other customary social relationships is a one-dimensional concept used on the handicap level ("survival role"), while family and marital role functioning are put in several disability categories. In essence, it is a different way of conceptualising and operationalising the same thing.

Another problem is that on the levels of both disability and handicap, social relationships and social functioning are to be assessed against normative standards and expectations, and therefore they are not value free, although that is claimed for the disability concept. A third problem is that much terminological confusion about handicap relates to the distinction between physical and social barriers outside the individual versus the inabilities of the individual.

What should be taken into account? The definition of handicap as a classification of circumstances differs from its actual measurement: the details of the handicap dimensions do not refer to circumstances but explicitly to the individual's abilities and competence.

So, the ICIDH is ambiguous and confusing with respect to social functioning, the use of the concepts of role, values and norms, and the issue of circumstances. Even its tri-axial character could be challenged. It remains to be seen whether the concept of handicap should be kept or whether another term should be introduced. Precise conceptual distinction is needed between disabilities on a functional or personal level and disabilities on the level of social relationships. Cooper (1993) made a significant contribution to this by redefining I, D and H, in terms of, respectively, a reduction in performance of a function in relation to an isolated task, a reduction in performance as a person in relation to the physical environment (personal disability), and a reduction in performance of a social role in relation to others (role handicap).

The conceptual framework of Nagi (1969, 1991) could be considered an alternative to the ICIDH model that is more coherent and consistent with respect to comparable, but slightly different, terms: active pathology (the condition involving interruption of normal processes and simultaneous efforts of the organism to regain a normal stage); impairment (loss or abnormality of anatomical, physiological, mental or emotional nature); functional limitations (functional impairment on the level of

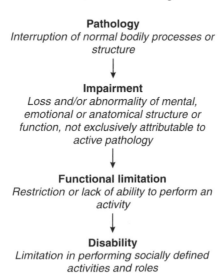

Pathology
Interruption of normal bodily processes or structure

↓

Impairment
Loss and/or abnormality of mental, emotional or anatomical structure or function, not exclusively attributable to active pathology

↓

Functional limitation
Restriction or lack of ability to perform an activity

↓

Disability
Limitation in performing socially defined activities and roles

Fig. 2. Nagi's model of disability

the organism as a whole); and disability (inability or limitation in performing socially defined roles and tasks expected within a socio-cultural and physical environment, such as those in the family or work/ employment, and education, recreation and self-care). The word handicap has been avoided, primarily because of the stigma attached to it. Disability in this model is explicitly focused on role functioning and it has become part of an extended model of disability and quality of life proposed by the US Committee on a National Agenda for the Prevention of Disabilities (Pope & Tarlov, 1991). I think it is worthwhile to gear these frameworks to one another (Fig. 8.2).

Social role theory

The category of social disabilities and social roles is of the utmost importance for psychiatry and mental health care. Functioning in social roles signifies the person's integration into the community. Sociologists, psychologists and anthropologists have used the concept of role to study both the individual and the collective within a single conceptual framework. Anthropologists such as Ralph Linton (1936) have traditionally treated role as a culturally derived blueprint for behaviour. In this sense it is an external constraint upon an individual and is a normative rather than a behavioural concept. Roles are always linked to status in a particular pattern or social structure, which consists of a network of social relations and communications. A role represents the dynamic aspect of a status. Linton and other anthropologists have made no distinction, however, between the behavioural and normative aspects of role. Actual and ideal behaviours are used to describe the people studied. The assumption is that there exists a uniform mode of behaviour with regard to status. Empirical research has shown that these assumptions are not valid and that consensus concerning status/role behaviour is lacking.

Psychologists such as Newcombe (see Gordon, 1966) have leaned heavily on interactional theory and were interested in roles more in relation to the self and to the personality. They treated role and status as given and not as variables. Role is defined as the subjective perception of direct interactions. This comes close to the symbolic interactionism that regards self-consciousness and the continuous interpretations of the actions of others as the motive for human action. The focus is on the individual response, based on the meaning attached to certain actions of other people. This interactionistic role concept, however, may not take proper account of the pathological changes in experiences and behaviour due to mental disorders.

In contrast, sociologists such as Parsons (1958), and many others, known as the structural functionalists, considered the reciprocal relationship or the socially preconditioned interaction of two or more persons as the core of the analysis. Parsons considered a role as the organised system of participation of an individual in a social system and defined it in terms of reciprocal orientations. Status and role are the building blocks or the means by which individuals are able to engage in the reciprocal relationship. The essential parts of such a relationship are expectations, which, according to Dahrendorf (1965), have the character of 'can', 'should' or 'must', implying the application of positive or negative sanctions in order to promote conformity to prevailing norms and values. Other people are important here to define whether an individual is behaving 'normally' or 'deviantly' or in a 'maladjusted' fashion.

But there is, unfortunately, no clear consensus regarding how to define a social role (see also Biddle, 1979). The following description, composed of elements common to most of the definitions, may be sufficient:

> A social role is a complex of expectations that people have as to the behaviour of a person who takes up a certain position in society.

A position is a location in a social structure that is associated with a set of social norms or expectations held in common by members of a social group. The group consists primarily of people with whom the individual frequently interacts, such as family members, friends or colleagues. There are many positions in the social structure of a group, an association, a profession, a community or society as a whole, with a corresponding number of social roles. Role performance refers to the actual behaviour of the individual in the context of a particular role.

Therefore, a social disability or a role disability is a deficiency that hinders the performance of activities and manifest behaviours, as these are expected in the context of a well-defined social role. It is important to understand that someone's behaviour should always be assessed against the background of how other people expect the individual to behave. Such an assessment, above all, pertains to the individual's capacity for interpersonal functioning.

Social role theory does not produce a standard classification of roles that should be taken into account in order to give an adequate description of the individual's overall functioning or integration into the community. We therefore rely on what researchers put into their schedules.

Classification of social functioning or social role performance

The number and content of roles in existing schedules vary. There are an overwhelming number of schedules and instruments, reviewed by Weissman (1975), Weissman *et al* (1981), Katschnig (1983), and Wing (1989), and by Hall (1980) specifically with respect of ward behaviour, Tyrer (1990) with respect to personality disorders, and Wallace (1984) and Rosen *et al* (1989) with respect to schizophrenia. There is, nevertheless, more or less agreement in various instruments on a number of roles:

- Groningen Social Disabilities Schedule (GSDS; Wiersma *et al*, 1988, 1990)
- Psychiatric Disability Assessment Schedule (DAS; World Health Organization, 1988)
- Role Activity Performance Scale (RAPS; Good-Ellis *et al*, 1987)
- Social Adjustment Scale (SAS; Weissman *et al*, 1971; Schooler *et al*, 1979)
- Social Behavior Assessment Schedule (SBAS; Platt *et al*, 1980)
- Social Role Adjustment Instrument (SRAI; Cohler *et al*, 1968)
- Standardized Interview to Assess Social Maladjustment (Clare & Cairns, 1978)
- Structured and Scaled Interview to Assess Maladjustment (SSIAM; Gurland *et al*, 1972).

A number of instruments are relevant in this respect (Hurry & Sturt, 1981). These are all better-known instruments described in the literature, with data on reliability and validity. It is striking that each instrument uses different terms to describe the role behaviours, half of them using terms with a negative connotation (maladjustment, disability) and half neutral terms (adjustment, performance). Nevertheless, their content looks to be largely the same, although there are big differences as to the precise wording, the description, the assessment, the anchor points, the scaling, and so on. Most instruments also measure other concepts, such as social support, psychiatric symptoms, the burden of the illness on the family, or satisfaction. There seems to be a consensus of opinion on the following areas of role behaviour:

- occupational role (work, education, household, regular activities)
- household role (participating and contributing to the household and its economic independence)
- marital role (emotional, sexual relationship with partner/ spouse)
- parental role (relationship with children, caring)
- family or kinship role (relationship with parents and siblings, extended family)
- social role (relationship in the community, with friends, acquaintances, neighbours)

- leisure activities and/or general interests
- self-care (personal grooming and appearance).

Each of these roles delineates an area of expected behaviours that determine to a large extent the level and quality or adequacy of the individual's functioning in the community. They describe general domains of roles and status that apply to everybody. Each area could be subdivided into smaller behavioural domains, such as instrumental tasks and affective or attitude aspects.

The description of expected behaviours could, of course, be different in various communities or cultures. For example, doing nothing is generally highly undesirable in Western countries but may be less so elsewhere. Taking part in the household (e.g. doing some cooking or household chores) may be quite different among men in various European countries. The applicability of the role concept is in principle not limited to time or place. It is very important to notice that the norms and values of the local community or of those with whom the person is interacting are decisive in the assessment. We should not assume general norms and values that apply to everybody. There is no general or objective standard of behaviour. Norms and values vary from community to community and the acceptability of a particular behaviour will sometimes be the result of negotiations between those involved.

So, ideal norms with respect to behaviour are not relevant here. Empirical research has shown that they are rarely applicable. Neither are statistical norms sufficient because they do not do justice to the differences between social environments. We prefer the norms of the 'reference group', which comprises people who, in social or other respects, are of great importance to the individual. (Reference group here is not taken in sociological terms, which implies that a person wants to be member of a group to which he or she does not belong.) This pertains to people in the close environment, such as the partner and other members of the family and to all those with whom the individual comes into direct contact while performing the different roles: colleagues at work, friends and neighbours. The composition of the reference group will depend partly on the particular role to be assessed of the many that can be considered.

Assessment and measurement of social or role disability

The following issues are crucial in the assessment of social or role disability and are based on the critical comments of several authors on existing schedules (see Platt *et al*, 1980; Katschnig, 1983; Link *et al*, 1990) and on our own work (Wiersma, 1986; De Jong & Van der Lubbe, 1994).

Independence of psychopathology

Considering the conceptual models of disabilities of the ICIDH or Nagi, there should be a clear distinction between signs and symptoms of psychopathology or psychological functioning, and social functioning (i.e. impairment, functional limitation, disability, and handicap). So, hearing voices or feeling depressed should not automatically lead to the assessment of a disability. Their measurement should be separated and not be mixed as in the Global Assessment of Functioning (GAF) scale (GAFS) of DSM–III–R (American Psychiatric Association, 1987). It should, however, also be kept in mind that social or role disability should demonstrably or plausibly be caused by physical, psychological or psychopathological impairments or functional limitations. The assessment has to take place in the context of the health experience or health problem: if no there is health problem, then there is no disability. One has to keep in mind that a person may not be working, not be married, have bad family relationships with the family, or have financial problems for other reasons than a mental illness or a personality disorder. The existence of such a problem does not in itself presuppose a mental health problem.

Actual role performance

The assessment of social or role disability should be based on the actual performance of activities, actual manifestation of behaviours, or actual execution of tasks over a certain period (e.g. the last month). The focus is on observable phenomena and not on inferences from abstract concepts such as competence or abilities that are assumed to be present.

Criteria of assessment

Each community or society at large has more or less defined criteria of eligibility for sickness benefits, disability pensions, sheltered work or living and social assistance for entering or exiting social roles, such as the marital role, the work role (disability pension) and the parental role. These norms and regulations define to a certain extent the level and quality of functioning and are the first guideline for the assessment. Further guidelines are the frequency of contacts, the number of completed tasks, the degree of conflict and the depth of involvement or strength of motivation. Important for the assessment of a role disability are criteria of frequency and duration of the deviations, the damage inflicted to the person him/herself or to others, and the desirability of help. This can mean that not fulfilling/occupying a social role implies a (severe or maximum) disability in role functioning. Examples would be not having a job owing to mental disorder, and therefore exempted from the obligation to look for work, or not fulfilling the parental role because of a divesting of parental authority.

Freedom of action or available opportunities

The reduction in or lack of performance should not result from personal or social circumstances that are beyond the control of the individual. An example is the hospitalised patient who cannot demonstrate certain behaviours because of the rules prevailing on the ward (e.g. visiting friends or family). Other examples of limited opportunities are the inaccessibility of the labour market, the stigma attached to mental illness, formal or informal rules precluding a patient or ex-patient from normal role fulfilment (civil rights, driving licence). It is evident that these factors should not lead to a disability *per se*. The assessment has to take into account the influence of such a circumstance while assessing role performance.

Sources of information

There are three main sources on which the assessment can be based: the patient, an informant (the partner or a parent or other family member) and an expert or mental health professional. Each source has its advantages and disadvantages, which influence the validity and reliability of the assessment. In consideration of the proposed assessment of role performance, it is preferred that several sources be used, not only one. The patient should always be asked, although the severity of symptoms may negatively influence any self-report of behaviour. The patient's own opinions are of importance in order to get informed about perceptions, feelings and satisfaction with social situations and the performed activities.

The informant – partner, parent or friend – is of course also influenced to a certain extent by the patient's symptoms. But factual information on the patient's behaviour is of great value in order to see the agreement on the report of the same behaviours or other behaviours not reported by the patient, and the evaluation or judgement of the behaviours. It must be noted that an informant is usually familiar with only some behaviours for some roles. It makes quite a difference whether the informant is the mother or a friend. It is important to find out the normative standards of the people with whom the patient interacts, although that may be difficult for certain groups, such as those who live alone.

The choice of an expert, usually a mental health professional and often a nurse or psychiatrist, may be obvious in case of the evaluation of a (hospital) treatment or of a long stay in the hospital. In the latter case they are then in contact with the patient the most, but it should be noted that there are disadvantages in using them as informants, such as the difference in education, the lack of opportunity to observe the patient outside the treatment setting, and different conceptions of normal and abnormal social behaviour.

From our research on the GSDS we found the influence of the informant on the ratings is substantial: there is an 8–29% change in the ratings compared with the ratings based on the patient's report only. It appears that in most cases greater disability was rated as a result.

Method of measurement

There are two principal means of measuring the disabilities, each with its advantages and disadvantages:

1   *Self-report (paper-and-pencil test).* This is easy and cheap to administer; no training is required and there is no interview bias. There is, however, a problem with illiterate or visually handicapped persons. Problems may be underreported as a result of symptoms, and in the case of serious mental disorder there may be a lack of proper understanding of the questions or even a lack of completion of the instrument. No allowance is made for the personal or social context, and by definition there is a lack of the opinion of others.

2   *Personal interview.* This may be either a standardised, respondent-based interview schedule or a semistructured investigator-based interview; both rely on an interview at least with the patient; the main differentiating characteristic is that in latter case the interviewer or the investigator determines the rating or score. These methods require training, are time-consuming, may suffer from interviewer bias and are relatively costly. The advantages are the direct observation of the patient's behaviour, the possibility of getting more precise information, and the flexibility of taking into account the personal context of the patient. For the assessment of social or role disabilities the semistructured interview is preferred, because it is the most flexible method.

Conclusions

Platt (1981) and Katschnig (1983) were rather pessimistic about the state of the art with respect to measuring social adjustment (because of the lack of agreement on social norms, unwarranted assumptions, variability of expectations, number of relevant roles and lack of validity). Progress in this field seems possible, to me, in the light of agreement on the disability concept, the (minimum) number of social roles, the allowance for relevant situational factors (freedom of action), the actual norms of the reference group, the application of criteria for assessment, and so on. Therefore, I would like to recall the definition of social or role disability:

- It is a restriction of the ability to perform activities (tasks) and to manifest behaviours as expected in the context of a social role.
- It is inferred from violations of or deviations from norms and expectations within the relevant reference group.
- It is caused by physical, psychological or psychopathological impairments.
- It does not result from personal or social circumstances beyond the control of the individual.

Our research on social disabilities (Wiersma *et al*, 1988, 1990; Kraaijkamp, 1992; De Jong & Van der Lubbe, 1994) has shown that the agreement on the assessment of social disabilities is high and that these assessments can be performed reliably (interrater and test–retest reliability). Proper assessments take the sociodemographic background of the patients adequately into account, differentiate between diagnostic and patient groups, have high internal and external validity and are sensitive to change.

Social role functioning deserves its own place in a classification of consequences of disease. It should not be mingled with other concepts such as social support, adverse social circumstances or quality of life. The revision of the ICIDH offers a good opportunity to solve a number of conceptual problems.

The extended model of disability (Fig. 8.3) that combines the conceptual framework of Nagi and the WHO/ICIDH as proposed by the Committee on a National Agenda for Prevention of Disabilities in the US (Pope & Tarlov, 1991) may be of some help here. The model contains, besides the concepts of pathology, impairment, functional limitation and disability described earlier, the notion of risk factors (biological, environmental and lifestyle risk factors) and quality of life, both in interaction with the disabling process. The risk factors may well solve the conceptual problem of handicap in the ICIDH. For example, some environmental risk factors deal with social expectations and opportunities in specific socio-cultural environments, such as paternalism, stigma, access to care, or women's work participation, and others with physical circumstances of the design of public places or lead paint. Lifestyle risk factors refer to smoking, excessive alcohol use, overeating and so on. These risk factors are important for identifying a mechanism for action or a prevention.

The model incorporates further the concept of quality of life, which unfortunately is not defined but loosely described as total well-being with reference to the World Health Organization's definition of health as a state of complete physical, mental, and social well-being, and not merely the absence of disease. It seems to me that using this concept does not clarify much and might give rise to new conceptual difficulties. The authors described as components of quality of life the performance of social roles, physical and emotional status, social interactions, intellectual functioning, economic status, subjective health status, and also aspects of personal well-being not related to health. Such a description will not help the theoretical formulation of an encompassing classification of disability and may even hinder the process of internal and external validation. We are in need of a good classification of disability and related factors, not vague concepts that again require the development of new instruments.

Ten years ago, social adjustment was said to be an umbrella concept encompassing skills, competence, integration, impairment, disability, inadequacy, and so on. Now it seems to have been replaced by 'quality of life', which is treated as a paradigm. It remains to be seen how fruitful this concept will be in theory and practice.

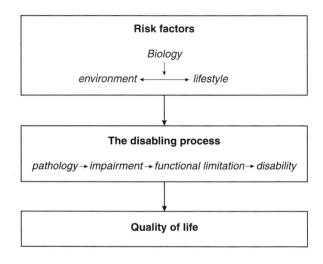

Fig. 8.3. Extended model of disability

References

AMERICAN PSYCHIATRIC ASSOCIATION (1987) *Diagnostic and Statistical Manual of Mental Disorders* (3rd edn, revised) (DSM–III–R). Washington, DC: APA.

BADLEY, E. M. (1993) An introduction to the concepts and classifications of the international classification of impairments, disabilities and handicaps. *Disability and Rehabilitation*, **15**, 161–178.

BIDDLE, B. J. (1979) *Role Theory: Expectations, Identities And Behaviors.* New York and London: Academic Press.

CLARE, A. W. & CAIRNS, V. E. (1978) Design, development and use of a standardised interview to assess social maladjustment and dysfunction in community studies. *Psychological Medicine*, **21**, 589–604.

COHLER, B., WOOLSEY, S., WEISS, J., *et al* (1968) Child rearing attitudes among mothers volunteering and revolunteering for a psychological study. *Psychological Reports*, **23**, 603–612.

COOPER, J. E. (1993) Draft papers of IDH–93. Unpublished manuscript. Geneva: World Health Organization.

DAHRENDORF, R. (1965) *Homo Sociologicus. Ein Versuch zur Geschichte, Bedeutung und Kritik der Kategorie der sozialen Rolle.* Cologne: Westdeutscher Verlag.

DE JONG, A. & VAN DER LUBBE, P. M. (1994) *Handleiding van de Groningse Vragenlijst over Sociaal Gedrag.* (*Manual of the Groningen Questionnaire about Social Behaviour.*) Groningen: Department of Social Psychiatry, University of Groningen.

ENDICOTT, J., SPITZER, R. L., FLEISS, J. L., *et al* (1976) The Global Assessment Scale: a procedure for measuring overall severity of psychiatric disturbance. *Archives of General Psychiatry*, **33**, 766–771.

GOOD-ELLIS, M. A., FINE, S. B., SPENCER, J. H., *et al* (1987) Developing a role activity performance scale. *The American Journal of Occupational Therapy*, **41**, 232–241.

GORDON, G. (1966) *Role Theory and Illness. A Sociological Perspective.* New Haven, CT: College and University Press.

GURLAND, B. J., YORKSTON, N. J., STONE, A. R., *et al* (1972) The Structured and Scaled Interview to Assess Maladjustment (SSIAM): description, rationale and development. *Archives of General Psychiatry*, **27**, 259–264.

HALL, N. J. (1980) Ward rating scales for long stay patients. A review. *Psychological Medicine*, **10**, 277–288.

HURRY, J. & STURT, E. (1981) Social performance in a population sample: relation to psychiatric symptoms. In: *What Is a Case?* (eds J. K. Wing, P. Bebbington & L. N. Robins), pp. 202–213. London: Grant McIntyre.

KATSCHNIG, H. (1983) Methods for measuring social adjustment. In *Methodology in Evaluation of Psychiatric Treatment* (ed. T. Helgason), pp. 205–218. Cambridge: Cambridge University Press.

KRAAIJKAMP, H. J. M. (1992) *Moeilijke Rollen. Psychometrisch Onderzoek naar de Betrouwbaarheid en Validitcit van de Groningse Sociale Beperkingenschaal bij Psychiatrische Patinten.* (*Difficult Roles. A Study into the Reliability and Validity of the Groningen Social Disabilities Schedule in Psychiatric Patients.*) Thesis, University of Groningen.

LINK, B. G., MESAGNO, F. P., LUBNER, M. E. & DOHRENWEND, P. (1990) Problems in measuring role strains and social functioning in relation to psychological symptoms. *Journal of Health and Social Behaviour*, **31**, 354–369.

LINTON, R. (1936) *The Study of Man.* New York: D. Appleton – Century Co.

NAGI, S. Z. (1969) *Disability and Rehabilitation.* Columbus: Ohio State University Press.

—— (1991) Disability concepts revisited: implications for prevention. In *Disability in America. Toward a National Agenda for Prevention* (eds A. M. Pope & A. R. Tarlov), Appendix A, pp. 309–327. Washington, DC: Institute of Medicine, National Academy Press.

PARSONS, T. (1958) Definitions of health and illness in the light of American values and social structure. In *Patients, Physicians, Illnesses* (ed. E. G. Jaco). Glencoe, IL: Free Press.

PLATT, S. (1981) Social adjustment as a criterion of treatment success: just what are we measuring? *Psychiatry*, **44**, 95–112.

——, WEYMAN, A., HIRSCH, S. R., *et al* (1980) The Social Behaviour Assessment Schedule (SBAS): rationale, contents, scoring and reliability of a new interview schedule. *Social Psychiatry and Psychiatric Epidemiology*, **15**, 43–55.

POPE, A. M. & TARLOV, A. R. (1991) *Disability in America. Toward a National Agenda for Prevention.* Washington, DC: Institute of Medicine, National Academy Press.

ROSEN, A., HADZI-PAVLOVIC, D. & PARKER, G. (1989) The Life-skills Profile: a measure assessing function and disability in schizophrenia. *Schizophrenia Bulletin*, **15**, 325–337.

SCHOOLER, N., HOGARTY, G. & WEISSMAN, M. (1979) Social Adjustment Scale II (SAS-II). In *Resource Materials for Community Mental Health Program Evaluators* (eds W. A. Hargreaves, C. C. Atkinson & J. E. Sorenson), pp. 290–303. Rockville, MD: Department of Health, Education and Welfare.

TYRER, P. J. (1990) Personality disorder and social functioning. In *Measuring Human Problems. A Practical Guide* (eds D. F. Peck & C. M. Shapiro), pp. 119–142. Chichester: Wiley.

WALLACE, C. J. (1984) Community and interpersonal functioning in the course of schizophrenic disorders. *Schizophrenia Bulletin*, **10**, 233–257.

WEISSMAN, M. M., PAYKEL, E. S. & SIEGEL, R. (1971) The social role performance of depressed women: comparisons with a normal group. *American Journal of Orthopsychiatry*, **41**, 390–405.

—— (1975) The assessment of social adjustment. A review of techniques. *Archives of General Psychiatry*, **32**, 357–365.

——, SHALOMSKAS, D. & JOHN, K. (1981) The assessment of social adjustment. An update. *Archives of General Psychiatry*, **38**, 1250–1258.

WIERSMA, D. (1986) Psychological impairments and social disabilities: on the applicability of the ICIDH to psychiatry. *International Rehabilitation Medicine*, **8**, 3–7.

——, DE JONG, A. & ORMEL, J. (1988) The Groningen Social Disabilities Schedule: development, relationship with the ICIDH and psychometric properties. *International Journal of Rehabilitation Research*, **11**, 213–224.

——, ——, KRAAIJKAMP, H. J. M., *et al* (1990) *GSDS–II. The Groningen Social Disabilities Schedule, Second Version. Manual, Questionnaire and Rating Form.* Department of Social Psychiatry, University of Groningen.

WING, J. K. (1989) The measurement of 'social disablement'. The MRC social behaviour and social role performance schedules. *Social Psychiatry and Psychiatric Epidemiology*, **24**, 173–178.

WORLD HEALTH ORGANIZATION (1980) *The International Classification of Impairments, Disabilities and Handicaps.* Geneva: WHO.

—— (1988) *Psychiatric Disability Assessment Schedule (DAS).* Geneva: WHO.

—— (1992) *The ICD–D Classification of Mental and Behavioural Disorders. Clinical Descriptions and Diagnostic Guidelines.* Geneva: WHO.

9 The Schedules for Clinical Assessment in Neuropsychiatry and the tradition of the Present State Examination

JOHN K. WING and TRAOLACH S. BRUGHA

The principles underlying the creation and long-term development of the Present State Examination (PSE), now incorporated with its glossary of definitions of symptoms and other components in a shell known as the Schedules for Clinical Assessment in Neuropsychiatry (SCAN), are derived from standards of clinical assessment gradually developed from the late eighteenth century onwards. A form of 'mental state examination' is now an established part of the standard curriculum in most medical schools. To conduct such an examination requires the clinician to meet a demanding list of requirements. The first essential is a sound grasp of clinical psychopathology. This confers an ability to recognise, and distinguish within and between, an extensive range of symptoms such as delusions, hallucinations, obsessional ruminations, irrational fears of harmless stimuli and feelings of excessive guilt. A technique of 'cross-examination', based on the glossary of differential definitions of symptoms, must be learned in the first place by observing practitioners experienced in interviewing their patients. It is only after completing a comprehensive clinical symptom base that diagnostic procedures should, if needed, be brought into play with the help of algorithms laid down in international standards, as well as those of any other system in local use. These specifics differentiate SCAN from methods such as fully structured questionnaires or self-report forms, which have other purposes.

The aims of SCAN

The overall aim of SCAN can be summarised very simply, in one sentence. It is to provide comprehensive, accurate and technically specifiable means of describing and classifying clinical phenomena in order to make comparisons. Making comparisons is at the heart of all clinical, educational and scientific activities.

The first, clinical, aim is to promote the use of high-quality clinical observation. The PSE (see below) is designed to allow a comparison of each respondent's experiences and behaviour against the examiner's glossary-defined concepts by a process of controlled clinical 'cross-examination'. The resulting outputs in the form of single symptoms, profiles, scores and rule-based categories of disorder can be compared with each other wherever in the world they are elicited. Thus they can be used as a comparable base for clinical audit, needs assessment and monitoring the progress of individual respondents. It is essential to understand that the SCAN database is not tied exclusively to systems such as ICD–10 or DSM–IV. All the items required for these internationally based systems, and the algorithms necessary to derive their diagnoses, are included. However, the SCAN database and glossary include large numbers of symptoms culled from the experience of its many authors, and from the literature of many decades, which are not tied to any particular system of categorisation.

The second aim is educational and developmental: to improve clinical concepts by teaching a common clinical language. This makes it feasible to compare and learn from different clinical schools. It is not necessary to agree with such a standard of reference in order to appreciate its value as a basis for communication, quantification and comparison. Differences between clinical schools of thought do exist and are taught. Comparison between them by means of a common standard of reference provides a basis for informed development. SCAN itself benefits from such comparisons. However, modifications must be made in carefully defined stages, following periods long enough to provide a substantial and generally agreed basis for change.

The third, scientific, aim is to accelerate the accumulation of knowledge. Using standard technical procedures in research projects makes the results more precise and comparable, thus leading to more rapid agreement on useful theoretical lines for further hypothesis testing. This is true of all types of scientific research – biological, epidemiological and psychosocial.

Together, the three aims can facilitate the accumulation of knowledge for clinical purposes of all kinds, including primary, secondary and tertiary prevention and high-quality health service management and planning.

The precursors of SCAN

The basic aims and rationale of the PSE were first conceived in studies carried out by the Medical Research Council's Social Psychiatry Research Unit in the late 1950s and early 1960s (Wing, 1960, 1961). A paper outlining the principles, based on studies of sections of symptoms associated with 'neurotic' and 'psychotic' disorders, was published by five clinicians (Wing *et al*, 1967). Most of the key characteristics of subsequent editions were anticipated in this paper. Three sample sections of the schedule derived from the studies (PSE–5), covering obsessional symptoms, delusions of bodily control and non-social speech, were included as an appendix to the paper and bear a close resemblance to their present-day counterparts.

Four revisions (the seventh to the present tenth editions), each related to major international research projects and systems of diagnosis, have amplified and improved the format while preserving the basic principles intact. Two projects were particularly influential. PSE–7 and PSE–8 were used in the US–UK Diagnostic Study (Cooper *et al*, 1972) and PSE–8 in the International Pilot Study of Schizophrenia (IPSS; World Health Organization, 1973, 1979). Reliability was satisfactory in both projects and in others conducted elsewhere (e.g. Kendell *et al*, 1968; Luria & McHugh, 1974; Cooper *et al*, 1977; Wing *et al*, 1977; Luria & Berry, 1979; Rogers & Mann, 1986; Lesage *et al*, 1991).

Both large international projects concentrated on the differential diagnosis between schizophrenia and other, particularly affective, disorders. In the US–UK study the same team of research psychiatrists interviewed patients who had been diagnosed as having schizophrenia or other (largely affective) disorders in hospitals in London and New York. The central result was substantial agreement in the London series, while clinicians in New York were far more likely to diagnose schizophrenia than the research team. This had no implications for validity in the strict sense but it did indicate that the boundaries of the disorder were, at that time, drawn so differently that the results of studies into causes, treatments and outcomes would not be comparable between New York and London if based on hospital diagnoses.

The IPSS investigators formed a larger and more diverse group than those of the US–UK study. They came from psychiatric departments in Arhus, Agra, Cali, Ibadan, London, Moscow, Prague, Taipei and Washington, DC. The results, however, were similar. The PSE symptom profiles showed that centres in Moscow and Washington used a broader definition of schizophrenia than the other seven. The case for an instrument such as the PSE was thus abundantly reinforced.

In addition, the experience of these projects indicated a need for three major improvements in the PSE:

- the glossary of differential definitions needed to be updated and expanded as a basis for training courses;
- additional schedules were needed to allow the rating of previous episodes of disorder and possible causes and pathologies;
- algorithms for deriving ICD–9 diagnostic categories (World Health Organization, 1978) from PSE item profiles needed to be created in order to give a standard of reference in addition to (not as a substitute for) clinical diagnosis, since at that time the international diagnostic systems did not provide 'official' algorithms.

These features were incorporated into PSE–9, which was short – only 140 items, derived from the 500 items of its predecessor. Each was given a differential definition in the glossary, which, together with a specified method of clinical examination, continued to be at the heart of the system. A syndrome checklist for previous episodes, an aetiology schedule, the CATEGO-4 computer program, and a computer-assisted version of the text were added, filling most of the gaps in the earlier systems. The principles were laid down in a reference manual (Wing *et al*, 1974).

Further innovations included a set of scales that allowed the ratings of specified groups of symptoms to be summed, and an Index of Definition (ID), which provided a means of differentiating eight levels of confidence that sufficient symptoms were present to allow a diagnosis of one of the 'functional' categories of ICD–9, an important indicator for general population studies (Wing, 1976; Wing *et al*, 1978). Three other additions were also found useful: a rating scale specifically to detect change, using PSE items for monitoring clinical progress over time (Tress *et al*, 1987), a technique for ascertaining lifetime prevalence (McGuffin *et al*, 1986), and a brief form using only 10 items to identify 'non-cases' with remarkable success (Cooper & MacKenzie, 1981).

Publishing the full PSE–9 and its accessories for the first time in 1974, after 15 years of development, provided an opportunity to state the aims of the system, summarise its limitations and advantages, and specify the relationships between the PSE text and glossary (Wing, 1983). These have not changed since. The interesting and difficult problems encountered during translation into many different languages have not changed either (Sartorius, 1998).

The PSE/CATEGO-4 system was used in numerous studies and translations in many corners of the world, both in sample population surveys and in experimental research (e.g. Henderson *et al*, 1979; Orley & Wing, 1979; Urwin & Gibbons, 1979; Knights *et al*, 1980; Bebbington *et al*, 1981; Okasha & Ashour, 1981; Sturt, 1981; Dean *et al*, 1983; Mavreas & Bebbington, 1988; Huxley *et al*, 1989; Brugha *et al*, 1990; Lehtinen *et al*, 1990, 1991, pp. 308–342; Pakaslahti, 1994).

One unexpected problem, appreciated only after long experience, was that many users tended to regard the computerised output from PSE–9 only in terms of a single diagnosis, rather than as a rich and varied psychometric profile. This was far from the authors' intention (Wing, 1983, 1994). A central principle is that the system cannot 'make a diagnosis' in the sense that a clinician can. Those who use it are responsible for interpreting the data according to their judgement of the adequacy of the interview, the quality of the data recorded, and the choice of outputs from the computer analysis. Most of these outputs are profiles of scores or 'pre-final' categories. A 'final' category should be derived and interpreted as a diagnosis only if the clinician so decides, but that decision is made by him or her, not by the PSE, and still less by the computer.

Rose (1992) has made the point that diagnosis "splits the world in two": those who have, and those who do not have, a disorder. But most problems have continuous distributions. The PSE was not originally designed as a diagnostic instrument, although in the course of its development as a comprehensive clinical tool it came to provide a database capable (in addition to its basic psychometric properties) of expanding to exploit the more exacting algorithms presented by the DSM series (American Psychiatric Association, 1994) and ICD–10 (World Health Association, 1993). Both systems will undoubtedly change in further editions, perhaps markedly. The symptoms of patients are much less likely to vary from those familiar now.

Preparation for SCAN

More than 15 years of experience with the PSE–9 system provided a mass of suggestions for improvement. Preparations for a tenth edition were started in 1980 in anticipation of ICD–10 (Jablensky *et al*, 1983). The major emphasis of collaborators and correspondents was on broadening the content, both by returning to the larger item pool of PSE–7 and PSE–8, and by adding new sections to cover somatoform, dissociative and eating disorders, alcohol and drug use, and cognitive impairments. Similar work was also begun in preparation for the use of DSM–III criteria in the Epidemiologic Catchment Area programme (Romanoski *et al*, 1988).

A second suggestion was that an extra rating point was needed to extend the 0–1–2 scales of severity used for most PSE–9 items, thus providing a mild or 'sub-clinical' level that would be useful in population surveys. There is some evidence that this could be useful, by allowing clinically inexperienced trainees to rate as present items that are only marginally significant clinically (Dean *et al*, 1983; Brugha *et al*, 1999*c*). It has, however, introduced a difficulty when comparing PSE–9 with PSE–10 studies. Users of PSE–9 had made it clear that they would wish relevant items in PSE–10 to be convertible into PSE–9 equivalents, so that the CATEGO computer programs could be applied to produce output comparable with data from earlier studies.

A third, very obvious, requirement was for a better technique for rating previous episodes of disorder, adding other items relevant to the history and to aetiology, and processing all the resulting information by means of one set of computer programs.

Finally, the widespread acceptance and use of DSM–III–R, and subsequently DSM–IV, meant that the databases must contain all the clinical and course criteria specified in those manuals, as well as those being developed for ICD–10, and that the new algorithms must contain all three sets of classifying rules. This was the right decision, but it enhanced the risk that it could be regarded as principally a diagnostic instrument, whereas the first intention remains to provide a broad and up-to-date clinical database fitted to serve much broader purposes. It also added to the delays.

Although an enhanced PSE–10 remained the major component, it was agreed that a new name would be needed to express the set of instruments now available and linked by software. 'SCAN' seemed a highly appropriate choice.

An early version of SCAN, containing an expanded PSE and glossary as its major components, was devised to meet these stringent requirements and was used in a study of long-stay day care in southeast London (Brugha *et al*, 1988). These experiences, together with suggestions from international reviewers, led to further additions and modifications (Wing *et al*, 1990). The February 1988 prototype was used in international field trials to test reliability between interviewer and observer and between two interviewers over time, and also its general practicality in use across a wide range of disorders. Subsequent changes in the sections dealing with the use of alcohol and other drugs, eating and obsessional disorders, and cognitive impairments led to further trials (Wing *et al*, 1998, chapter 8). SCAN was redesigned in the light of all the results and a sequence of further drafts ensued. All contained the updated Item Group Checklist and Clinical History Schedule as well.

Finally, many additions were needed to cover the development and successive publication of algorithms for the major international diagnostic systems. All the new items and instructions (including course criteria and attributions of cause) in ICD–10 diagnostic criteria for research and the texts of DSM–III–R and DSM–IV had to be included. A computer-assisted PSE (CAPSE) was devised and went through similar modifications. In the event, three consecutive versions of SCAN were published by the World Health Organization: one printed by Design Locker (World Health Organization Division of Mental Health, 1992) but not used in formal trials; one by the American Psychiatric Association Press (version 2.0; World Health Organization Division of Mental Health, 1994); the third printed by the World Health Organization Division of Mental Health (1999). This last is the definitive version 2, and it incorporates PSE–10.2 and CAPSE–2.

The structure of SCAN

The full list of SCAN version 2 components is as follows:

- The SCAN manual, comprising –
    PSE–10.2 (sections 1–25)
    Item Group Checklist (IGC) (section 26)
    Clinical History Schedule (CHS) (section 27)
- The SCAN glossary
- The computer-assisted PSE–10.2 (CAPSE–2 with WHO SCAN I-Shell)
- The SCAN training materials
- The SCAN reference manual (Wing *et al*, 1998).

The tenth edition of the Present State Examination

The largest part of the SCAN manual is PSE–10.2, taking up the first 25 of its 27 sections. Each section is devoted to a particular type of symptom or sign or other clinical feature. The phenomena of disorders in sub-chapters F0–F5 of ICD–10 and their equivalents in DSM–III–R and DSM–IV are all included, as part of the comprehensive database, as follows:

- F0, dementia, including symptomatic mental disorders
- F1, mental and behavioural disorders due to psychoactive substance use
- F2, schizophrenia, schizotypal and delusional disorders
- F3, mood disorders
- F4, neurotic, stress-related and somatoform disorders
- F50–51, eating disorders, non-organic sleep disorders.

Some sections have optional checklists attached, covering items related to disorders that require specific time relationships, for example to psychosocial trauma, as in the stress and adjustment disorders. Other checklists allow a more extended list of items to be rated than is provided for in the main text, for example an extra list of somatoform symptoms.

A repeat caveat must be attached to this description, to reinforce earlier statements that PSE–10.2 contains numerous items that are not present in the two international systems, and that the complete database is intended to support projects independently of whether a diagnosis is or is not required.

Item Group Checklist (IGC, section 26)

The IGC provides a simple means of rating information obtained from case records and informants, including the respondent's account of previous episodes. The item groups are not diagnostic syndromes and do not contain the items necessary for all the algorithms for ICD or DSM disorders. The resulting classification is therefore approximate compared with that of the PSE, but it is a useful supplement and can substitute in situations where the PSE cannot be fully completed.

Users of the IGC must have been trained in the use of PSE–10 and its glossary, and have become completely familiar with the structure of SCAN. This provides a substantial degree of operationalisation for rating item groups, each of which is composed of designated PSE–10 items.

Clinical History Schedule (CHS, section 27)

The CHS is an optional section but is recommended because of the opportunity it offers to match personal details and historical information against data recorded elsewhere in SCAN. It also provides the investigator with an opportunity to record any relevant points on ICD–10 sub-chapters F1 (dementias), F6 (personality disorders) and F9 (disorders with onset in childhood), which are not covered in detail in the PSE. Interviewing the patient is not generally suited to eliciting the problems associated with these disorders. For example, a full developmental history, which is essential for the diagnosis of autistic spectrum disorders, such as Asperger's syndrome, is not included.

The SCAN glossary

The glossary is at the heart of the SCAN system. It consists of differential definitions of items in the SCAN text, that is, not only definitions of what an item signifies but also of what it excludes. This 'item concept' is learned during training and thereafter carried in the examiner's mind. Virtually every item in SCAN is defined in the glossary, not only those representing symptoms but those concerned with time relationships, precipitants, clinical course, attribution of cause, and so on. It provides a common clinical language, in which interviewers, whatever their own school of thought and wherever in the world they are working, can communicate with each other and make useful comparisons.

Computer applications

Computer programs are provided to facilitate data entry, data analysis and output of the results for individual respondents. Data analysis is both top-down, in terms of rule-based categories such as the disorders in ICD–10, but also bottom-up, in the sense that the items, item groups and dimensional scores provide alternative descriptive profiles. The computer applications can provide an immediate output as each interview is completed. In its present form, the SCAN I-Shell also provides a standard statistical output (in SPSS–PC) and outputs from ICD–10 and DSM–IV. Up-to-date details can be obtained from the Division of Mental Health and Prevention of Substance Abuse, World Health Organization, Geneva 27, and from SCAN websites: http://www.who.ch\msa\scan; http://www.psy.med.rug.nl/0018.

SCAN training

Training centres recognised by the World Health Organization (because they have a critical mass of staff experienced in the use of SCAN for clinical and research purposes and knowledgeable about translation problems) have been set up worldwide, for example in China, Denmark, Luxembourg, Germany, India, Russia, Spain, the UK and the USA. A core element is standard in all centres but details are adapted to local circumstances. Further information can be obtained from the World Health Organization's Division of Mental Health, as above.

Further work

The developmental version of SCAN (printed as SCAN–2.0) was used in a number of community surveys, most notably to interview people screened from a first-stage UK national sample to identify people with all grades of mental illness (Jenkins *et al*, 1997). A further study compared two lay administered diagnostic interviews (CIDI and CISR) with SCAN–1 in a representative random sample of adults in 2000 households (Brugha *et al*, 1999*a,b*). The target disorders were current anxiety, depressive and obsessional disorders. As similar studies have suggested, the results show that fixed interview schedules, allowing no informed cross-questioning, have poor concordance with instruments like SCAN.

Because of the successive changes made between the prototype and the field trials, further studies will be required to establish current reliability, structure and usefulness. In particular, work is needed on test–retest reliability in the general population and in primary care, together with work on sections that have not been fully tested, such as the somatoform, stress and adjustment disorders. International projects are coordinated by the World Health Organization. Other developments include versions dedicated to particular research settings, such as the survey form referred to above, and a short form more suited to service and professional training purposes.

The importance of high-quality psychiatric epidemiological data has been emphasised by the report on the Global Burden of Disease from the World Bank (Murray & Lopez, 1997). The use of mathematical modelling techniques will make it possible for high-quality data from SCAN reappraisal interviews to re-weigh and estimate prevalence rates originally derived from large-scale surveys (Kessler, 1999; Brugha *et al*, 2001). Close collaboration between developers of semistructured and fully structured survey measures therefore continues to be necessary.

References

AMERICAN PSYCHIATRIC ASSOCIATION (1994) *Diagnostic and Statistical Manual of Mental Disorders* (4th edn) (DSM–IV). Washington, DC: APA.

BEBBINGTON, P. E., HURRY, J., TENNANT, C., *et al* (1981) Epidemiology of mental disorders in Camberwell. *Psychological Medicine*, **11**, 561–580.

BRUGHA, T. S., WING, J. K., BREWIN, C. R., *et al* (1988) The problems of people in long-term psychiatric day-care. An introduction to the Camberwell High Contact Survey. *Psychological Medicine*, **18**, 443–456.

——, BEBBINGTON, P. E., MACCARTHY, B., *et al* (1990) Gender, social support and recovery from depressive disorders: a prospective clinical study. *Psychological Medicine*, **20**, 147–156.

——, JENKINS, R., TAUB, N.A.,*et al* (2001)A general population comparison of the Composite International Diagnostic Interview (CIDI) and the Schedules for Clinical Assessment in Neuropsychiatry (SCAN). *Psychological Medicine*, in press.

——, ——, JENKINS, R., *et al* (1999*a*) Cross validation of a household population survey diagnostic interview: a comparison of CIS–R with SCAN ICD–10 diagnostic categories. *Psychological Medicine*, **29**, 1029–1042.

—, — & —(1999*b*) A difference that matters: comparisons of structured and semi-structured diagnostic interviews of adults in the general population. *Psychological Medicine*, **29**, 1013–1020.

—, NIENHUIS, F. J., BAGCHI, D., *et al* (1999*c*) The survey form of SCAN: the feasibility of using experienced lay survey interviewers to administer a semi-structured systematic clinical assessment of psychotic and non-psychotic disorders. *Psychological Medicine*, **29**, 703–712.

COOPER, J. E., KENDELL, R. E., GURLAND, B. J., *et al* (1972) *Psychiatric Diagnosis in New York and London*. London: Oxford University Press.

—, COPELAND, J. R. M., BROWN, G. W., *et al* (1977) Further studies on interviewer training and inter-rater reliability of the PSE. *Psychological Medicine*, **7**, 517–523.

— & McKENZIE, S. (1981) The rapid prediction of low scores on a standardized psychiatric interview (PSE). In *What Is a Case?* (eds J. K. Wing, P. Bebbington & L. N. Robins). London: Grant McIntyre.

DEAN, C., SURTEES, P. G. & SASHIDHARAN, S. P. (1983) Comparison of research diagnostic systems in an Edinburgh community sample. *British Journal of Psychiatry*, **142**, 247–256.

HENDERSON, S., DUNCAN-JONES, P., BYRNE, D. G., *et al* (1979) Psychiatric disorder in Canberra. A standardized study of prevalence. *Acta Psychiatrica Scandinavica*, **60**, 355–374.

HUXLEY, P., RAVAL, H., KORER, J., *et al* (1989) Psychiatric morbidity in the clients of social workers. Clinical outcome. *Psychological Medicine*, **19**, 189–198.

JABLENSKY, A., SARTORIUS, N., HIRSCHFELD, R., *et al* (1983) Diagnosis and classification of mental disorders and alcohol- and drug-related problems. A research agenda for the 1980s. *Psychological Medicine*, **13**, 907–921.

JENKINS, R., LEWIS, G., BEBBINGTON, P., *et al* (1997) The national psychiatric morbidity surveys of Great Britain – initial findings from the household survey. *Psychological Medicine*, **27**, 775–789.

KENDELL, R. E., EVERITT, B., COOPER, J. E., *et al* (1968) Reliability of the PSE. *Social Psychiatry*, **3**, 123–129.

KESSLER, R. C. (1999) The WHO International Consortium in Psychiatric Epidemiology. Initial work and future directions. *Acta Psychiatrica Scandinavica*, **99**, 2–9.

KNIGHTS, A., HIRSCH, S. R. & PLATT, S. D. (1980) Clinical change as a function of brief admission to hospital in a controlled study using the PSE. *British Journal of Psychiatry*, **137**, 170–180.

LEHTINEN, V., LINDHOLM, T., VEIJOLA, J., *et al* (1990) The prevalence of PSE–CATEGO disorders in a Finnish adult population cohort. *Social Psychiatry and Psychiatric Epidemiology*, **25**, 187–192.

—, JOUKAMAA, M., JYRKINEN, T., *et al* (1991) *Mental Health and Mental Disorders in the Finnish Adult Population*. Helsinki: Social Institute.

LESAGE, A. D., CYR, M. & TOUPIN, J. (1991) Reliable use of the PSE by psychiatric nurses of psychotic and non-psychotic patients. *Acta Psychiatrica Scandinavica*, **83**, 121–124.

LURIA, R. E. & McHUGH, P. R. (1974) Reliability and clinical utility of the Wing PSE. *Archives of General Psychiatry*, **30**, 866–871.

— & BERRY, R. (1979) Reliability and descriptive validity of the PSE syndromes. *Archives of General Psychiatry*, **36**, 1187–1195.

MAVREAS, V. G. & BEBBINGTON, P. E. (1988) Greeks, British Greek Cypriots and Londoners. A comparison of morbidity. *Psychological Medicine*, **18**, 433–442.

McGUFFIN, P., KATZ, R. & ALDRICH, J. (1986) Past and present state examination. The assessment of 'lifetime ever' psychopathology. *Psychological Medicine*, **16**, 461–466.

MURRAY, C. J. L. & LOPEZ, A. D. (1997) Alternative projections of mortality and disability by cause, 1990–2020. Global burden of disease study. *Lancet*, **349**, 1498–1504.

OKASHA, A. & ASHOUR, A. (1981) Psycho-demographic study of anxiety in Egypt. The PSE in its Arabic version. *British Journal of Psychiatry*, **139**, 70–73.

ORLEY, J. & WING, J. K. (1979) Psychiatric disorders in two African villages. *Archives of General Psychiatry*, **36**, 513–520.

PAKASLAHTI, A. (1994) Predictors of working disability in first admission schizophrenic patients. *Psychiatrica Fennica*, **25**, 150–168.

ROGERS, B. & MANN, S. A. (1986) The reliability and validity of PSE assessments by lay interviewers. A national population survey. *Psychological Medicine*, **16**, 689–700.

ROMANOSKI, A. J., NESTAD, G., CAHAL, R., *et al* (1988) Inter-observer reliability of a 'Standard Psychiatric Examination' for case ascertainment (DSM–III). *Journal of Nervous and Mental Disease*, **176**, 63–71.

ROSE, G. (1992) *The Strategy of Preventive Medicine*. Oxford: Oxford University Press.

SARTORIUS, N. (1998) Cross-cultural and language problems. In *Diagnosis and Clinical Measurement in Psychiatry. An Instruction Manual for the SCAN System* (eds J. K. Wing, N. Sartorius & T. B. Üstün), pp. 44–57. Cambridge: Cambridge University Press.

STURT, E. (1981) Hierarchical patterns in the distribution of psychiatric symptoms. *Psychological Medicine*, **11**, 783–794.

TRESS, K. H., BELLENIS, C., BROWNLOW, J. H., *et al* (1987) The PSE change rating scale. *British Journal of Psychiatry*, **150**, 201–207.

URWIN, P. & GIBBONS, J. L. (1979) Psychiatric diagnosis in self poisoning patients. *Psychological Medicine*, **9**, 501–507.

WING, J. K. (1960) The measurement of behaviour in chronic schizophrenia. *Acta Psychiatrica et Neurologica*, **35**, 245–254.

—— (1961) A simple and reliable sub-classification of chronic schizophrenia. *Journal of Mental Science*, **107**, 862–875.

—— (1976) A technique for studying psychiatric morbidity in in-patient and out-patient series and in general population samples. *Psychological Medicine*, **6**, 665–671.

—— (1983) Use and misuse of the PSE. *British Journal of Psychiatry*, **143**, 111–117.

—— (1994) Relevance of psychiatric epidemiology to clinical psychiatry. *International Review of Psychiatry*, **6**, 259–264.

——, BIRLEY, J. L. T., COOPER, J. E., *et al* (1967) Reliability of a procedure for measuring and classifying 'present psychiatric state'. *British Journal of Psychiatry*, **113**, 499–515.

——, COOPER, J. E. & SARTORIUS, N. (1974) *The Description and Classification of Psychiatric Symptoms. An Instruction Manual for the PSE and CATEGO System*. London: Cambridge University Press.

——, NIXON, J. M., MANN, S. A., *et al* (1977) Reliability of the PSE (ninth edition) used in a population survey. *Psychological Medicine*, **7**, 505–516.

——, MANN, S. A., LEFF, J. P., *et al* (1978) The concept of a 'case' in psychiatric population surveys. *Psychological Medicine*, **8**, 203–217.

——, BABOR, T., BRUGHA, T., *et al* (1990) SCAN: Schedules for Clinical Assessment in Neuropsychiatry. *Archives of General Psychiatry*, **47**, 589–593.

——, SARTORIUS, N. & ÜSTÜN, T. B. (eds) (1998) *Diagnosis and Clinical Measurement in Psychiatry. A Reference Manual for the SCAN System*. Cambridge: Cambridge University Press.

WORLD HEALTH ORGANIZATION (1973) *The International Pilot Study of Schizophrenia (IPSS)*. Geneva: WHO.

—— (1978) *International Classification of Diseases* (9th edn) (ICD–9). Geneva: WHO.

—— (1979) *Schizophrenia. An International Follow-Up Study*. Geneva: WHO.

—— (1993) *The ICD–10 Classification of Mental and Behavioural Disorders: Diagnostic Criteria for Research*. WHO: Geneva.

WORLD HEALTH ORGANIZATION DIVISION OF MENTAL HEALTH (1992) *SCAN: Schedules for Clinical Assessment in Neuropsychiatry, Version 1*. Geneva: WHO.

—— (1994) *SCAN: Schedules for Clinical Assessment in Neuropsychiatry, Version 2*. Washington, DC: American Psychiatric Association Press.

—— (1999) *SCAN Schedules for Clinical Assessment in Neuropsychiatry Version 2 Revised (2.1)*. Geneva: World Health Organization.

10   The costs of mental health care: paucity of measurement

PAUL McCRONE and SCOTT WEICH

The supply of resources in an economy is limited. However, the demand for resources is generally unlimited. This is particularly the case with health care; if the technology and expertise to treat people exist, then there will be a demand for such resources. If the technology and expertise do not exist, then there will be a demand for their provision. Scarcity of resources leads to competing alternatives, and in the health care arena policy makers and clinicians are confronted with having to decide how resources should be allocated. What should guide decision makers in this task of resource allocation? Obviously we would expect treatments and interventions to be looked at favourably if they are known to produce good outcomes. However, it is also necessary to know what the costs of achieving these outcomes are, and this is particularly relevant given the high and increasing cost of health care. But economics should not be concerned with simply cutting costs. Costs are, in effect, proxies for units of production. More units of production could well result in improved outcomes. Therefore, the more expensive option may be the preferred one. If an evaluation does not include a cost component, then inefficient services may go undetected and resources will be used inappropriately. Both high-quality outcome data and cost data are therefore required to advise policy makers and clinicians as to the best use of their limited resources. This chapter examines the extent to which costs have been calculated in an appropriate way in mental health care evaluations.

Cost measurement has been undervalued in many studies. Sometimes costs have been omitted. In other cases not all relevant costs have been collected. Costs are frequently measured incorrectly or not interpreted correctly. When they have been measured, it has often been in an *ad hoc* fashion. Hardly any costing instruments have been published and described. One exception in the UK is the Client Service Receipt Interview (Beecham & Knapp, 1992; Beecham, 1995).[1] This is unfortunate, as costs are one of the few measures that have regularly exhibited large variations among treatment interventions.

We need to be sure that the cost data being collected are appropriate. Although cost measurement has been performed imperfectly in many evaluations, a number of programmes and projects have sought to incorporate a cost–benefit or cost-effectiveness analysis into their evaluations. Without an adequate measurement of cost, the usefulness of such analyses will not be fully realised. Indeed, the very term 'cost-effective' has often been poorly understood and misused (Doubilet *et al*, 1986). The aim of this chapter is to examine evaluations that have included an economic element. From these studies we can deduce what services were considered relevant for the purposes of costing. A growing number of studies include an economic component and it is beyond the scope of this review to include them all. As such, the focus is on general adult mental health services, thereby excluding services specifically provided to children, elderly people, people with eating disorders and people with substance misuse disorders. Also excluded are studies that have evaluated pharmacological interventions. Compared with the previous edition of this book, we have now included studies examining the costs of routine mental health services (as opposed to experimental interventions) and also evaluations of psychological therapies.

Even after excluding the above categories of studies, the range that could be included remains vast and it is inevitable that many studies will have been omitted. This is therefore not a systematic review, but it is hoped that it does present a good overview of what costs are included in evaluations of different interventions. Readers wishing to gain a more thorough understanding of the literature in specific areas would do well to consult some of the reviews that are available (e.g. Gabbard *et al*, 1997; Latimer, 1999; Knapp *et al*, 1999).

Cost

Definition

It is important to have an understanding of the concept of cost before calculating it. Cost is often referred to as *opportunity cost*, which is the

---

[1] This is now known as the Client Service Receipt Inventory. Those interested in using the questionnaire should contact the Centre for the Economics of Mental Health, Institute of Psychiatry, De Crespigny Park, Denmark Hill, London SE5 8AF.

value of resources in their best alternative use. This is a definition used by economists in general. Health economists are no exception: "The cost of a unit of a resource is the benefit that would be derived from using it in its best alternative use" (Drummond, 1980: p. 2). Essentially then, a cost occurs because, with the existence of scarcity, some opportunities have to be missed. For many products and services it is assumed that an appropriate proxy for opportunity cost is the market value of the product. However, for some products there is no market price and, therefore, an opportunity cost must be imputed.

How should cost be measured?

Cost can refer to an entire service, or to the cost of any one individual using the service. It would be advantageous to know what the cost is of one more person using the service, as decisions are often made about expanding or reducing services. If there is spare capacity (such as unused hospital beds) the extra cost may be small. Higher costs are incurred if a service is already operating at full capacity. Considering these *marginal costs* is intrinsically correct. They are, though, difficult to calculate. In the long run (a period over which the structure of a service can alter) *average costs* are assumed to approximate marginal costs. Most studies in mental health care focus upon potential policy-changing schemes and, therefore, examining average costs is appropriate.

The timescale over which costs are measured is crucial. It is important to choose a length of time that would be representative of service receipt. Six months to a year should be acceptable, although this does depend on the particular programme being evaluated. In addition, different service components require particular costing procedures. For an outline of costing methods, the reader is referred to Allen & Beecham (1993).

Components of cost packages

All relevant costs should be examined to assess the economic impact of a mental health care intervention (Glass & Goldberg, 1977; Drummond, 1980; Weisbrod, 1981; Rubin, 1982; Knapp & Beecham, 1990; Clark *et al*, 1993; Manning, 1999). It is rare that mental health service users will have contact with only one particular agency and services often will have effects on each other via interagency cooperation, and substitution and complementary effects. The implementation of a mental health programme could, for example, potentially decrease psychiatric service costs but increase those falling on social services departments or general practitioners. Indeed, overall costs may be higher than initially, but if only psychiatric service costs were calculated the results could show that the new programme was less costly. Thus it is important to capture the economic costs of both the psychiatric service intervention *and* the non-psychiatric service inputs. There may also be indirect effects of a mental health care intervention. A further category, non-measured costs, includes aspects of care that are either too difficult to cost or where it would be inappropriate to cost them on the grounds of ethics.[2]

A cost instrument should capture information that would enable comprehensive costs to be calculated. It is realised, though, that there are limits as to how comprehensive a cost evaluation should be. Collecting data on every possible cost may result in accuracy of measurement being sacrificed. It may sometimes be preferable to ensure that the major costs are measured with utmost accuracy, with perhaps less emphasis being placed upon minor services (Challis *et al*, 1993). Knapp & Beecham (1993) suggest that in mental health care evaluations it may be possible to cost a 'reduced list' of services, but they do urge caution in this, in case important service inputs are neglected.

Psychiatric service costs

When contacts are made with specialist mental health providers, direct psychiatric service costs are incurred. Examples of these are indicated in Table 10.1. Many studies calculate only these costs. This may appear reasonable. Patients in hospital will often not be using services that are provided by other agencies. In addition, staff conducting the research may be concerned only with the costs incurred by their service. These costs are relatively straightforward, and less time-consuming to calculate than full costs. However, there will inevitably be other cost implications of mental health care programmes, particularly when they are based in the community. To ignore these other costs reduces the impact and usefulness of an economic evaluation, and can make conclusions regarding cost-effectiveness invalid.

Non-psychiatric service costs

People with mental health problems often use services from a wide range of agencies. Table 10.2, though not an exhaustive list, reveals that the

---

[2] In the previous edition of this book we referred to non-psychiatric service inputs as indirect costs. We have now followed convention and refer to these as direct costs, with indirect costs relating to what we previously called hidden costs.

TABLE 10.1
Examples of psychiatric service costs

Psychiatric hospital	Community
In-patient	Community psychiatric nurse
Out-patient	Psychiatrist home visit
Day patient	Community mental health centre
Depot clinic	Crisis house
Emergency clinic	Respite house
Psychologist	Drop-in/day centre
Occupational therapy	

range of non-psychiatric services is extensive. We have disaggregated these costs as follows: other health services (community and hospital), law and order agencies, social services, educational services, employment services, voluntary sector services, and accommodation.

Indirect costs

Indirect costs are not readily observable and it is unusual for payments to be made which are of equivalent value. Three main types of indirect cost are identified in Table 10.3. The burden on families is reflected by the cost of informal care. Time may need to be taken off work to care for a family member with a mental health problem, or leisure time may need to be given up.

Many patients are also unemployed. There are costs associated with this lost employment. From the point of view of the user, there is the absence of earnings. In addition, the whole of society suffers from reduced production. The degree of this depends on the workings of the labour market. It may be that lost employment opportunities are not included in cost evaluations, as they will be the same whatever the intervention – that is, clients will remain unemployed. However, the aim of many involved in mental health care is to help people to become rehabilitated, which should increase their employment prospects; thus the costs of lost employment are still relevant. The financial gains made from employment, in the form of earnings, are often included in cost–benefit analyses (where outcomes are monetised).

Finally, the costs of time and travelling, which are incurred when services are used, should ideally be considered in a cost evaluation. The opportunity cost of this time is determined by what the patient would have been doing otherwise – clearly this is difficult to value and is usually omitted.

TABLE 10.2
Categories of non-psychiatric service costs

General category	Services
Community health services	General practitioner Home visits by general practitioner Optician Chiropodist Family planning clinic District nurse Domiciliary nurse Dentist
Hospital services	In-patient Out-patient Day patient Accident and emergency Physiotherapy Dental services
Law and order	Police Probation service Court Solicitor Legal aid Prison
Social services	Social worker Home visit by a social worker Home help Meals on wheels Social security officer Counsellor
Education	Evening classes
Employment	Job centre Job club Disablement rehabilitation officer Careers advice
Voluntary services	Counselling Bereavement service Samaritans Voluntary day centres Churches
Accommodation	Supported residential care Private accommodation

TABLE 10.3
Categories of indirect costs

Category	Examples
Informal care	Lost employment of friends and relatives Lost leisure time of friends and relatives
User time	Travelling Waiting
Lost employment	Time off work due to mental health problem Foregone potential employment Lost production to economy

Welfare benefits

Costs arise because a productive activity has taken place, for example the provision of a particular service. Welfare benefits are not a means of production and therefore not a cost. They are a transfer payment from one group of economic agents (taxpayers) to another (recipients). The cost to taxpayers is offset by the gain to recipients and hence there is no residual cost (excluding the costs of administering the benefits system). However, to the individual service user welfare benefits are a definite gain, and to the rest of society they are a diversion of funds, even if this is deemed to be appropriate. The level of benefits may also be an indication of the cost of living (Knapp, 1991). It is useful for studies to record the receipt of welfare benefits, even if this is not essential for the costing process.

Areas in which costing has been undertaken

Many areas of mental health care have undergone economic evaluation and costs have frequently been reported. It should be stressed that reporting costs alone is as dangerous as omitting them altogether – the cost element should be viewed in the context of a full evaluation. Here we are concerned with what costs have been collected, not what these costs actually were. Table 10.4 summarises the studies under different headings. Some studies fit neatly into the categories of Table 10.4, while others could arguably be placed elsewhere. No one evaluation covers all relevant areas of cost. The more sophisticated evaluations are discussed below. Readers are advised to refer to these papers when undertaking similar studies. Some studies that examine only direct costs are sometimes valuable in their costing of such services.

TABLE 10.4
Summary of studies including economic evaluation

Study	PS	OHS	LO	SS	ED	EMP	VOL	ACC	IC	LEM	TT	WB
Hospital discharge												
Rothbard *et al* (1998)	+											
Beecham *et al* (1997)	+	+		+			+	+				
Beecham *et al* (1996)	+	+		+	+	+		+				
Knapp *et al* (1990)	+	+	+	+	+			+			+	
Häfner & an der Heiden (1989)	+					+	+					
Muller & Caton (1983)	+	+		+						+		
Murphy & Datel (1976)	+	+		+				+				+
Cassell *et al* (1972)	+								+			
Residential/home-based care												
Chisholm *et al* (1997)	+	+		+				+				
Beecham *et al* (1993)	+	+	+	+		+		+				
Bedell & Ward (1989)	+							+				
Bond *et al* (1989)	+							+				
Hyde *et al* (1987)	+	+	+	+				+				
Rappaport *et al* (1987)	+							+				
Wherley & Bisgaard (1987)	+							+				
Dickey *et al* (1986a)	+	+	+	+				+				
Linn *et al* (1985)	+							+				
Weisman (1985)	+							+				
Mosher *et al* (1975)	+							+				
Sheehan & Atkinson (1974)	+							+				
After-care												
Tyrer *et al* (1998)	+	+	+	+								
Wiersma *et al* (1991)	+	+										
Linn *et al* (1979)	+											

TABLE 10.4 (contd...)

Study	PS	OHS	LO	SS	ED	EMP	VOL	ACC	IC	LEM	TT	WB
Alternative hospital-based services												
O'Shea et al (1998)	+							+	+			
Creed et al (1997)	+	+								+		
Scott (1995)	+			+								
Grizenko & Papineau (1992)	+											
Moscarelli et al (1991)	+											
Marinoni et al (1988)	+	+		+					+			
Dick et al (1985)	+	+									+	
Gudeman et al (1983)	+							+	+			
Schulz et al (1983)	+											
Goldberg & Jones (1980)	+	+		+		+	+		+			+
Jones et al (1980)	+	+		+		+	+		+			+
Endicott et al (1978)	+			+								
Levenson et al (1977)	+											
Washburn et al (1976)	+											
Glick et al (1974)	+											
May (1971)	+											
Case management/assertive outreach												
Rosenheck & Neale (1998)	+	+	+					?				
Essock et al (1998)	+	+	+							+		+
Knapp et al (1994, 1998)	+	+	+	+		+		+				
Hu & Jerrell (1998)	+	+	+	+				+	+			+
Ford et al (1997)	+	+		+	+			+				
Wolff et al (1997)	+					+		+				
Quinlivan et al (1995)	+							+				
Rosenheck et al (1995)	+	+		+				+				

Table continues over

Key to costs: PS = psychiatric services, OHS = other health services, LO = law and order, SS = social services, ED = education, EMP = employment, VOL = voluntary costs, ACC = accommodation costs, IC = informal care, LEM = lost employment, TT = time and travelling, WB = welfare benefit receipt.

Table 10.4 (contd...)

Study	PS	OHS	LO	SS	ED	EMP	VOL	ACC	IC	LEM	TT	WB
Case management/assertive outreach (continued)												
McCrone et al (1994)	+	+	+	+	+	+	+	+				+
Burns et al (1993)	+	+		+								
Burns & Raftery (1991)	+	+										
Kivlahan et al (1991)	+											
Hu & Jerrell (1991)	+	+	+	+				+	+		+	+
Bond et al (1988)	+	+	+	+				+				
Franklin et al (1987)	+											
Dickey et al (1986b)	+	+	+	+				+				
Fenton et al (1984)	+											
Hoult et al (1983)	+											
Mueller & Hopp (1983)	+					+						
Weisbrod et al (1980)	+	+	+	+					+			+
Psychological treatments												
Lave et al (1998)	+	+										
Kuipers et al (1998)	+	+		+				+			+	
Healey et al (1998)	+	+	+	+	+	+						
Antonuccio et al (1997)	+	+								+	+	
Rund et al (1994)	+			+								
Xiong et al (1994)	+									+	+	
Scott & Freeman (1992)	+											
Tarrier et al (1991)	+			+				+				
Cardin et al (1985)	+	+	+	+								+
Ginsberg et al (1984)	+	+		+					+	+		
Mangen et al (1983)	+	+							+		+	+

TABLE 10.4 (contd...)

Study	PS	OHS	LO	SS	ED	EMP	VOL	ACC	IC	LEM	TT	WB
Routine care												
Amaddeo et al (1998)	+			+				+				
McCrone et al (1998)	+	+	+	+				+	+			
Haro et al (1998)	+			+	+	+		+	+	+		
Dickey & Scott (1997)	+					+		+				
Suleiman et al (1997)	+	+		+	+			+	+	+		
Lang et al (1997)	+	+		+		+	+	+				
Salize & Rössler (1996)	+	+		+		+		+				
Others												
Clarkson et al (1999)	+	+	+	+	+	+		+	+			
Hoff & Rosenheck (1998)	+	+	+	+								
Merson et al (1996)	+	+	+	+	+	+						
Jerrell & Hu (1996)	+	+	+	+				+	+			+
Goldberg et al (1996)	+	+		+						+	+	
Gournay & Brooking (1995)	+	+							+	+	+	+

Key to costs: PS = psychiatric services, OHS = other health services, LO = law and order, SS = social services, ED = education, EMP = employment, VOL = voluntary costs, ACC = accommodation costs, IC = informal care, LEM = lost employment, TT = time and travelling, WB = welfare benefit receipt.

Hospital closure and discharge studies

There has long been a trend towards deinstitutionalisation in the UK and other nations (Thornicroft & Bebbington, 1989). This has major economic implications. As hospitals close and people are placed in the community the cost burden on local agencies may rise. This has led to cost comparisons between long-stay hospital care and community provision.

In the UK, the closure of the Friern and Claybury hospitals and discharge of patients into the community has been evaluated. The economic component (Knapp *et al*, 1990; Beecham *et al*, 1997) was comprehensive in its costing. It involved the calculation of psychiatric service costs, and also those falling on a number of other agencies. Client travel costs were also calculated, and benefit receipt information was recorded. Informal care and lost employment were not costed though. This latter cost may be important. In a discharge study from the United States (Muller & Caton, 1983) the costs of foregone employment were calculated, and these proved to be extremely high.

An attractive aspect of costing reprovision programmes is the possibility of predicting the costs of future patient discharges (Murphy & Datel, 1976; Knapp *et al*, 1992). An accurate and comprehensive calculation of cost is a precondition for the gains of this exercise to be realised.

Residential and home-based treatment as alternatives

In many settings there is a reluctance to admit patients to hospital if this can possibly be avoided. This has been reflected by the introduction of alternative residential placements for potential in-patients. Evaluation is required to ascertain whether these alternatives are more efficient than traditional hospital care.

An evaluation of crisis housing stands out in its comprehensive approach to costing. Quarterway House was a residential alternative to in-patient care for patients with chronic schizophrenia deemed to be unsuitable for normal community placements. A two-year cost evaluation of the project was undertaken (Dickey *et al*, 1986*a*). Cost data were collected for psychiatric and non-psychiatric services. Omitted were costs associated with education, employment and voluntary services. Indirect costs were not included. An examination of domestic care in two different facilities also explored a wide range of costs (Beecham *et al*, 1993). However, because of the nature of the residential provision, few outside services were required.

After-care

Often, choices regarding after-care must be made. The economic costs of 50 schizophrenic patients randomised to day treatment or standard after-care have been evaluated (Wiersma *et al*, 1991). Although not described in detail, day treatment included case management, day hospital care and short-term domiciliary care. Cost data were limited to average primary and secondary treatment costs.

In the UK, a system of 'care programming' – a concept that espouses coordinated and effective community care – was evaluated by Tyrer *et al* (1998). A sample of patients who had been in hospital within the previous three years was recruited from three areas of London. Patients cared for by hospital-based teams were compared with those cared for by those based in the community. The main measure of interest was symptoms, but with much emphasis also placed on economic costs. Costs were fairly comprehensively measured and included those pertaining to the psychiatric services, general health services, the criminal justice system and social services. Indirect costs were omitted because the authors felt that they would not contribute greatly to the total and would not differ much across groups.

Alternative hospital-based services

It remains appropriate to treat some people in hospital for their mental health problems. However, the particular way in which hospitals provide care need not be fixed, and different methods should be explored. Again, careful examination of costs must be undertaken.

Psychiatric units based in general hospitals have been considered as an alternative to traditional mental hospitals. One prominent study compared these two possibilities in the Manchester area (Goldberg & Jones, 1980; Jones *et al*, 1980). The authors gathered costs relating to psychiatric and non-psychiatric services.

Day treatment and out-patient contacts have also been compared with in-patient episodes for non-psychotic psychiatric patients in a randomised trial at three Scottish centres (Dick *et al*, 1985). In addition to psychiatric service costs, general practice costs and travelling costs were also measured. However, many other inputs were not measured. More recently, in Manchester, Creed *et al* (1997) compared costs and outcomes of day hospital care with in-patient care. They measured psychiatric service costs and other health service and social service costs as well as loss of patients' income. Travel costs and foregone carers' income were also costed, although the time spent caring and the time spent travelling were not (even though the actual time was recorded).

A study in Boston reported on the reorganisation of acute hospital services with the aim of reducing admission and increasing the use of a day hospital by introducing a dormitory for homeless patients

(Gudeman *et al*, 1983). Monetary costs were measured for accommodation and all mental health services and costs to families were estimated.

The Italian mental health care system underwent major reforms during the late 1970s. From 1978 psychiatric hospitals were not allowed to admit patients – in-patients would be cared for in general hospitals. An evaluation measured the costs of managing psychotic patients in the community (Marinoni *et al*, 1988). Cost comparisons were made between patients in contact with the mental health services and those who had dropped out of care. Again, psychiatric and non-psychiatric costs were measured, as well as informal care contacts.

Case management/assertive outreach

The move to community provision has often taken the form of implementing case management programmes. This is a method of allowing for the continuation and coordination of care. Usually an individual will act as the case manager for a number of users. Case management is not rigidly defined and it takes many forms. Consequently, its cost implications are unpredictable and should be examined. Recently there has been a refocus towards assertive outreach schemes, which target patients most in need of service inputs, often with the overriding desire to prevent hospital admission.

One of the more thorough cost evaluations of a case management system was that carried out of a community mental health service in Wisconsin (Weisbrod *et al*, 1980). The community initiative, which included assertive home-based care, was compared with traditional provision. Cost information was gathered for the psychiatric services, other services and informal care. This study has been replicated to different degrees in a number of countries (Hoult *et al*, 1983; Fenton *et al*, 1984). One of these replications was in London (Marks *et al*, 1994). The economic component of this study (Knapp *et al*, 1994) measured costs to most key agencies, but did not measure informal care costs or those arising from lost employment.

A number of other forms of case management have been implemented and evaluated. The problem of applying model programmes to other settings was illustrated by Bond *et al* (1988). Patients at risk of rehospitalisation, in three centres, were randomised to home-based assertive case management or to a control condition consisting of all other public mental health services. The range of costs measured was relatively comprehensive. They included direct psychiatric service costs, residential costs and law enforcement costs.

In Greenwich, London, community psychiatric nurses became case managers in a departure from generic community psychiatric nursing care. The economic evaluation of the new service (McCrone *et al*,

1994) involved the assessment of patients who were randomly allocated to the new community support team or to the traditional team acting as a control. Costs were measured for psychiatric inputs and a wide range of other services. Indirect costs were not calculated.

In two randomised cost-effectiveness studies in California, Hu & Jerrell (1991) set out a method for comparing different models of case management, and public capitation funding, coupled with assertive community treatment. Comprehensive cost measures were described for both studies covering psychiatric treatment and a range of non-psychiatric services. Additionally, informal care and travelling time were costed. The same authors later reported on costs of three case management interventions (Hu & Jerrell, 1998). Most service costs were measured as were welfare benefits.

Psychological treatments

As can be seen from the above studies, there is much emphasis placed on the settings and structure in which care is provided. Evaluations that have examined *specific therapies* have often been concerned with those of a pharmacological nature, which are not dealt with here. Alternatives to pharmacological therapies have also been assessed, although few evaluations have contained an economic component. There are, though, some exceptions.

The cost-effectiveness of behavioural therapy provided to families of patients discharged from hospital following an acute schizophrenic illness was studied by Cardin *et al* (1985). Patients at high risk of relapse were randomly allocated to receive either family therapy or individual supportive psychotherapy. Costs were measured relatively comprehensively, and included the value of earnings gained. Welfare benefits were also included.

Cognitive–behavioural therapy used in the care of patients with psychosis who had treatment-resistant conditions was evaluated by Kuipers *et al* (1998). In this study, costs of services used by patients receiving therapy were compared with those used by patients receiving a standard service. Psychiatric services, other health services and social services were included, as was accommodation.

Healey *et al* (1998) calculated the costs of services used by patients receiving a psychological intervention designed to improve their compliance with treatment. Included were psychiatric services, general health services, criminal justice services, social services, education services and employment services. Accommodation costs were not included.

Out-patients in south London with diagnoses of neurosis or personality disorder were allocated to continued out-patient care or to treatment from a community psychiatric nurse, which involved problem solving and medication assistance (Mangen *et al*, 1983). Costs were measured widely, and included direct services, social service input, travel time and welfare benefits. Cost measurement excluded foregone earnings, on the grounds that no differences were found on measures of social functioning.

Ginsberg *et al* (1984) evaluated patients with specific neurotic disorders referred by their general practitioner as suitable for psychotherapy. They were randomly allocated to immediate nurse-led treatment or to a waiting-list control group. Cost data were derived for forgone earnings and family burden, as well as medical and social support costs.

Routine care

While most evaluations are of specific interventions, often introduced under experimental conditions, a number of studies have examined the effectiveness and costs of routine mental health services. In London, two catchment area services were compared, one of which contained a team focusing on long-term care and the other a team focusing on acute service provision. Most key psychiatric and non-psychiatric service costs were calculated, as well as informal care costs (McCrone *et al*, 1998). A similar range of services were costed in an assessment of services in Edinburgh (Lang *et al*, 1997).

Other interventions

A community-based service for patients experiencing psychiatric emergencies was compared with a service based in hospital by Merson *et al* (1996). This study measured a wide range of psychiatric and non-psychiatric service costs, but did not include accommodation or informal care costs.

Patients who have a substance misuse disorder in addition to another mental health problem may well require a high level of service inputs. Jerrell & Hu (1996) measured the costs of three different programmes designed to care for dual-diagnosis patients and included a wide range of service inputs, including informal care. They also recorded the level of welfare benefits received.

Conclusions

Cost information is vital for a complete and worthwhile evaluation of a mental health care intervention. However, cost calculations have, with exceptions such as those discussed above, often been poorly performed and many areas of service provision which are affected have been neglected. Clearly, there is a need for stringent methods of costing.

Indeed, well thought out costing frameworks have been proposed (Weisbrod, 1981; Knapp & Beecham, 1990; Drummond *et al*, 1997). However, many of the recommendations mooted have not as yet been acted upon. Ignoring the importance of accurate costings can, at best, reduce the impact of wider evaluation and, at worst, provide wrong information to policy makers that would be to the detriment of all.

References

ALLEN, C. & BEECHAM, J. (1993) Costing services: ideals and reality. In *Costing Community Care: Theory and Practice* (eds A. Netten & J. Beecham), pp. 25–42. Aldershot: Ashgate.

AMADDEO, F., BEECHAM, J., BONIZZATO, P., *et al* (1998) The cost of community-based psychiatric care for first-ever patients. A case register study. *Psychological Medicine*, **28**, 173–183.

ANTONUCCIO, D. O., THOMAS, M. & DANTON, W. G. (1997) A cost-effectiveness analysis of cognitive behavior therapy and fluoxetine in the treatment of depression. *Behavior Therapy*, **28**, 187–210.

BEDELL, J. & WARD, J. (1989) An intensive community-based treatment alternative to state hospitalization. *Hospital and Community Psychiatry*, **40**, 533–535.

BEECHAM, J. (1995) Collecting and estimating costs. In *The Economic Evaluation of Mental Health Care* (ed. M. Knapp), pp. 61–82. Aldershot: Arena.

—— & KNAPP, M. (1992) Costing psychiatric interventions. In *Measuring Mental Health Needs* (eds G. Thornicroft, C. Brewin & J. Wing), pp. 163–183. London: Gaskell.

——, CAMBRIDGE, P., HALLAM, A., *et al* (1993) The costs of domus care. *International Journal of Geriatric Psychiatry*, **8**, 827–831.

——, KNAPP, M., McGILLOWAY, S., *et al* (1996) Leaving hospital II: The cost-effectiveness of community care for former long-stay psychiatric hospital patients. *Journal of Mental Health*, **5**, 379–394.

——, HALLAM, A., KNAPP, M., *et al* (1997) Costing care in hospital and in the community. In *Care in the Community: Illusion or Reality?* (ed. J. Leff), pp. 93–108. Chichester: Wiley.

BOND, G. R., MILLER, L. D., KRUMWIED, R. D., *et al* (1988) Assertive case management in three CMHCs: a controlled study. *Hospital and Community Psychiatry*, **39**, 411–418.

——, WITHERIDGE, T. F., WASMER, D., *et al* (1989) A comparison of two crisis housing alternatives to psychiatric hospitalization. *Hospital and Community Psychiatry*, **40**, 177–183.

BURNS, T. & RAFTERY, J. (1991) Cost of schizophrenia in a randomized trial of home-based treatment. *Schizophrenia Bulletin*, **17**, 407–410.

——, ——, BEADSMOORE, A., *et al* (1993) A controlled trial of home-based acute psychiatric services. II: Treatment patterns and costs. *British Journal of Psychiatry*, **163**, 55–61.

CARDIN, V., McGILL, C. & FALLOON, I. (1985) An economic analysis: costs, benefits, and effectiveness. In *Family Management of Schizophrenia: A Study of Clinical, Social, Family, and Economic Benefits* (ed. I. Falloon), pp. 115–123. Baltimore: Johns Hopkins University Press.

CASSELL, W. A., SMITH, C. M., GRUNBERG, F., *et al* (1972) Comparing costs of hospital and community care. *Hospital and Community Psychiatry*, **23**, 17–20.

CHALLIS, D., CHESTERMAN, J. & TRASKE, K. (1993) Case management: costing the experiments. In *Costing Community Care: Theory and Practice* (eds A. Netten & J. Beecham), pp. 143–161. Aldershot: Ashgate.

CHISHOLM, D., KNAPP, M., ASTIN, J., *et al* (1997) The mental health residential care study: the costs of provision. *Journal of Mental Health*, **6**, 85–99.

CLARK, R. E., DRAKE, R. E. & TEAGUE, G. B. (1993) The costs and benefits of case management. In *Case Management for Mentally Ill Patients* (eds M. Harris & H. C. Bergman), pp. 217–235. Langorne: Harwood.

CLARKSON, P., MCCRONE, P., SUTHERBY, K., *et al* (1999) Outcomes and costs of a community support worker service for the severely mentally ill. *Acta Psychiatrica Scandinavica*, **99**, 196–206.

CREED, F., MBAYA, P., LANCASHIRE, S., *et al* (1997) Cost effectiveness of day and inpatient psychiatric treatment: results of a randomised controlled trial. *British Medical Journal*, **314**, 1381–1385.

DICK, P., CAMERON, L., COHEN, D., *et al* (1985) Day and full time psychiatric treatment: a controlled comparison. *British Journal of Psychiatry*, **147**, 246–250.

DICKEY, B., CANNON, N. L., MCGUIRE, T. G., *et al* (1986a) The Quarterway House: a two-year cost study of an experimental residential program. Hospital and Community Psychiatry, 37, 1136–1143.

——, MCGUIRE, T. G., CANNON, N. L., *et al* (1986b) Mental health cost models: refinements and applications. *Medical Care*, **24**, 857–867.

—— & SCOTT, J. (1997) An international comparison of cost and outcomes of psychiatric care: research and policy implications. *Journal of Mental Health*, **6**, 251–263.

DOUBILET, P., WEINSTEIN, M. C. & MCNEIL, B. J. (1986) Use and misuse of the term 'cost effective' in medicine. *New England Journal of Medicine*, **314**, 253–256.

DRUMMOND, M. (1980) *Principles of Economic Appraisal in Health Care*. Oxford: Oxford University Press.

——, O'BRIEN, B., STODDART, G. L., *et al* (1997) *Methods for the Economic Evaluation of Health Care Programmes*. Oxford: Oxford University Press.

ENDICOTT, J., HERZ, M. I. & GIBBON, M. (1978) Brief verses standard hospitalization: the differential costs. *American Journal of Psychiatry*, **135**, 707–712.

ESSOCK, S. M., FRISMAN, L. K. & KONTOS, N. J. (1998) Cost-effectiveness of assertive community treatment teams. *American Journal of Orthopsychiatry*, **68**, 179–190.

FENTON, F. R., TESSIER, L., STRUENING, E. L., *et al* (1984) A two-year follow-up of a comparative trial of the cost-effectiveness of home and hospital psychiatric treatment. *Canadian Journal of Psychiatry*, **29**, 205–211.

FORD, R., RAFTERY, J., RYAN, P., *et al* (1997) Intensive case management for people with serious mental illness – site 2: Cost-effectiveness. *Journal of Mental Health*, **6**, 191–199.

FRANKLIN, J. L., SOLOVITZ, B., MASON, M., *et al* (1987) An evaluation of case management. *American Journal of Public Health*, **77**, 674–678.

GABBARD, G. O., LAZAR, S. G., HORNBERGER, J., *et al* (1997) The economic impact of psychotherapy: a review. *American Journal of Psychiatry*, **154**, 147–155.

GINSBERG, G., MARKS, I. & WATERS, H. (1984) Cost–benefit analysis of a controlled trial of nurse therapy for neuroses in primary care. *Psychological Medicine*, **14**, 683–690.

GLASS, N. J. & GOLDBERG, D. (1977) Cost–benefit analysis and the evaluation of psychiatric services. *Psychological Medicine*, **7**, 701–707.

GLICK, I. D., HARGREAVES, W. A. & GOLDFIELD, M. D. (1974) Short vs long hospitalization. *Archives of General Psychiatry*, **30**, 363–369.

GOLDBERG, D. & JONES, R. (1980) The costs and benefits of psychiatric care. In *The Social Consequences of Psychiatric Illness* (eds L. Robins, P. Clayton & J. Wing), pp. 55–70. New York: Brunner/Mazel.

——, JACKSON, G., GATER, R., *et al* (1996) The treatment of common mental disorders by a community team based in primary care: a cost-effectiveness study. *Psychological Medicine*, **26**, 487–492.

GOURNAY, K. & BROOKING, J. (1995) The community psychiatric nurse in primary care: an economic analysis. *Journal of Advanced Nursing*, **22**, 769–778.

GRIZENKO, N. & PAPINEAU, D. (1992) A comparison of the cost-effectiveness of day treatment and residential treatment for children with severe behaviour problems. *Canadian Journal of Psychiatry*, **37**, 393–400.

GUDEMAN, J. E., SHORE, M. F. & DICKEY, B. (1983) Day hospitalization and an inn instead of inpatient care for psychiatric patients. *New England Journal of Medicine*, **308**, 749–753.

HÄFNER, H. & AN DER HEIDEN, W. (1989) Effectiveness and cost of community care for schizophrenic patients. *Hospital and Community Psychiatry*, **40**, 59–63.

HARO, J. M., SALVADOR-CARULLA, L., CABASÉS, J., *et al* (1998) Utilisation of mental health services and costs of patients with schizophrenia in three areas of Spain. *British Journal of Psychiatry*, **173**, 334–340.

HEALEY, A., KNAPP, M., ASTIN, J., *et al* (1998) Cost-effectiveness evaluation of compliance therapy for people with psychosis. *British Journal of Psychiatry*, **172**, 420–424.

HOFF, R. A. & ROSENHECK, R. A. (1998) Long-term patterns of service use and cost among patients with both psychiatric and substance abuse disorders. *Medical Care*, **36**, 835–843.

HOULT, J., REYNOLDS, I., CHARBONNEAU-POWIS, M., *et al* (1983) Psychiatric hospital versus community treatment: the results of a randomised trial. *Australian and New Zealand Journal of Psychiatry*, **17**, 160–167.

HU, T-W. & JERRELL, J. (1991) Cost-effectiveness of alternative approaches in treating severely mentally ill in California. *Schizophrenia Bulletin*, **17**, 461–468.

—— & —— (1998) Estimating the cost impact of three case management programmes for treating people with severe mental illness. *British Journal of Psychiatry*, **173** (suppl. 36), 26–32.

HYDE, C., BRIDGES, K., GOLDBERG, D., *et al* (1987) The evaluation of a hostel ward: a controlled study using modified cost–benefit analysis. *British Journal of Psychiatry*, **151**, 805–812.

JERRELL, J. M. & HU, T-W. (1996) Estimating the cost impact of three dual diagnosis treatment programs. *Evaluation Review*, **20**, 160–180.

JONES, R., GOLDBERG, D. & HUGHES, B. (1980) A comparison of two different services treating schizophrenia: a cost–benefit approach. *Psychological Medicine*, **10**, 493–505.

KIVLAHAN, D. R., HEIMAN, J. R., WRIGHT, R. C., *et al* (1991) Treatment cost and rehospitalization rate in schizophrenic outpatients with a history of substance abuse. *Hospital and Community Psychiatry*, **42**, 609–614.

KNAPP, M. (1991) The direct costs of the community care of chronically mentally ill people. In *Evaluation of Comprehensive Care of the Mentally Ill* (eds H. Freeman & J. Henderson), pp. 142–173. London: Gaskell.

—— & BEECHAM, J. (1990) Costing mental health services. *Psychological Medicine*, **20**, 893–908.

—— & —— (1993) Reduced list costings: examination of an informed short cut in mental health research. *Health Economics*, **2**, 313–322.

——, ——, ANDERSON, J., *et al* (1990) The TAPS project. 3: Predicting the community costs of closing psychiatric hospitals. *British Journal of Psychiatry*, **157**, 661–670.

——, —— & GORDON, K. (1992) Predicting the community cost of closing psychiatric hospitals: national extrapolations. *Journal of Mental Health*, **1**, 315–325.

——, ——, KOUTSOGEORGOPOULOU, V., *et al* (1994) Service use and costs of home-based versus hospital-based care for people with serious mental illness. *British Journal of Psychiatry*, **165**, 195–203.

——, MARKS, I., WOLSTENHOLME, J., *et al* (1998) Home-based versus hospital-based care for serious mental illness. Controlled cost-effectiveness study over four years. *British Journal of Psychiatry*, **172**, 506–512.

——, ALMOND, S. & PERCUDANI, M. (1999) Costs of schizophrenia. In *Schizophrenia* (eds M. Maj & N. Sartorius), pp. 407–482. Chichester: Wiley.

KUIPERS, E., FOWLER, D., GARETY, P., *et al* (1998) London–East Anglia randomised controlled trial of cognitive–behavioural therapy for psychosis: III. Follow-up and economic evaluation at 18 months. *British Journal of Psychiatry*, **173**, 61–68.

LANG, F. H., FORBES, J. F., MURRAY, G. D., *et al* (1997) Service provision for people with schizophrenia: I. Clinical and economic perspective. *British Journal of Psychiatry*, **171**, 159–164.

LATIMER, E. A. (1999) Economic impacts of assertive community treatment: a review of the literature. *Canadian Journal of Psychiatry*, **44**, 443–454.

LAVE, J. R., FRANK, R. G., SCHULBERG, H. C., *et al* (1998) Cost-effectiveness of treatments for major depression in primary care practice. *Archives of General Psychiatry*, **55**, 645–651.

LEVENSON, A. J., LORD, C. J., SERMAS, C. E., *et al* (1977) Acute schizophrenia: an effacious outpatient treatment approach as an alternative to full-time hospitalization. *Diseases of the Nervous System*, **38**, 242–245.

LINN, M. W., CAFFEY, E. M., KLETT, C. J. *et al* (1979) Day treatment and psychotropic drugs in the aftercare of schizophrenic patients. *Archives of General Psychiatry*, **36**, 1055–1066.

——, GUREL, L., WILLIFORD, W. O., *et al* (1985) Nursing home care as an alternative to psychiatric hospitalization. *Archives of General Psychiatry*, **42**, 544–551.

MANGEN, S. P., PAYKEL, E. S., GRIFFITH, J. H., *et al* (1983) Cost-effectiveness of community psychiatric nurse or out-patient psychiatric care of neurotic patients. *Psychological Medicine*, **13**, 407–416.

MANNING, W. G. (1999) Panel on cost-effectiveness in health and medicine recommendations: identifying costs. *Journal of Clinical Psychiatry*, **60** (suppl. 3), 54–58.

MARINONI, A., GRASSI, M., EBBLI, D., *et al* (1988) Cost-effectiveness of managing chronic psychotic patients: Italian experience under the new psychiatric law. In *Costs and Effects of Managing Chronic Psychotic Patients* (eds D. Schwefel H. Zöllner & P. Potthoff), pp. 126–161. Berlin: Springer-Verlag.

MARKS, I., CONNOLLY, J., MUIJEN, M., *et al* (1994) Home-based versus hospital-based care for people with serious mental illness. *British Journal of Psychiatry*, **165**, 179–194.

MAY, P. R. A. (1971) Cost efficiency of treatments for the schizophrenic patient. *American Journal of Psychiatry*, **127**, 118–121.

McCRONE, P., BEECHAM, J. & KNAPP, M. (1994) Community psychiatric nurses in an intensive community support team: cost-effectiveness comparisons with generic CPN care. *British Journal of Psychiatry*, **165**, 218–221.

——, THORNICROFT, G., PHELAN, M., *et al* (1998) Utilisation and costs of community mental health services. PRiSM Psychosis Study 5. *British Journal of Psychiatry*, **173**, 391–398.

MERSON, S., TYRER, P., CARLEN, D., *et al* (1996) The cost of treatment of psychiatric emergencies: a comparison of hospital and community services. *Psychological Medicine*, **26**, 727–734.

MOSCARELLI, M., CAPRI, S. & NERI, L. (1991) Cost evaluation of chronic schizophrenic patients during the first 3 years after the first contact. *Schizophrenia Bulletin*, **17**, 421–426.

MOSHER, L. R., MENN, A. & MATTHEWS, S. M. (1975) Soteria: evaluation of a home-based treatment for schizophrenia. *American Journal of Orthopsychiatry*, **45**, 455–467.

MUELLER, J. & HOPP, M. (1983) A demonstration of the cost benefits of case management services for discharged mental patients. *Psychiatric Quarterly*, **55**, 17–24.

MULLER, C. F. & CATON, C. L. M. (1983) Economic costs of schizophrenia: a postdischarge study. *Medical Care*, **21**, 92–104.

MURPHY, J. G. & DATEL, W. E. (1976) A cost–benefit analysis of community verses institutional living. *Hospital and Community Psychiatry*, **27**, 165–170.

O'SHEA, E., HUGHES, J., FITZPATRICK, L., *et al* (1998) An economic evaluation of inpatient treatment verses day hospital care for psychiatric patients. *Irish Journal of Psychological Medicine*, **15**, 127–130.

QUINLIVAN, R., HOUGH, R., CROWELL, A., *et al* (1995) Service utilization and costs of care for severely mentally ill clients in an intensive management program. *Psychiatric Services*, **46**, 365–371.

RAPPAPORT, M., GOLDMAN, H., THORNTON, P., *et al* (1987) A method for comparing two systems of acute 24-hour psychiatric care. *Hospital and Community Psychiatry*, **38**, 1091–1095.

ROSENHECK, R., NEALE, M., LEAF, P., *et al* (1995) Multisite experimental cost study of intensive psychiatric community care. *Schizophrenia Bulletin*, **21**, 129–140.

ROSENHECK, R. A. & NEALE, M. S. (1998) Cost-effectiveness of intensive psychiatric community care for high users of inpatient services. *Archives of General Psychiatry*, **55**, 459–466.

ROTHBARD, A. B., CHINNAR, A. P., HADLET, T. P., *et al* (1998) Cost comparison of state hospital and community-based care for seriously mentally ill adults. *American Journal of Psychiatry*, **155**, 523–529.

RUBIN, J. (1982) Cost measurement and cost data in mental health settings. *Hospital and Community Psychiatry*, **33**, 750–754.

RUND, B. R., MOE, L., SOLLIEN, T., *et al* (1994) The Psychosis Project: outcome and cost-effectiveness of a psychoeducational treatment programme for schizophrenic adolescents. *Acta Psychiatrica Scandinavica*, **89**, 211–218.

SALIZE, H. J. & RÖSSLER, W. (1996) The cost of comprehensive care of people with schizophrenia living in the community. A cost evaluation from a German catchment area. *British Journal of Psychiatry*, **169**, 42–48.

SCHULZ, R. I., GREENLEY, J. R. & PETERSON, R. W. (1983) Management, cost, and quality of acute inpatient psychiatric services. *Medical Care*, **21**, 911–928.

SCHWEFEL, D., ZÖLLNER, H. & POTTHOFF, P. (1988) *Costs and Effects of Managing Chronic Psychotic Patients*. Darmstadt: Springer-Verlag.

SCOTT, A. I. F. & FREEMAN, C. P. L. (1992) Edinburgh primary care depression study: a treatment outcome, patient satisfaction, and cost after 16 weeks. *British Medical Journal*, **304**, 883–887.

SCOTT, J. (1995) A 12-month pilot evaluation of a British partial hospitalization program. *International Journal of Mental Health*, **24**, 60–69.

SHEEHAN, D. & ATKINSON, J. (1974) Comparative costs of state hospital and community-based inpatient care in Texas: who benefits most? *Hospital and Community Psychiatry*, **25**, 242–244.

SULEIMAN, T. G., OHAERI, J. U., LAWAL, R. A., *et al* (1997) Financial cost of treating out-patients with schizophrenia in Nigeria. *British Journal of Psychiatry*, **171**, 364–368.

TARRIER, N., LOWSON, K. & BARROWCLOUGH, C. (1991) Some aspects of family interventions in schizophrenia. II: Financial considerations. *British Journal of Psychiatry*, **159**, 481–484.

THORNICROFT, G. & BEBBINGTON, P. (1989) Deinstitutionalisation – from hospital closure to service development. *British Journal of Psychiatry*, **155**, 739–753.

TYRER, P., EVANS, K., GANDHI, N., *et al* (1998) Randomised controlled trial of two models of care for discharged psychiatric patients. *British Medical Journal*, **316**, 106–109.

WASHBURN, S., VANNICELLI, M., LONGABAUGH, R., *et al* (1976) A controlled comparison of psychiatric day treatment and inpatient hospitalization. *Journal of Consulting and Clinical Psychology*, **44**, 665–675.

WEISBROD, B. A. (1981) A guide to benefit–cost analysis, as seen through a controlled experiment in treating the mentally ill. *Journal of Health Politics, Policy and Law*, **7**, 808–845.

——, TEST, M. A. & STEIN, L. I. (1980) Alternative to mental hospital treatment: II. Economic benefit–cost analysis. *Archives of General Psychiatry*, **37**, 400–405.

WEISMAN, G. (1985) Crisis-orientated residential treatment as an alternative to hospitalization. *Hospital and Community Psychiatry*, **36**, 1302–1305.

WHERLEY, M. & BISGAARD, S. (1987) Beyond model programs: evaluation of a countywide system of residential treatment programmes. *Hospital and Community Psychiatry*, **38**, 852–857.

WIERSMA, D., KLUITER, H., NIENHUIS, F. J., *et al* (1991) Costs and benefits of day treatment with community care for schizophrenic patients. *Schizophrenia Bulletin*, **17**, 411–419.

WOLFF, N., HELMINIAK, T. W., MORSE, G. A., *et al* (1997) Cost-effectiveness evaluation of three approaches to case management for homeless mentally ill clients. *American Journal of Psychiatry*, **154**, 341–348.

XIONG, W., PHILLIPS, M. R., HU, X., *et al* (1994) Family-based intervention for schizophrenic patients in China: a randomised controlled trial. *British Journal of Psychiatry*, **165**, 239–247.

11 Uses and limits of randomised controlled trials in mental health service research

RUTH TAYLOR and
GRAHAM THORNICROFT

This chapter begins by outlining the theoretical requirements of an adequate evaluation of any intervention in medicine. The randomised controlled trial (RCT) fulfils these requirements and we summarise the power this experimental design holds in overcoming methodological difficulties, and its consequent value in assessing alternative clinical interventions. There are, however, important differences between the paradigms in medicine, where the RCT has been most extensively used and developed, and its use in evaluating psychiatric care. These differences arise from the nature of what is being evaluated, and they produce two types of problem in using the RCT design, which are conceptual and technical.

Conceptual problems arise from the social and political context of mental health services. While researchers in mental health service provision have had to tackle technical problems, they have often failed to recognise difficulties at the conceptual level. RCT designs have been attempted in other fields of public services research, but in such fields these conceptual difficulties have been recognised and extensively discussed, for example in the penal system. These conceptual problems can place specific limitations on the information that an RCT can give about alternative methods of psychiatric care.

Theoretical aspects of evaluation

Evaluation is essentially a process that aims to reach a conclusion about the value of an intervention, and in the field of mental health services it involves considering the effectiveness of a particular treatment or type of service. There are two basic components to the evaluation of any system: the identification of the goals of an intervention; and a method to decide how far that intervention achieves these goals. In evaluating community mental health services, both these components produce particular methodological problems. Essentially what the researcher wants to show is that there is a causal relationship between the intervention used and a specific outcome. Ideally, a closed system should be designed that comprises intervention, specified outcome, and a knowledge of all other factors that might be relevant to the outcome, that is all possible confounding factors.

To determine a causal connection, an evaluation must fulfil certain criteria in its design:

- The patient group must be characterised.
- The intervention must be standardised and clearly described.
- The outcome must be clearly identified in advance and measurable.
- Intervening variables must be known and controlled for.

The randomised controlled trial

A method of evaluation that best fulfils these requirements and that is widely used in medical research is the RCT. In critically examining RCT studies it is important to consider internal and external validity (Braun *et al*, 1981; Häfner & an der Heiden, 1989). Internal validity is defined as the extent to which the study design ensures that changes in one variable can be explained by changes in another variable, and external validity refers to the applicability of the results to conditions outside the study setting. An advantage of the RCT is that, if properly conducted, its internal validity is high.

The current prevailing view on RCTs within medicine as a whole is illustrated by the opening statement in a paper on RCTs in the *Lancet*, "Randomised clinical trials are the sine qua non for evaluating treatment in man" (Korn & Baumrind, 1991). Within psychiatry there is now a substantial literature that testifies to the fact that the RCT is regarded as the 'gold standard' for answering questions about treatment efficacy (Kraemer & Pruyn, 1990; Leber, 1991).

Pocock (1983) gives a detailed account of the use, design and analysis of RCTs. This design is extremely powerful and one of its major advantages is that it controls for the many confounding variables that may exist. It also eliminates the problematic effects of spontaneous remission, regression to the mean, and the placebo effect, all of which can produce improvement that may be incorrectly attributed to the treatment. A further important advantage provided by the RCT is that, if blindness is maintained, the results are independent of any bias from the clinicians involved in giving treatment or from the researchers conducting the study.

The RCT design has been extensively used for comparing two drug treatments. The RCT method in medicine as a whole, and in psychiatry in particular, has been based on evaluating the efficacy of new drugs. Leber (1991) states that, in the view of the Food and Drug Administration in the USA, there is simply no acceptable alternative to the RCT in assessing drug efficacy. However, the method has been taken up enthusiastically in evaluating other treatments, for example the psychotherapies (Andrews, 1989) and in evaluating alternatives to hospital treatment in psychiatry.

Technical difficulties with RCTs evaluating community mental health services

Achieving random allocation

A difficulty occurs when random allocation of patients is not possible. An example of this is a patient who is potentially suicidal or homicidal, where clinicians involved in the trial may feel it is unsafe to allocate such a patient to a community rather than a hospital treatment. This problem may be dealt with by stipulating exclusion criteria, but this ensures that only a particular and selected patient population is included in such RCTs and that the more challenging patients are never studied. The results of RCTs may not therefore be generalised to the true wider population of patients in need of psychiatric care.

Most of the early evaluations of community care in the international literature used an RCT design. Although important in providing the foundation of evidence for the value of community care, the careful review by Braun *et al* (1981) of these early studies of alternatives to hospital care illustrates well many of the technical difficulties of using RCTs in this setting. The majority of studies did claim to have randomly allocated patients, but this was achieved often by resorting to exclusion criteria that removed from the study patients who would present problems for random allocation. All except two of the studies excluded important patient groups, the major exclusions being homicidal or suicidal behaviour, patients with severe or chronic disorders, and those with no family or surrogate family support. In addition, many studies excluded patients with organic brain disorder or a diagnosis of primary drug or alcohol misuse.

Another review, by Kiesler (1982), revealed similar limitations, with only two of 10 RCTs of alternative care having no exclusion criteria, and many studies (e.g. Pasamanick *et al*, 1967) having very restrictive inclusion criteria or excluding a high proportion of patients before randomisation (78% of the total pool excluded in one study!). The population of patients included in such studies is therefore far from representative of the general population of patients with psychiatric disorder. The external validity of these RCTs can be said to be extremely low and their claims that community care approaches are superior may apply to only a rather select group of less challenging patients.

More recently, the three most important studies of alternatives to hospital care that have tried to overcome the methodological deficiencies of earlier work were those by Stein & Test (1980) in Madison in the USA, the evaluation by Hoult *et al* (1984) in Sydney, and the evaluation of the Daily Living Programme in London (Muijen *et al*, 1992). For example, the comparison by Stein & Test (1980) of an intensive community treatment – the Training in Community Living (TCL) model – with hospital care using an RCT study is widely quoted because it seems to have overcome many of the obstacles to RCTs in this field. It achieved complete random allocation, and the authors specifically comment that no patients were excluded on the basis of severity of illness. However, although the exclusion criteria were few, there is no mention of how patients requiring compulsory detention or homicidal or suicidal patients were managed, and there was a lack of data on the frequency of various diagnoses, which constrains the generalisability of the study.

A UK RCT (Burns *et al*, 1993) compared home-based with hospital-based acute psychiatric care for all patients referred. No patients were excluded on the grounds of diagnosis or severity of illness; however, there was a very high rate of exclusion after random allocation, with 48% failing to become study subjects. The authors comment that long-term, severely disabled patients were underrepresented in their eventual sample.

Studies of day-hospital versus in-patient care further illustrate potentially serious problems in conducting RCTs. Platt *et al* (1980) found such difficulties in using an RCT design to compare day-hospital and in-patient care that they abandoned their project. This occurred because doctors would allow only 10% of patients to be allocated, many patients being regarded as mandatory in-patients because they were too ill or suicidal. Creed *et al* (1990) reported a prospective RCT of day-patient versus in-patient psychiatric treatment for all acutely ill patients presenting for admission, and although they did not have major exclusion criteria they found that 42% of patients could not be allocated. An RCT study of day-hospital care compared with in-patient care (Dick *et al*, 1985) was again plagued by the difficulty of achieving random allocation, and even though they were considering only a rather select group of non-psychotic patients, out of 242 patients who were considered for allocation to the study, 101 were deemed too ill.

Intention-to-treat analysis

A further problem, related to the difficulty of achieving random allocation, is where patients who have been enrolled in a study subsequently withdraw from it (e.g. if they require formal admission because of the nature of their disturbance). Newell (1992) draws attention to this problem and its solution by using an 'intention-to-treat' analysis. This is a concept that is widely accepted but not always applied in practice, and it involves including in the analysis all patients who were allocated to a particular treatment option, even if they were subsequently withdrawn from, or dropped out of, the study. This is frequently relevant in comparing alternative care settings, for example where patients become a risk to themselves or others and require in-patient admission, and therefore withdrawal from a community treatment group.

Patient consent and motivation

Before participation in an RCT, patients need to be informed about the study, and give their consent to enter it. The most disabled patients give their consent less often and so by their own choice may be excluded from such studies. This is another problem that may bias evaluation studies in favour of the less severely ill patients and so limit our ability to generalise from them.

A related issue is that of patient motivation, which in the RCT studies discussed so far has never been taken into account. Brewin & Bradley (1989) draw attention to the importance of which treatment a patient prefers in what they call 'participative' interventions. They include among these deinstitutionalisation programmes for the chronically mentally ill, where clearly the patients' motivation will influence outcome. They argue that it is vital that patients are fully informed about both treatment options, but even if they then still agree to random allocation they may have a preference for one treatment over the other, and this will influence the enthusiasm with which they engage in the treatment. Brewin & Bradley consequently criticise research evaluations of participative treatments that are designed as though they were drug trials, and so take no account of the psychological processes involved.

Blindness

We have seen that blindness is a crucial component in the design of an RCT – blindness of the subjects, of the clinicians giving the treatment, and of the researcher making outcome ratings. As the intervention in mental health evaluation usually consists of a specific approach to service provision, it is generally impossible for patients, their relatives, clinicians or the researchers to remain blind as to which intervention the patient is receiving. This is particularly important because it means that such research is open to researcher and clinician bias. Since this field is subject to close political and public scrutiny, there is a problem that ideologically committed clinicians may pursue research to confirm their preconceived convictions about the value of alternatives to hospitalisation. A related difficulty is that since both experimenters and patients will always know which group they are in, the Hawthorne effect may operate, whereby patients and their relatives benefit from non-specific factors to do with being studied, and therefore the results may be biased towards the experimental intervention.

Nature of the experimental condition

In other areas of medicine or psychiatry the 'treatment' is a specifiable single intervention, be it simply a particular drug or a more complex but nevertheless known and quantifiable therapy. In contrast, the interventions in community mental health usually consist of a particular innovative service provision, such as care in a day hospital instead of hospital admission. There is a tendency in evaluating different services to overlook this complexity and treat the alternatives as if they were simple unified entities. This is flawed, because the multifaceted nature of the interventions means that there will be many different factors that could have contributed to a particular outcome.

Researchers in the field have responded to this problem by producing ever-more restrictive criteria defining a particular type of intervention (Deci *et al*, 1995; Teague *et al*, 1998). This is exemplified by the heated debate about the ingredients of assertive community treatment (ACT) (Marshall *et al*, 1999; Thornicroft *et al*, 1999). However, since there is no one single intervention, it is not possible to know which aspects of a package of care are effective. A more productive approach to this problem may be to try to ascertain which parts of a care package are effective and to target interventions more specifically.

Nature of the control condition

The review by Braun *et al* (1981) clearly illustrates these difficulties in describing how many studies failed adequately to describe the interventions used and what the control condition comprised. In the Daily Living Programme study (Muijen *et al*, 1992) precise details of the interventions used by staff are not given, although there is mention of family sessions and an emphasis on practical help. Nor are details given of the care provided in the control condition, other than that the patients received "standard hospital care". Indeed, there may often be far less homogeneity between control conditions than between experimental conditions of similar interventions, so reducing the comparability of studies for the purposes of meta-analysis.

Another problem with the control condition is that it may alter during the course of the study. This may be unavoidable because interventions take place in the real world, where political and economic change will produce a constant shift in the type of services delivered to patients.

Measuring outcomes

A major requirement in using an RCT design is that the outcomes be specified and measurable. Since 'mental health' is neither operationally defined nor an easily measurable domain, it is necessary to choose indicators of mental health to use as outcome measures. Further, in severe mental illness the goal of achieving mental health may not be valid and more realistic aims may be to lessen symptoms (impairment), to improve a patient's functioning (lessen disability), or to improve quality of life. Many of the early studies in this area used indicators of outcome that reflect this assumption, such as lengths of stay in hospital and readmission rates (Häfner & an der Heiden, 1991). As evaluative research has evolved, there has been a shift towards measures of symptoms and social function. More recently, more subjective, patient-centred outcome measures such as quality of life (Oliver, 1991) and satisfaction with services (Ruggeri & Dall'Agnola, 1993) have become prominent, and other chapters in this volume summarise many of the relevant outcome measures available.

Ethical aspects

In any setting, RCTs pose a range of ethical issues. Some researchers in the field suggest that random allocation of patients to what are presumed inferior or placebo treatments is becoming increasingly difficult to justify (e.g. Häfner & an der Heiden, 1991). In the evaluation of mental health services it could be argued that if, on humanitarian grounds, patients should be treated in the least restrictive settings, then it is unethical for the purposes of research to offer some patients care in an institution when it is already known that for the majority of patients it is possible to offer community-based care. This issue may lead staff in community mental health teams to fail to cooperate in some research projects. The counter-argument is that it is in fact unethical to proffer treatments to patients unless they have been subject to scrutiny using the most rigorous methods of scientific evaluation.

Internal and external validity

There is often a tendency for there to be a trade-off between internal and external validity, since in order to achieve the rigour demanded by the RCT design (i.e. to achieve high internal validity) the resulting study may apply to only a rather select group of patients under particular experimental circumstances, and so have low external validity. Newcombe (1988) discusses the practical difficulties psychiatric treatments present to the execution of an RCT, but feels that these are merely technical and can be overcome with sufficient ingenuity and dedication. But even if an ideal RCT could be conducted in the field of service evaluation, it would involve conducting an experiment within what is essentially a social situation, and this produces further conceptual issues, which are addressed below.

Conceptual issues in RCTs for mental health services

Other limitations of RCTs are not due to specific technical problems in achieving the rigour demanded by their design, but arise because of factors quite specific to the nature of evaluating systems of psychiatric care that are intrinsically social and political in nature. Minimal attention has been drawn to this fundamental difference between mental health service evaluation and the evaluation of a particular drug or surgical technique. Similar problems are most frequently encountered in sociological research, where they have long been recognised.

RCTs in institutional settings

In discussing an evaluation of a new treatment regimen, within an approved school for adolescents, using an RCT, Clarke & Cornish

(1972) outline the numerous difficulties encountered, which they regard as inevitable when attempting such a trial within an institutional setting, and most of these are also germane to the mental health services setting. They suggest that any penal treatment setting is not an isolated system but exists as part of a wider social system. Thus the isolated system in which inputs, outputs and intervening variables are all known or controlled for, on which the RCT depends, is often not achievable in such real-life settings. For example, they noted that the selection criteria for the inclusion of boys in the new treatment house led to a 'creaming off' of less challenging boys into the study, and this had an effect on both staff and boys' morale in the control house, and on the way this house was run. The success of the new treatment may be offset by negative effects in other directions, such as increasing staff tensions and turnover, which may make it impossible to complete the evaluation. Similar considerations may apply to mental health services: experimental programmes may select out a particular group of often less-difficult patients (as was illustrated in the previous section) and may attract more enthusiastic staff, producing disruptive effects on the morale and resources in the standard service.

An additional limitation Clarke & Cornish encountered was in enlisting the cooperation of practitioners whose fears of losing prestige, power and responsibility, or of being found to be ineffective or inefficient, may cause the experiment to be seen as a personal or professional threat. It can be imagined that in psychiatry similar concerns may exist in professionals used to working in institutional settings, who fear the consequences of examining their work too closely or the loss of power that a shift to the community provision of mental health services may bring.

The limitations of the RCT in evaluating innovative mental health services

The RCT has a central role in mental health research, where its high internal validity can lend scientific weight to assertions that a particular new alternative treatment strategy works. However, we must not ignore its limitations, which arise from the nature of the system within which it is being used. First, many of the experimental programmes evaluated by RCTs have been intensive and have demanded extremely high levels of dedication and commitment from the staff involved, but because of their experimental nature they have been time limited. Although staff were able to provide the high level of care demanded over a short, defined period, often benefiting from charismatic understanding, and with the goal of proving an experimental point to maintain morale, this may be more difficult in an ongoing routine service. This point may be countered only by evidence that community care works when it is provided as an ongoing part of a standard psychiatry service. The RCT methodology is not able to provide such evidence.

Second, the experimental approach makes the methodological assumption that a closed system can be created in which all factors influencing the outcome can be either eliminated in their effect by randomisation or controlled for in study design or analysis. This assumption often does not hold, as the reality is that patients exist in a wider society and factors in that society, such as housing policy or unemployment, can have a profound influence on mental health.

Third, as Goldberg (1991) has pointed out, RCTs alone do not create new health policy, but only allow us to compare existing alternative interventions. Leber (1991), in discussing RCTs to evaluate psychiatric drugs, makes the similar point that, if the goal is the generation of new ideas and hypotheses, RCTs can limit inventiveness, and the importance of controls is not as great as when we want to answer specific questions about existing alternative drugs.

Finally, but importantly, the experimental approach to evaluation is expensive. It requires the setting up of a specific intervention, the employment of an independent research team to evaluate it, and the intervention often has to be finished at the end of the study, as funds do not exist to continue. This can be demoralising for the staff and patients involved, particularly if the intervention was shown to be successful. The wait for results to filter through to planners and politicians can be frustrating for all concerned. An alternative strategy to the RCT is to use what Häfner & an der Heiden (1991) describe as 'naturalistic' designs, which offer a way of dealing with the complexity of factors involved in such systems.

Conclusions

This chapter has shown that, although the RCT is often seen within evidence-based medicine as the ultimate test of treatment efficacy, there are important technical and conceptual problems that limit its use in evaluating alternative mental health services. Despite this, it has resulted in good research, and has provided evidence that psychiatric care can be successfully provided outside hospital settings for substantial numbers of patients. The problems produced in trying to conduct these trials have also thrown some light on the types of patients for whom such alternative treatment settings are not possible. It is important to be aware in considering the results of such studies that even if they have achieved a reasonable degree of internal validity, their external validity may be limited. This is because they have been forced to include a rather select group of patients and the nature of the intervention may be atypical in its quality and the enthusiasm with which it is applied. Even if increasingly sophisticated study designs overcome some of the technical difficulties, the problems posed by evaluating something that is part of and interacts with a wider social system will remain.

While the RCT will undoubtedly continue to have an important part to play, particularly when we are concerned with establishing a strictly causal connection between a specific intervention and an outcome, it is suggested here that we should consider other study designs in order to examine better the complexity of processes involved in providing mental health care. An alternative strategy to the RCT is to use what Häfner & an der Heiden (1991) describe as more naturalistic studies, which offer a way of dealing with the complexity of factors involved in such systems. These new approaches will not provide such direct information about an intervention and its outcome, but may enable us to take a realistic look at the way in which community services work for different groups of patients and help us to gain some understanding of the complex but important blend of factors involved, and so enhance the generalisability of the results.

References

ANDREWS, G. (1989) Evaluating treatment effectiveness. *Australian and New Zealand Journal of Psychiatry*, **23**, 181–186.

BRAUN, P., KOCHANSKY, G., SHAPIRO, R., *et al* (1981) Overview. Deinstitutionalisation of psychiatric patients: a critical review of outcome studies. *American Journal of Psychiatry*, **138**, 736–749.

BREWIN, C. & BRADLEY, C. (1989) Patient preferences and randomised controlled trials. *British Medical Journal*, **299**, 313–315.

BURNS, T., BEADSMOORE, A., BHAT, A. V., *et al* (1993) A controlled trial of home-based acute psychiatric services. I: Clinical and social outcome. *British Journal of Psychiatry*, **163**, 49–54.

CLARKE, R. V. G. & CORNISH, D. B. (1972) *The Controlled Trial in Institutional Research – Paradigm or Pitfall for Penal Evaluators?* London: HMSO.

CREED, F., BLACK, D., ANTHONY, P., *et al* (1990) Randomised controlled trial of day patient versus inpatient psychiatric treatment. *British Medical Journal*, **300**, 1033–1037.

DECI, P. A., SANTOS, A. B., HIOTT, D. W., *et al* (1995) Dissemination of assertive community treatment programs. *Psychiatric Services*, **46**, 676–678.

DICK, P., CAMERON, L., COHEN, D., *et al* (1985) Day and full time psychiatric treatment: a controlled comparison. *British Journal of Psychiatry*, **147**, 246–250.

GOLDBERG, D. (1991) Cost effectiveness studies in the treatment of schizophrenia: a review. *Social Psychiatry and Psychiatric Epidemiology*, **26**, 139–142.

HÄFNER, H. & AN DER HEIDEN, W. (1989) The evaluation of mental health care systems. *British Journal of Psychiatry*, **155**, 12–17.

—— & —— (1991) Evaluating effectiveness and cost of community care for schizophrenic patients. *Schizophrenia Bulletin*, **17**, 441–451.

HOULT, J., ROSEN, A. & REYNOLDS, I. (1984) Community orientated treatment compared to psychiatric hospital orientated treatment. *Social Science and Medicine*, **18**, 1005–1010.

KIESLER, C. A. (1982) Mental hospitals and alternative care: non institutionalisation as a potential public policy for mental patients. *American Psychologist*, **37**, 349–360.

KORN, E. L. & BAUMRIND, S. (1991) Randomised clinical trials with clinician-preferred treatment. *Lancet*, **337**, 149–153.

KRAEMER, H. C. & PRUYN, J. P. (1990) The evaluation of different approaches to randomized clinical trials. *Archives of General Psychiatry*, **47**, 1163–1169.

LEBER, P. (1991) The future of controlled clinical trials. *Psychopharmacology Bulletin*, **27**, 3–8.

MARSHALL, M., BOND, G., STEIN L. I., *et al* (1999) PRiSM Psychosis Study. Design limitations, questionable conclusions (Editorial). *British Journal of Psychiatry*, **175**, 501–503.

MUIJEN, M., MARKS, I., CONNOLLY, J., *et al* (1992) Home based care and standard hospital care for patients with severe mental illness: a randomised controlled trial. *British Medical Journal*, **304**, 749–754.

NEWCOMBE, R. G. (1988) Evaluation of treatment effectiveness in psychiatric research. *British Journal of Psychiatry*, **152**, 696–697.

NEWELL, D. J. (1992) Intention-to-treat analysis: implications for quantitative and qualitative research. *International Journal of Epidemiology*, **21**, 837–841.

OLIVER, J. P. J. (1991) The Social Care Directive: development of a quality of life profile for use in community services for the mentally ill. *Social Work and Social Sciences Review*, **3**, 5–45.

PASAMANICK, B., SCARPITTI, F. R. & DINITZ, S. (1967) *Schizophrenics in the Community: An Experimental Study in the Prevention of Hospitalisation.* New York: Appleton-Century-Crofts.

PLATT, S. D., KNIGHTS, A. C. & HIRSCH, S. R. (1980) Caution and conservatism in the use of psychiatric day hospital: evidence from a research project that failed. *Psychiatry Research*, **3**, 123–132.

POCOCK, S. J. (1983) *Clinical Trials: A Practical Approach.* New York: Wiley.

RUGGERI, M. & DALL'AGNOLA, R. (1993) The development and use of the Verona Expectations for Care Scale (VECS) and the Verona Service Satisfaction Scale (VSSS) for measuring expectations and satisfaction with community-based psychiatric services in patients, relatives and professionals. *Psychological Medicine*, **23**, 511–524.

STEIN, L. I. & TEST, M. A. (1980) Alternative to mental hospital treatment: 1. Conceptual model, treatment program and clinical evaluation. *Archives of General Psychiatry*, **37**, 392–397.

TEAGUE, G. B., BOND, G. R. & DRAKE, R. E. (1998) Program fidelity in assertive community treatment: development and use of a measure. *American Journal of Orthopsychiatry*, **68**, 216–232.

THORNICROFT, G., BECKER, T., HOLLOWAY, F., *et al* (1999) Community mental health teams: evidence or belief? *British Journal of Psychiatry*, **175**, 508–513.

12 Psychiatric assessment instruments developed by the World Health Organization: an update

NORMAN SARTORIUS
and ALEKSANDAR JANCA

Over the past 30 years the World Health Organization (WHO) has produced a number of assessment instruments intended for national and cross-cultural psychiatric research. WHO instruments have been tested and used in many collaborative studies involving more than 100 centres in different parts of the world. This chapter represents an updated review of the main WHO instruments for the assessment of: psychopathology; disability, quality of life and satisfaction; services; and environment, and risks to mental health. The principles used in the development of WHO instruments, their translation and their use across cultures and settings are discussed.

The WHO occupies a unique position in the field of health care and represents a neutral platform that can be used to bring about international collaboration in research. Over the years, the WHO has gained experience in the management of international collaborative research projects and has produced reliable methods for their conduct in different cultures and settings (Sartorius, 1989). The development of cross-culturally applicable and reliable methods for the assessment of problems related to mental health has been one of the major activities in the WHO's Mental Health Programme. Many of these methods have been described in scientific publications, released for general use and applied in various research projects worldwide (Sartorius, 1993). This chapter outlines the basic characteristics of the main instruments produced and used in the studies coordinated by the WHO Mental Health Programme. The specific characteristics of the instruments described – such as their format, area of assessment, main users, training requirements and available translations – are summarised in Tables 12.1–12.4, and are discussed below. More details about these and other WHO instruments can be found in the catalogue of assessment instruments used in the studies coordinated by the WHO Mental Health Programme (Janca & Chandrashekar, 1993), available from the WHO on request.

Instruments for the assessment of psychopathology

Alcohol Use Disorders Identification Test

The Alcohol Use Disorders Identification Test (AUDIT; Babor *et al*, 1989) is a brief structured interview aimed at identifying people whose alcohol consumption has become harmful to their health. It consists of 10 questions: three on the amount and frequency of drinking, three on drinking behaviour and four on problems or adverse psychological reactions related to alcohol. The instrument can be interviewer- or self-administered, and the average administration time is 1–2 minutes. If the respondent is defensive or uncooperative, the clinical screening procedure (CSP) may be used to complement AUDIT. The CSP contains a listing of indirect questions and clinical signs likely to indicate the harmful consequences of alcohol use.

AUDIT has been tested in a WHO collaborative project on the early detection of people with harmful alcohol consumption. High reliability of the constituent scales, as well as high face validity and the ability to distinguish light drinkers from those with harmful drinking, has been reported (Saunders & Aasland, 1987; Saunders *et al*, 1993*a,b*).

Composite International Diagnostic Interview

The Composite International Diagnostic Interview (CIDI; WHO, 1993*a*) is a highly standardised diagnostic instrument for the assessment of mental disorders according to the definitions and criteria of ICD–10 (WHO, 1992) and DSM–III–R (American Psychiatric Association, 1987). A version of CIDI accommodating DSM–IV criteria (American Psychiatric Association, 1994) was released in 1995.

CIDI is primarily intended for use in epidemiological studies of mental disorders in general populations. The instrument consists of fully spelled-out questions and of a probing system aimed at assessing

TABLE 12.1
WHO instruments for the assessment of psychopathology

Instrument	Format	Area	User	Training	Languages
Alcohol Use Disorder Identification Test	Structured	Harmful alcohol use	Health or research worker	Not required	English, Japanese, Norwegian, Romanian, Spanish
Composite International Diagnostic Interview	Structured	ICD–10, DSM–III–R and DSM–IV mental disorders	Lay interviewer	Essential	Arabic, Chinese, Dutch, English, French, German, Greek, Icelandic, Italian, Japanese, Kannada, Russian, Serbian, Spanish
ICD–10 Symptom Checklist for Mental Disorders	Semistructured	ICD–10 mental disorders	Psychiatrist or psychologist	Not required	Chinese, English, Estonian, German, Italian, Japanese, Kannada, Portuguese, Russian, Spanish
International Personality Disorder Examination	Semistructured	ICD–10, DSM–III–R and DSM–IV personality disorders	Psychiatrist or psychologist	Essential	Dutch, English, Estonian, French, German, Greek, Hindi, Japanese, Kannada, Norwegian, Swahili, Tamil
Schedules for Clinical Assessment in Neuropsychiatry	Semistructured	Symptoms and signs of mental disorders	Psychiatrist or psychologist	Essential	Chinese, Danish, Dutch, English, French, German, Greek, Italian, Kannada, Portuguese, Spanish, Turkish, Yoruba

Table 12.1 (contd...)

Instrument	Format				
Standardized Assessment of Depressive Disorders	Semistructured	Depressive disorders	Psychiatrist or psychologist	Essential	Bulgarian, Farsi, French, German, Hindi, Japanese, Polish, Turkish
Schedules for Clinical Assessment of Acute Psychotic States	Semistructured	Acute psychotic states	Psychiatrist or psychologist	Essential	Czech, Danish, English, Hindi, Yoruba
Social Description	Semistructured	Social history	Social worker or psychologist	Essential	Chinese, Czech, Danish, English, Hindi, Russian, Spanish, Yoruba
Self-Reporting Questionnaire	Questionnaire	Neurotic and psychotic symptoms	Self-administered	Not applicable	Amharic, Arabic, Bahasa (Malaysia), Bengali, Eglish, French, Hindi, Italian, Kiswahili, Njanja Lusaka, Portuguese, Spanish, Tagalog

Table 12.2
WHO instruments for the assessment of disability, burden and quality of life

Instrument	Format	Area	User	Training	Languages
WHO Psychiatric Disability Assessment Schedule	Semistructured	Disability due to mental and other disorders	Psychiatrist, psychologist, or social worker	Essential	Arabic, Bulgarian, Chinese, Croatian, Danish, English, French, German, Hindi, Japanese, Russian, Serbian, Spanish, Turkish, Urdu
WHO Short Disability Assessment Scale	Rating scale	Disability due to mental and/or physical disorders	Psychiatrist or psychologist	Not required	Arabic, Chinese, Czech, Danish, Dutch, English, German, Hindi, Italian, Japanese, Kannada, Portuguese, Romanian, Russian, Spanish
WHO Psychological Impairments Rating Schedule	Semistructured	Psychological and behavioural deficits	Psychiatrist or psychologist	Essential	Arabic, Bulgarian, Croatian, English, French, German, Serbian, Turkish
Broad Rating Schedule	Semistructured	Psychotic symptoms and related disability	Psychiatrist or psychologist	Not required	Bulgarian, Chinese, Czech, Danish, English, German, Hindi, Japanese, Russian, Yoruba
Family Interview Schedule	Structured	Family perception of patient	Psychiatrist, psychologist, social worker or nurse	Essential	Bulgarian, Chinese, Czech, Danish, English, German, Hindi, Japanese, Russian, Yoruba

TABLE 12.2 (contd...)

Instrument	Format	Area	User	Training	Languages
Social Unit Rating	Semistructured	Burden of mental illness on the family	Lay interviewer	Essential	Arabic, English, French, Hindi, Portuguese, Spanish
Burden Assessment Schedule	Questionnaire	Burden on care-givers	Self-administered	Not applicable	English, Hindi
WHO Quality of Life Assessment Instrument	Questionnaire	Quality of life	Self-administered	Not applicable	Croatian, Dutch, English, French, Russian, Shona, Spanish, Tamil
Subjective Well-Being Inventory	Questionnaire	Feelings of well-being	Self-administered	Not applicable	English, Hindi

TABLE 12.3
WHO instruments for the assessment of services

Instrument	Format	Area	User	Training	Languages
Pathways Interview Schedule	Semistructured	Sources of care	Health or research worker	Not required	Arabic, Bahasa (Indonesia), Chinese, Czech, English, French, Japanese, Kannada, Korean, Portuguese, Spanish, Turkish, Urdu
Checklists for Quality Assurance in Mental Health Care					
Mental Health Policy Checklist	Semistructured	Mental health care (policy)	Health or administrative worker	Not required	Chinese, English, French, Italian, Portuguese, Spanish
Mental Health Programme Checklist	Semistructured	Mental health care (programme)	Health or administrative worker	Not required	Chinese, English, French, Italian, Portuguese, Spanish
Primary Health Care Facility Checklist	Semistructured	Mental health care (primary-care facility)	Health or administrative worker	Not required	Chinese, English, French, Italian, Portuguese, Spanish
Outpatient Mental Health Facility Checklist	Semistructured	Mental health care (out-patient facility)	Health or administrative worker	Not required	Chinese, English, French, Italian, Portuguese, Spanish
Inpatient Mental Health Facility Checklist	Semistructured	Mental health care (in-patient facility)	Health or administrative worker	Not required	Chinese, English, French, Italian, Portuguese, Spanish

TABLE 12.3 (contd...)

Instrument	Format	Area	User	Training	Languages
Residential Facility for the Elderly Mentally Ill Checklist	Semistructured	Mental health care (residential facility for the elderly mentally ill)	Health or administrative worker	Not required	Chinese, Czech, Danish, English, Hindi, Russian, Spanish, Yoruba
WHO Child Care Facility Schedule	Semistructured	Quality of child care facility	Health or administrative worker	Not required	English, French, Greek, Portuguese

TABLE 12.4
WHO instruments for the assessment of environment, risks and qualitative research

Instrument	Format	Area	User	Training	Languages
Axis III Checklist	Semistructured	Contextual factors	Psychiatrist or psychologist	Not required	Arabic, Chinese, Czech, Danish, Dutch, English, German, Hindi, Italian, Japanese, Kannada, Portuguese, Romanian, Russian, Spanish
Interview Schedule for Children	Semistructured	Child's psycho-social environment	Psychiatrist, psychologist, social worker or nurse	Not required	English, German, Portuguese, Slovenian, Spanish
Parent Interview Schedule	Semistructured	Child's psycho-social environment	Psychiatrist, psychologist, social worker or nurse	Not required	English, German, Portuguese, Slovenian, Spanish
Home Risk Card	Semistructured	Child's home risk factors	Health or research worker	Not required	English, Hindi
Qualitative research instruments					
Exploratory Translation and Back-Translation Guidelines	Guide	Linguistic equivalence	Health or research worker	Not required	English, Greek, Kannada, Korean, Romanian, Spanish, Turkish, Yoruba

TABLE 12.4 (contd...)

Instrument	Format	Area	User	Training	Languages
Key Informant Interview Schedule	Semistructured	Cultural aspects of mental health	Anthropologist or ethnographer	Essential	English, Greek, Kannada, Korean, Romanian, Spanish, Turkish, Yoruba
Focus Group Interview Guide	Guide	Cultural aspects of mental health	Anthropologist or ethnographer	Essential	English, Greek, Kannada, Korean, Romanian, Spanish, Turkish, Yoruba

the clinical significance and psychiatric relevance of reported phenomena. No clinical judgement is required in coding and recording respondents' answers, and the schedule can be competently administered by a lay or clinician interviewer after a week's training. The average administration time is 90 min.

CIDI is accompanied by a set of supporting materials, including manuals and computer programs for data entry and scoring of ICD–10 and DSM–III–R diagnoses.

A number of versions and modules of CIDI have been produced for specific research purposes (Janca *et al*, 1994*a*), including a computerised version of CIDI (CIDI-Auto; WHO, 1993*c*) and the Substance Abuse Module (Robins *et al*, 1990). CIDI has been extensively tested in two field trials involving 20 centres, 12 languages and about 1200 respondents. The field trials results show that the instrument is generally acceptable, appropriate and a reliable diagnostic tool for use across cultures and settings (Robins *et al*, 1988; Cottler *et al*, 1991; Wittchen *et al*, 1991; Janca *et al*, 1992).

ICD–10 Symptom Checklist for Mental Disorders

The ICD–10 Symptom Checklist for Mental Disorders (Janca *et al*, 1994*b*) is a semistructured instrument intended for clinicians' assessment of psychiatric symptoms and syndromes in the F0–F6 categories of ICD–10. The instrument requires the clinician user to examine the patient or case notes in order to be able to rate the presence or absence of symptoms that are necessary to make a firm diagnosis in the ICD–10 system. The Checklist also lists symptoms and states that, according to ICD–10 criteria, have often been found to be associated with the syndrome (e.g. alcohol misuse in patients with mania) or should be assessed independently from the syndrome (e. g. mental retardation in patients with organic mental disorder). The symptom lists are accompanied by instructions intended to help the user consider differential diagnoses. The recording of the onset, severity and duration of the syndrome, as well as the number of episodes (where applicable), is also provided for. The Checklist is accompanied by the ICD–10 Symptom Glossary for Mental Disorders (Isaac *et al*, 1994). The Glossary provides brief definitions of the symptoms and terms used in the Checklist.

The ICD–10 Symptom Checklist for Mental Disorders was used at one of the sites participating in the ICD–10 field trials, and preliminary results show good psychometric properties for the instrument. The average administration time is 15 minutes, and the interviewer/observer reliability is acceptable ($\kappa = 0.72$; Janca *et al*, 1993).

International Personality Disorder Examination

The International Personality Disorder Examination (IPDE; WHO, 1993*b*) is a semistructured interview schedule designed for the assessment of personality disorders according to ICD–10 and DSM–III–R/DSM–IV criteria. It is designed for use by clinicians who have received the appropriate training.

The IPDE covers the following six areas of the respondent's personality and behaviour: work, self, interpersonal relationships, affects, reality testing and impulse control. The last six items in the schedule are scored without questioning and are based on the interviewer's observation of the respondent during the interview. The IPDE requires that a behaviour or a trait be present for at least five years before it should be considered a manifestation of personality or a symptom of personality disorder and that at least one criterion of personality disorder be fulfilled before the age of 15 years. Information about the respondent obtained by reliable informants can also be recorded and is used in the final scoring of the diagnosis. The final scoring, which may be done clerically or by computer, is used in making ICD–10 and DSM–III–R diagnoses; a dimensional score can also be calculated.

Because of the length of the interview (it takes two to three hours to administer) the IPDE has recently been produced in two versions, one for ICD–10 and the other for DSM–IV diagnoses. Both versions of the instrument are accompanied by a user manual, screener, hand-scoring sheets and computer-scoring programs.

The IPDE has been tested in a WHO-coordinated field trial in which 14 centres from 11 countries participated. The results indicate good acceptability, high interrater reliability and satisfactory temporal stability for the criteria and diagnoses assessed by the interview (Loranger *et al*, 1991, 1994).

Schedules for Clinical Assessment in Neuropsychiatry

The Schedules for Clinical Assessment in Neuropsychiatry (SCAN; WHO, 1994 – see also Chapter 9) are a semistructured clinical interview schedule designed for clinicians' assessment of the symptoms and course of adult mental disorders. SCAN comprises an interview schedule, namely the tenth edition of the Present State Examination (PSE; see Wing *et al*, 1974, for a full account of the ninth edition), a glossary of differential definitions, Item Group Checklist (IGC) and Clinical History Schedule (CHS). SCAN consists of two parts. Part 1 covers non-psychotic symptoms such as physical health, worrying, tension, panic, anxiety and phobias, obsessional symptoms, depressed mood and ideation, impaired thinking, concentration, energy, interests, bodily functions, weight, sleep, eating disorders, and alcohol and drug misuse. Part 2 covers psychotic and cognitive disorders, as well as abnormalities of behaviour, speech and affect. When using SCAN, the clinician interviewer (e.g. psychiatrist or clinical psychologist) decides whether a symptom has been present during the specified time and to what degree of severity. One or two periods are selected to cover the main phenomena necessary for diagnosis. The periods usually include the 'present state' (i.e. the month before examination) and the 'lifetime before' (i.e. any time previously). Another option is to rate the 'representative episode', which may be chosen because it is particularly characteristic of the patient's illness. The average administration time of SCAN is 90 minutes. The glossary is an essential part of SCAN and provides differential definitions of SCAN items and a commentary on the SCAN text. A reference manual for SCAN facilitates the use of the instrument (Wing *et al*, 1998).

A set of computer programs (CATEGO) is used for processing SCAN data and for the scoring and diagnoses according to ICD–10 and DSM–IV criteria. A computerised version of SCAN (CAPSE) is also available. It assists the interviewer in applying SCAN and allows direct entry of ratings at the time of the interview. Questions and ratings are displayed on the screen; if needed, SCAN glossary definitions can also be referred to.

SCAN has been tested in WHO-organised field trials involving 20 centres in 14 countries. The results indicate good feasibility and reliability of the instrument, comparable to those obtained in testing the PSE–9 (Wing *et al*, 1990).

Standardized Assessment of Depressive Disorders

The Standardized Assessment of Depressive Disorders (SADD) is a structured clinical interview schedule aimed at assessing the symptoms and signs of depressive disorders. Part 1 covers the basic socio-demographic data about the patient. Part 2 contains a checklist of 39 symptoms and signs characteristic of depression, accompanied by a glossary that provides definitions of symptoms and signs to be assessed, as well as a listing of possible probes and examples of answers for each symptom. The checklist also includes a number of open-ended questions for recording rare or culture-specific symptoms of depression, as well as items related to the history of the patient (e.g. number of previous episodes, precipitating factors, presence of mental disorders in relatives). Part 3 of the instrument serves to record the diagnosis and severity of the patient's condition. The ratings in SADD refer to the week preceding the interview and to any other time before the current episode. The administration of the instrument takes a short time if the clinician has examined the patient previously.

If the case is 'fresh', the time taken to obtain the necessary information and rate it is longer (i.e. 45–60 minutes).

SADD has been tested in the WHO Collaborative Study on the Standardized Assessment of Depressive Disorders and has been found to be easy to use and acceptable to both psychiatrists and patients. The reliability of the socio-demographic, symptom checklist and history sections of the instrument has been found to be high (Sartorius *et al*, 1980, 1983).

Schedule for Clinical Assessment of Acute Psychotic States

The Schedule for Clinical Assessment of Acute Psychotic States (SCAAPS) is a semistructured interview schedule for clinicians' recording of information about patients with acute psychotic states. Such information is collected from different sources, such as the clinical interview of the patient, key informants and medical records. The instrument also offers the possibility of recording the follow-up diagnostic evaluation of the patient.

SCAAPS consists of six parts. Part A contains the screening criteria for acute psychotic states (e.g. onset of symptoms within three months of the initial assessment); Part B comprises items related to the psychiatric history and social description of the patient; Part C contains a 19-item symptom check-list covering symptoms from worrying and anxiety to symptoms reflecting stressful life events; Part D serves to record the initial diagnostic evaluation and the results of the one-year follow-up assessment; Part E covers the treatment, course and outcome of the disorder; Part F is intended for narrative summaries of the initial examination, and three-month and one-year follow-up. The average duration of the SCAAPS interview is 120 minutes.

The instrument has been used in the WHO Collaborative Studies on Acute Psychoses and has been found to be a cross-culturally appropriate tool for collecting data about acute psychotic states in different parts of the world (Cooper *et al*, 1990).

Social Description

The Social Description (SD) is a schedule with open-ended questions aimed at collecting information in a systematic manner about the social history of the psychiatric patient. The schedule is intended for research purposes, and can be used by social workers or clinicians. It covers the following areas: residence and household; education; work activities; children; marital status; education and occupation of the spouse; education and occupation of the parents; education and occupation of the head of the current household; religion; patient's childhood setting; daily and leisure activities; birth order of the patient and siblings; a thumbnail sketch by the interviewer, who has to rate on a five-point scale the current socio-economic status of the patient, the patient's family background and the patient's current social isolation within the framework of his/her culture. The average administration time of the instrument is 120 minutes.

The SD has been used in the WHO International Pilot Study of Schizophrenia and has been found to be a useful means for collecting the social history of patients in different cultures and settings (WHO, 1973). It has been used in a modified form in several other WHO studies, such as the Collaborative Determinants of Outcome of Severe Mental Disorders (Jablensky *et al*, 1992).

Self-Reporting Questionnaire

The Self-Reporting Questionnaire (SRQ) is an instrument designed for screening for the presence of psychiatric illness in patients in primary care. It can be self-administered or interviewer-administered with illiterate or semi-literate patients, and its administration time is 5–10 minutes. It consists of 24 questions, 20 of which are related to neurotic symptoms and four to psychotic symptoms. Each of the 24 questions is scored 1 or 0: a score of 1 indicates that the symptom was present during the past month; a score of 0 indicates that it was absent. Depending on the criteria, culture and language, different cut-off scores are selected in different studies, but most often 7 indicates the probable existence of a psychological problem. The SRQ is accompanied by a recently produced user's guide (Beusenberg & Orley, 1994), which describes the instrument, its use and scoring, and also summarises the results of reliability and validity studies.

The SRQ has been tested in over 20 studies (including the WHO Collaborative Study on Strategies for Extending Mental Health Care and the WHO Study on Mental Disorders in Primary Health Care) and has been found to be an appropriate, reliable and valid case-finding tool for use in primary care, particularly in developing countries (Harding *et al*, 1980, 1983; WHO, 1984).

Instruments for the assessment of disability, burden and quality of life

WHO Psychiatric Disability Assessment Schedule

The WHO Psychiatric Disability Assessment Schedule (WHO/DAS) is a semistructured instrument designed for the evaluation of the social functioning of patients with mental disorders. Such an evaluation can be done by a psychiatrist, psychologist or social worker. The information about the functioning of the patient is collected from the patient, key informant(s) or written records. The instrument has been developed in accordance with the principles underlying the WHO International Classification of Impairments, Disabilities and Handicaps (WHO, 1980; see also Chapter 8).

The WHO/DAS consists of 97 items grouped in five parts. Part 1 comprises items related to the patient's overall behaviour, and includes ratings of self-care, underactivity, slowness and social withdrawal. Part 2 serves to assess the patient's social role performance, and covers participation in household activities, marital role, parental role, sexual role, social contacts, occupational role, interests and information, and behaviour in emergencies or out-of-the-ordinary situations. Part 3 is intended for the assessment of the patient's social functioning in the hospital, including ward behaviour, nurses' opinions, occupations and contact with the outside world. Part 4 covers modifying factors related to the patient's dysfunction (specific assets, specific liabilities, home atmosphere and outside support). Part 5 comprises a global evaluation of the patient and is followed by a summary of the ratings and scoring, respectively. Items in Parts 1 and 2 of DAS are rated on a six-point scale: no dysfunction, minimal dysfunction, obvious dysfunction, serious dysfunction, very serious dysfunction, and maximum dysfunction. The patient's current functioning (past month) is to be rated against the presumed 'average' or 'normal' functioning of a person of the same sex, comparable age and similar socio-economic background. The average administration time of the WHO/DAS is 30 minutes. A guide to its use and an explanation of certain key terms (e.g. psychological burden, social skills, impairment) accompany the instrument.

The WHO/DAS has been tested and used in the WHO Collaborative Study on the Assessment and Reduction of Psychiatric Disability and has been found to be a reliable and valid tool for the assessment and cross-cultural comparison of psychiatric disability (Jablensky *et al*, 1980). A revised version of the instrument (WHO/DAS–II) is being produced as a companion to the ongoing revision of the International Classification of Impairments, Activities and Participation (WHO, 1997*a*).

WHO Short Disability Assessment Schedule (WHO/DAS-S)

The WHO/DAS-S has been developed as a component of the multiaxial presentation of the ICD–10 Classification of Mental and Behavioural Disorders (WHO, 1997*b*). It is a simple scale intended for the recording of the clinicians' assessment of disablement caused by mental and physical disorders. The ratings refer to specific areas of functioning, such as personal care (e.g. personal hygiene, dressing, feeding), occupation (e.g. function in paid activities, studying, home-making), family and household (e.g. interaction with spouse, parents, children and other relatives), and the broader social context (e.g. performance in relation to community members, participation in leisure and other social activities). The scale provides anchor-point definitions for six ratings ranging from 0 (no dysfunction) to 5 (maximum dysfunction). It takes five minutes to administer if the clinician knows and has examined the patient.

The WHO/DAS-S has been tested in WHO-coordinated field trials of the ICD–10 multi-axial classification, which involved about 70 centres from more than 25 countries. The field trial results indicate good acceptance of the instrument by clinicians belonging to different psychiatric schools and traditions (Janca *et al*, 1996*a*).

WHO Psychological Impairments Rating Schedule

The WHO Psychological Impairments Rating Schedule (WHO/PIRS) is a semistructured instrument intended for clinicians' assessment of selected areas of psychological and behavioural deficits in patients with functional psychotic disorder. The main areas covered by the instrument concern negative symptoms, social skills and communication, and an overall impression of the patient and his/her personality. WHO/PIRS should be administered after a PSE interview, preferably by the same clinician. The average administration time is 25 minutes.

The instrument consists of 97 items grouped in 10 sections. Part A includes items and scales for rating observed behaviour. Part B includes a pattern assembly, three Rorschach cards and a letter-deletion test aimed at eliciting the patient's performance when presented with standard tasks.

The WHO/PIRS has been used in the WHO Collaborative Study on Impairments and Disabilities Associated with Schizophrenic Disorders and has been found to be a reliable assessment tool (test–retest reliability, $\kappa = 0.79$; Jablensky *et al*, 1980).

Broad Rating Schedule

The Broad Rating Schedule (BRS) has been developed for use in a long-term follow-up study of patients given the diagnosis of schizophrenia, and serves to summarise the follow-up findings. The BRS uses information from all available sources, including the patient, informant and medical or other records. The severity of psychotic symptoms and disabilities is rated for the previous month on a scale ranging from absent to severe. Symptoms, as well as disabilities, are also rated on a modified version of the DSM–III–R Global Assessment of Functioning (GAF) Scale, which ranges from 1 (persistent danger of severely hurting oneself or others, or persistent inability to function in almost all areas) to 90 (absent or minimal symptoms, or good functioning in all areas, interested and involved in a wide range of activities, etc.). The instrument also contains sections on subjects lost to follow-up and deceased subjects. The ratings of these sections are based on the best judgement of the clinician using all available information. The BRS should be rated after completion of the interview with the patient and informant and a review of the records. Clinicians do not need specific training in the use of the schedule.

Family Interview Schedule

The Family Interview Schedule (FIS) is a structured instrument for the assessment of family members' perception of the patient's psychiatric problems and their consequences for the patient and family. It is also an instrument developed for use in the WHO Long-Term Follow-Up Study of Schizophrenia. The source of information for the FIS should be a permanent member of the patient's family.

The FIS is divided into the following sections: I, symptoms and social behaviour; II, impact; III, stigma; IV, service providers; V, attribution. The section on symptoms and social behaviour covers the day-to-day behaviour and responsibilities of the patient in the past month (e.g. helping with household chores). The section on impact ascertains the involvement of family members in helping the patient as well as their difficulties in managing and coping with problems caused by the patient's psychiatric problems. The section on stigma consists of a list of experiences the family member has had because of the patient's psychiatric problems (e.g. that neighbours treated him or her differently). The section concerning service providers is aimed at assessing the help provided to the patient and the family by doctors, nurses and other relevant care-givers. The section on attribution is intended to record the family member's views (based on the information obtained from care-givers) on causes of the patient's psychiatric problems.

The FIS is accompanied by a visual analogue measure, ranging from 'almost never or not at all' to 'almost always or a lot'. Administration takes 30–45 minutes. The user (psychiatrist, psychologist, social worker or nurse) should be trained in the administration of the instrument.

Social Unit Rating

The Social Unit Rating (SUR) is a semistructured interview aimed at recording the effect of an illness on the patient's immediate living group. The instrument consists of 20 items, covering basic socio-demographic information about the patient (e.g. occupation, education, employment), time residing in a given area, time residing in the present household, composition of the social unit, main sources of income, total weekly income and sources of help for the social unit. The rest of the items in the instrument relate to the pre-illness status of the social unit and to the effect of the patient's illness on the social unit.

Any lay interviewer can administer the SUR after appropriate training. The administration time of the instrument is 30–45 min. The SUR has been used in the WHO Collaborative Study on Strategies for Extending Mental Health Care and has been found to be a useful means for the assessment of the effects of mental illness on the family or household of the patient (Giel *et al*, 1983).

Burden Assessment Schedule

This 20-item questionnaire is aimed at assessing and quantifying the subjective role burden as perceived by the care-givers and in particular the spouses of chronic psychotic patients. The following areas of concern (which reflect care-givers' main feelings about their care-giving role) are covered by the instument: impact on well-being, on marital relationships and on relations with others, appreciation for caring and perceived severity of the disease. Each question related to these areas of concern is rated on a scale ranging from 'not at all' to 'very much', and an example of such a question is: "Does caring for the patient make you feel tired and exhausted?" The Burden Assessment Schedule was developed and tested in India using an ethnographic exploration method that demonstrated good acceptability and reliability of the instrument (Sell *et al*, 1998).

WHO Quality of Life Assessment Instrument

The WHO Quality of Life Assessment Instrument (WHOQOL) allows an enquiry into the perception of individuals of their own position in life in the context of the culture and value systems in which they live and in relation to their goals, expectations, standards and concerns. The instrument covers the following six broad domains of quality of life: physical well-being, psychological well-being, level of independence, social relationships, environment and spiritual domain. Within each domain a series of facets of the quality of life summarises that particular domain. For example, the psychological domain includes the facets: positive feelings; thinking, learning, memory and concentration; self-esteem; body image and appearance; and negative feelings. Response scales in the instrument are concerned with the intensity, frequency and subjective evaluation of states, behaviour and capacities. The WHOQOL provides a quality-of-life profile that consists of an overall quality-of-life score, scores for each of the broad domains of the quality of life, scores for individual facets of the quality of life and, within facets, separate scores for the recording of the subject's perception of his or her condition and quality of life.

The WHOQOL is being developed in the framework of a WHO collaborative project on quality-of-life measures involving numerous centres in different cultural settings. One of the main goals of the project is to assess the psychometric properties of the instrument such as its reliability, validity and cross-cultural sensitivity (WHOQOL Group, 1994).

Subjective Well-Being Inventory

The Subjective Well-Being Inventory (SUBI) is a questionnaire for the assessment of subjective well-being. It can be self- or interviewer-administered and is designed for research purposes. It consists of 40 items designed to measure feelings of well-being (or lack of it) as experienced by an individual in relation to concerns such as health or family. The items in SUBI represent the following factors in the structure of subjective well-being: general well-being – positive effect; expectation–achievement congruence; confidence in coping; transcendence; family group support; social support; primary group concern; inadequate mental mastery; perceived ill-health; deficiency in social contacts; general well-being – negative effect. SUBI is accompanied by the 'stepwise ethnographic exploration' procedure, which can be used to assess whether SUBI is appropriate for use in the cultural setting in which the study will take place.

The instrument has been used in research projects carried out by the WHO Regional Office for South-East Asia and has been found to be culturally applicable for the quantitative measurement of subjective well-being (Sell & Nagpal, 1992).

Instruments for the assessment of services

Pathways Interview Schedule

The Pathways Interview Schedule is a semistructured instrument designed for the systematic gathering of information on the routes and sources of care used by patients before they see a mental health professional. The instrument can be administered by a psychiatrist, psychologist, social worker or nurse, and its average administration time is 10 minutes. An instruction manual describing how to use the instrument is available.

The Pathways Interview Schedule consists of seven sections. Section A covers basic information about the centre and the mental health professional. In Section B the basic information about the patient is recorded (e.g. age, sex, marital status, social position, history of care by any mental health service). Section C covers the details of the first carer (e.g. who he/she was, who suggested that care, the main problem presented, when it began, the main treatment offered, duration of the patient's journey to the first carer). Sections D, E and F cover similar details of the second, third and fourth carers. Section G is intended for the diagnosis of the patient according to the assessment by the mental health professional.

The instrument has been used in the WHO Study on Pathways to Psychiatric Care and has been found to be a simple and inexpensive method of studying a psychiatric service and routes followed by patients seeking care for psychiatric disorders (Gater *et al*, 1990, 1991).

Checklists for Quality Assurance in Mental Health Care

The Checklists for Quality Assurance in Mental Health Care are a set of checklists accompanied by glossaries designed to assist in the development of programmes of quality assurance in mental health care. They are based on recommendations of a group of experts in the field of mental health care and have been tested in a field trial that included 10 countries in all the WHO regions (Bertolote, 1994).

The following checklists and glossaries are available.

The Mental Health Policy Checklist is an instrument aimed at assessing national mental health policies and assisting in the development of national programmes of quality assurance in mental health. It has 21 items enquiring about issues such as the existence of a written mental health policy and operational programmes. The rest of the items are grouped into the following categories: decentralisation, intersectoral action, comprehensiveness, equity, continuity, community participation and periodic reviews of mental health policy. The average administration time is 75 minutes. The instrument can also be used to assess the policy of smaller population units (e.g. a federal state).

The Mental Health Programme Checklist is an instrument aimed at assessing countries' mental health programmes and assisting in the development of programmes of quality assurance in mental health. It consists of 32 items covering several main areas such as whether there are written national, regional and local mental health programmes, the range of actions for the promotion of mental health, treatment, rehabilitation and prevention of mental disorders. The rest of the items are grouped into the following sections: plan of work, monitoring and evaluation, and community participation in the planning, implementation and evaluation of mental health actions/programmes. A glossary provides descriptions of these items. The average completion time of the checklist is 30 minutes.

The Primary Health Care Facility Checklist is an instrument for the assessment of primary care facilities delivering mental health care and for assistance in the development of programmes of quality assurance of mental health care in such facilities. The instrument consists of a checklist, glossary, scoring instructions and list of references. The checklist has 42 items covering physical environment (e.g. reasonable space available, adequate supply of basic drugs); administrative arrangements (e.g. written procedures regarding the confidentiality of patient and staff records); care process (e.g. treatment plans are written down for each patient and followed by all staff); interaction with families (e.g. family members are encouraged to be involved in the patient's treatment programme); outreach (e.g. contact is regularly made with other health facilities, social agencies, patients' employers). The average completion time is 60 minutes.

The Outpatient Mental Health Facility Checklist is an instrument used to assess out-patient mental health facilities in a given country or set-up, and to assist in the development of programmes of quality assurance in mental health in such facilities. The instrument consists of a checklist, glossary and scoring instructions. The checklist comprises 53 items and covers areas such as physical environment (e.g. the facility has been officially inspected and meets local standards for the protection of the health and safety of patients and staff); administrative arrangements (e.g. a written policy on the philosophy and model of care is available and priorities have been defined); care process (e.g. every patient is evaluated in terms of biological, psychological and social functioning); interaction with families (e.g. home visits for improving the caring and coping skills of families of selected patients are carried out); outreach (e.g. a standard information form is always sent to another facility whenever a patient is referred to it). The average completion time is 60 minutes.

The Inpatient Mental Health Facility Checklist is used to assess in-patient mental health facilities in a given country or set-up, and to assist in the development of programmes of quality assurance in mental health in such facilities. The instrument consists of 77 items covering areas such as physical environment, administrative arrangements, staffing, care process, interaction with families, discharge and follow-up. A glossary provides descriptions of items to be assessed. Scoring instructions are also available. The average completion time is 20 minutes.

The Residential Facility for the Elderly Mentally Ill Checklist is used to assess residential facilities for the elderly mentally ill in a given set-up and to assist in the development of programmes of quality assurance in mental health in such facilities. It consists of 69 items that cover the physical environment, administrative arrangements, care process, and interaction with families and community. The glossary provides a description of these items and instructions for their scoring are also given. The average completion time is 75 minutes.

WHO Child Care Facility Schedule

The WHO Child Care Facility Schedule (WHO CCFS; WHO, 1990*a*) is an observer-rating schedule aimed at assessing the quality of child care in day-care programmes for children. It can be administered by a researcher or administrative worker, who should be familiar with recording and rating procedures. The average administration time is 90 mintues.

The instrument consists of 80 items, covering the following areas that define quality of child care: physical environment (e.g. the indoor environment is spacious enough for the number of children present and is attractive and pleasant); health and safety (e.g. the facility meets local standards for protection of the health and safety of children in group settings); nutrition and food (e.g. meal times are used by staff to promote good nutrition); administration (e.g. at least annually, staff conduct a self-study to identify strengths and weaknesses of the programme); staff–family interaction (e.g. parents and other family members are encouraged to be involved in the programme in various ways and there are no rules prohibiting their unannounced visits); staff–children interaction (e.g. staff respect the cultural backgrounds of the children and adapt the learning situation to preserve their heritage and acquaint other children with the cultural legacy of all members of the group); observable child behaviour (e.g. children respect the needs, feelings and property of others, take turns, share toys); curriculum (e.g. the daily schedule is planned to provide a variety of activities – indoor and outdoor, quiet and active, etc.).

The WHO CCFS contains a glossary that defines each of the items to be observed and rated. The instrument is also accompanied by a user manual and a list of relevant references. Field studies of WHO CCFS have been carried out in Greece, the Philippines and Nigeria and the instrument has been found to be cross-culturally acceptable and reliable in terms of a level of percentage agreement between raters (Tsiantis *et al*, 1991).

Instruments for the assessment of environment and risks

Axis III Checklist

The Axis III Checklist instrument has been produced in the framework of the development of the ICD–10 multi-axial schema (WHO, 1997*b*) and is intended for clinicians' assessment of axis III, that is, contextual (environmental/circumstantial and personal lifestyle/life management) factors contributing to the presentation or course of the ICD–10 mental and/or physical disorder(s) recorded on axis I of the schema. The contextual factors listed under axis III represent a selection of ICD–10 Z00–Z99 categories, "Factors influencing health status and contact with health services" (Chapter XXI of ICD–10). The following groups of contextual factors are covered by axis III and assessed by the Checklist: negative events in childhood (e.g. removal from home in childhood, Z61.1); problems related to education and literacy (e.g. underachievement in school, Z55.3); problems related to the primary support group, including family circumstances (e.g. disruption of family by separation or divorce, Z63.5); problems related to the social environment (e.g. social exclusion and rejection, Z60.4); problems related to housing or economic circumstances (e.g. homelessness, Z59.0); problems related to (un)employment (e.g. change of job, Z56.1); problems related to physical environment (e.g. occupational exposure to risk factors, Z57); problems related to psychosocial or legal circumstances (e.g. imprisonment or other incarceration, Z65.1); problems related to a family history of diseases or disabilities (e.g. family history of mental or behavioural disorders, Z81); lifestyle and life management problems (e.g. burn-out, Z73.0).

The Axis III Checklist is included in the ICD–10 Multiaxial Diagnostic Formulation Form, and the clinician is required to tick all applicable categories of Z factors and specify Z codes for each. A listing of contextual factors and the respective ICD–10 Z codes is given as an appendix to the Form. The average administration time of the Axis III Checklist is 10 minutes. The instrument has been tested in the multi-centre international field trials of the multi-axial presentation of ICD–10 and has been found to be useful and easy to use by clinicians in different parts of the world (Janca *et al*, 1996*b*).

Interview Schedule for Children

The Interview Schedule for Children (ISC; WHO, 1991) is a semi-structured instrument for the systematic collection of information on a child's psychosocial environment. The instrument has been developed as a companion to the psychosocial axis (axis V) of the WHO Multiaxial Classification of Child and Adolescent Psychiatric Disorders (WHO, 1988). The ISC is accompanied by a glossary that provides descriptions of items and diagnostic guidelines for axis V (associated abnormal psychosocial situations). However, to ensure the smooth flow of the interview, the items in the ISC are in a different order from those of the glossary. The items in the ISC are as follows: abnormal immediate environment; stressful events/situations resulting from child's disorder/disability; societal stressors; chronic interpersonal stress associated with school/work; acute life events; abnormal qualities of upbringing; abnormal intrafamilial relationships; inadequate or distorted intrafamilial communication; mental disorder, deviance or handicap in the child's primary support group.

The relevant codes for each category have to be inserted into each individual section and the results are transferred to a summary page. It is, however, recommended that the coding and scoring should not be done until the interview has been completed. The instrument is intended for psychiatrists, psychologists, social workers and nurses, and its administration takes 60 minutes (Van Goor-Lambo *et al*, 1990).

Parent Interview Schedule

The Parent Interview Schedule (PIS; WHO, 1990*b*) is a semistructured instrument for the systematic collection of information about the child's psychosocial environment so that appropriate codings can be made on the psychosocial axis (axis V) of the WHO Multiaxial Classification of Child and Adolescent Psychiatric Disorders (WHO, 1988). The instrument is accompanied by a glossary and diagnostic guidelines for the assessment of items. As in the ISC, the relevant codes have to be inserted in each individual section and the results should be transferred to the summary page after the interview. Items in the PIS are identical with those in the ISC, and their order in the schedule and glossary is different to ensure the smooth flow of the interview.

The instrument is intended for psychiatrists, psychologists, social workers and nurses, and its administration takes 60 minutes. The preliminary results of the axis V field trials (Van Goor-Lambo *et al*, 1990) were used in the preparation of the PIS version that is being tested at present.

Home Risk Card

The Home Risk Card is a listing of risk factors that, if present at the home of a child, may indicate that both child and family need extra help and special attention. The risk factors covered by the instrument include: mother's age (under 17 years); number of children under three years (more than two); mother/carer ignorant about the child's needs and unresponsive to health messages (e.g. cannot answer questions about the child that mothers normally can answer); mother/carer mentally disordered or severely depressed (e.g. looks desperate, hopeless, cries easily); mother/carer neglectful or uninterested in the well-being/development of the child (e.g. shouts or hits the child for trivial reasons during home visit); disorganised, uncleaned house; father known to be delinquent (e.g. arrested by police), alcoholic or otherwise mentally disordered; severe marital discord (e.g. physical violence between parents); abject poverty (e.g. no change of clothing).

The Home Risk Card guides the user in noting facts about the child and household that may indicate that intervention is warranted. The recorded information should also be inserted into the child's weight card and serve as a reminder to the health professional about the child's need for extra help and attention.

A brief set of instructions helps the user in the application of the Card, which usually takes 5–10 minutes to complete. The Home Risk Card has been used in a project organised by the WHO Regional Office for South-East Asia and has been found to be a useful guide for the assessment of home risk factors in this region (Sell & Nagpal, 1992).

Qualitative research instruments

A guide providing a general overview of the concepts, methods and tools commonly used in qualitative research has been produced by WHO (Hudelson, 1994). It is an introductory guide for programme managers, project directors, researchers and others who need to make decisions concerning when and how to conduct research for programme development purposes. This guide gives an overview of qualitative research and its potential uses; provides descriptions of the most common data collection methods used in qualitative research, specifying their strengths and weaknesses; discusses issues of sampling, study design and report writing in qualitative research; and gives examples of several qualitative research designs used by health programmes.

For the WHO Cross-cultural Applicability Research (CAR) study on diagnostic criteria and instruments for the assessment of alcohol and drug misuse and dependence, a set of qualitative research methods and instruments has been developed (Room *et al*, 1996). These include the following three instruments.

The Exploratory Translation and Back-Translation Guidelines is a set of specified procedures for conducting a careful translation and back-translation of an instrument so as to ensure its equivalence in different languages and cultures. The exploratory translation and back-translation method used in the WHO CAR study comprises a series of step-by-step procedures summarised in Table 12.5.

The Key Informant Interview Schedule is a semistructured, exploratory, ethnographic interview schedule that covers phenomena relevant to ICD–10 and DSM–III–R definitions and criteria for substance misuse disorders (e.g. withdrawal, tolerance, loss of control). The questions follow a 'funnel-type' structure: general topics are first discussed and then more detailed questions about specific issues are asked.

The informant's answers are noted on the schedule verbatim. However, to ensure accuracy of the notes, the key informant interviews should be tape-recorded whenever possible or an observer

TABLE 12.5
Steps in the development of equivalent versions of instruments in different languages

Step	Procedure
1	Establishment of a (bilingual) group of experts belonging to the culture in which the instrument was developed and the culture in which it will (also) be used.
2	Examination of the conceptual structure of the instrument by the expert group.
3	Translation of items into the target language (or formulation of items in both languages if the instrument is produced anew).
4	Examination of translation by bilingual group.
5	Examination of the translation in unilingual groups (i.e. groups of individuals who do not know the source language of the instruments and therefore cannot guess the meaning of badly formulated items). The unilingual groups are usually moderated by a member of the bilingual expert group.
6	Back-translation of the text, possibly amended by the unilingual group.
7	Examination of the back-translation by a bilingual group informed by its members about the contents of discussion in the unilingual groups. Participation of members of the bilingual group in the designing of the studies to establish the metric properties (e.g. validity, reliability, sensitivity) of the instrument.

should be present while the interviewer asks questions and both should take notes.

The Key Informant Interview Schedule developed for the WHO CAR study has been applied in nine centres representing distinct cultures and has been found to be an appropriate method for eliciting information on culture-specific characteristics of substance use and misuse in different parts of the world (Bennett *et al*, 1993).

The Focus Group Interview Guide is a brief interview guide specifying the main topics for discussions on various aspects of culture-specific characteristics of psychoactive substance use and misuse. According to the WHO CAR study protocol, the following topics have been explored by this method: what is normal and abnormal use of alcohol or drugs; what are the meanings of the various diagnostic terms related to the concept of alcohol or drug dependence; what are the similarities and differences between alcohol and drug misuse and alcohol and drug addiction; which prevention and intervention strategies are most likely to be effective against alcohol- or drug-related problems in the culture?

A set of instructions for the selection, composition and moderation of focus groups accompanies the list of discussion topics. Techniques of recording, reconstructing, managing and analysing the information obtained through the focus groups are also specified.

Discussion

All the WHO instruments have been developed in the context of collaborative and cross-cultural studies. In some instances an instrument that was already in use in one cultural setting was selected as the initial draft, which was then developed further; in other instances the development of the instrument started from a draft produced by an international group of experts representing several cultural settings and disciplines. All the instruments exist in more than one language and the vast majority have been used in more than one country. This was not accidental: the WHO has in fact made it its aim to produce instruments for cross-cultural and collaborative work that will serve as part of a common language helping researchers and other experts from different countries to understand one another, to work together and to compare the results of their studies even when these are not performed at a particular time following a commonly agreed protocol.

The decision to develop instruments suitable for international, cross-cultural and collaborative work had several consequences. First, the development of the instruments took more time than it would take to develop an instrument for use in a single country or language.

Second, certain characteristics of patients, their socio-cultural surroundings and the health services that they receive are so different that it is not possible to assess them using the same instrument. In such instances guidelines about the assessment were provided, while the formulation of specific items and other measurement tasks were entrusted to groups of experts who were fully acquainted with the circumstances.

Third, the development of instruments required additional funds for face-to-face meetings of the experts involved. These meetings (usually conducted at the participating centres) proved to have important consequences and benefits for the process of instrument development. The discussions of the results of the field trials and other aspects of the research necessary to produce the instrument and assess its psychometric characteristics gave invaluable insights into the differences between cultures and into the feasibility of investigations in different settings. The meetings also served as an important motivator to continue the often tedious work required over a long period. An effort was made on each occasion to bring together the centre heads and younger investigators, for whom attendance at such meetings was of particular importance.

Fourth, certain constraints were imposed on the instruments by the structure of the languages in which they were produced. Certain concepts have no natural 'home' in other languages and enquiring about them can therefore be both time-consuming and difficult. In such instances it is usually best to sacrifice an item or section rather than to make part of the instrument awkward to use and complicate the training of interviewers. When this is not acceptable, it is usually necessary to return to the beginning and consider whether it is possible to obtain information about the topic of interest in another manner, not using assessment instruments of the type described here.

Fifth, cross-cultural differences can best be overcome if the assessments are carried out by individuals who are familiar with the culture and well trained in the use of the instruments. Most of the instruments that the WHO has developed are therefore semistructured and have been proposed for application by a well-trained member of the same culture. The use of semistructured interviews, however, requires more intensive training than is the case for fully standardised instruments. This is a disadvantage that is less grave than the very much more intensive training necessary when non-structured assessment methods are chosen. Furthermore, semistructured instruments share some of the advantages of the fully structured instruments (e.g. the systematic coverage of all areas of interest, simpler data processing).

Sixth, issues such as copyright, translation rights and modification procedures have to be designed with a view to covering the different centres and languages in which the instrument has been produced.

The WHO instruments have been developed in collaboration with groups of experts in many countries. Their contribution to the production of the instruments has been invaluable, and it is certain that without their selfless and enthusiastic collaboration it would not have been possible to develop the many materials – instruments and results of scientific investigations – that have been made available over the years. In the course of this work over the past three decades most of the centres that have participated have made many international contacts, gained new insights about other cultures, increased their expertise in cross-cultural work and learned about the most convenient ways of international collaboration. The network of centres that has come into existence and that continues to work on instruments (and collaborate in research) has been an excellent by-product of the work on instrument development.

Another by-product of the work on instruments and of other WHO-coordinated international and cross-cultural collaborative research has been the formulation of guidelines concerning ethical aspects of collaboration in the field of mental health across national borders (Sartorius, 1990). One of the principles developed is that collaboration in research – in view of the high investments and various potential disadvantages of short-term international collaborative projects – should be structured in a manner that will make it highly probable that the collaborative network will continue after the project has been completed. This has been realised in the instance of the WHO network, which continues its collaborative links between all centres – including those that are at present not actively involved in any particular studies.

The technology of translation used in the development of WHO instruments deserves a brief mention. The method that has been developed rests on various previous methods used to ensure equivalence of translation in collaborative mental health research (Sartorius, 1979) but has parts that have not been systematically used before. The steps used to produce equivalent versions in different languages are shown in Table 12.5. The procedure shown is an approximation of the process described in more detail elsewhere (Sartorius, 1998; Sartorius & Kuyken, 1994). The features that deserve attention at this point are the decision to incorporate an examination of the translation by a unilingual group and the existence of bilingual/bicultural groups that can guide the process of producing equivalent versions of the instrument in different languages.

The instruments described in this chapter cover the needs for data collection in a number of areas of psychiatric investigation. Other areas, however, also require attention, and it is to be hoped that the

WHO will continue working on the development of instruments for these. Among them are:

- Instruments that could be used to assess the stigma of psychiatric illness and its changes under the influence of various interventions that the health services or that society as a whole might undertake to diminish it.
- Instruments that would be useful to measure the tolerance of individuals to their own diseases and the diseases in those who surround them.
- Instruments that might help us to assess conditions and states such as 'burn-out' and 'malaise' and their impact on the productivity of the individuals who suffer from them and of the community as a whole.
- Instruments that could help us to assess features of the community relevant to the provision of mental health care (e.g. the capacity of the community to accept sick and disabled members).
- Instruments that could better describe the needs of individuals and communities.
- Instruments we could use in the assessment of states that are at the borderline of normality (e.g. mild cognitive disorders, subthreshold mental disorders).
- Instruments that could be used in international studies of impairments, disabilities and handicaps defined in terms of the second revision of the International Classification of Impairments, Disabilities and Handicaps.

The difficulties of producing an instrument satisfying all the metric requirements and dealing with an area of assessment that should be investigated because of its public health importance pale in comparison with the difficulty of ensuring that the instrument is well known, properly updated, sufficiently well learned and widely applied. It is probably to this second task that the majority of efforts should be directed if we are to contribute to a better understanding among all those concerned with mental illness and with ways of helping patients, their families and communities.

References

AMERICAN PSYCHIATRIC ASSOCIATION (1987) *Diagnostic and Statistical Manual of Mental Disorders* (3rd edn, revised) (DSM–III–R). Washington, DC: APA.
—— (1994) *Diagnostic and Statistical Manual of Mental Disorders* (4th edn) (DSM–IV). Washington, DC: APA.

BABOR, T. F., DE LA FUENTE, J. R., SAUNDERS, J. B., *et al* (1989) *AUDIT, the Alcohol Use Disorders Identification Test. Guidelines for Use in Primary Health Care*. Geneva: WHO.

BENNETT, L. A., JANCA, A., GRANT, B. F., *et al* (1993) Boundaries between normal and pathological drinking: a cross-cultural comparison. *Alcohol Health and Research World*, **17**, 190–195.

BERTOLOTE, J. (1994) *Quality Assurance in Mental Health Care: Checklists and Glossaries, Vol. I*. Geneva: WHO.

BEUSENBERG, M. & ORLEY, J. (1994) *A user's guide to the Self-Reporting Questionnaire (SRQ)*. Geneva: WHO.

COOPER, I. E., JABLENSKY, A. & SARTORIUS, N. (1990) WHO collaborative studies on acute psychoses using the SCAAPS schedule. In *Psychiatry: A World Perspective, Vol. 1. Classification and Psychopathology, Child Psychiatry, Substance Use* (eds C. N. Stefanis *et al*), pp. 185–192 (International Congress Series). Amsterdam: Excerpta Medica.

COTTLER, L. B., ROBINS, L. N., GRANT, B. F., *et al* (1991) The CIDI-Core substance abuse and dependence questions: cross-cultural and nosological issues. *British Journal of Psychiatry*, **159**, 653–658.

GATER, R., GOLDBERG, D. & SARTORIUS, N. (1990) The WHO Pathways to Care Study. In *Psychiatry: A World Perspective, Vol. 4. Social Psychiatry Ethics and Law: History of Psychiatry, Psychiatric Education* (eds C. N. Stefanis *et al*), pp. 75–78 (International Congress Series). Amsterdam: Excerpta Medica.

——, DE ALMEIDA, E., SOUSA, B., *et al* (1991) The pathways to psychiatric care: a cross-cultural study. *Psychological Medicine*, **21**, 761–764.

GIEL, R., DE ARANGO, M. V., BABIKIR, A. H., *et al* (1983) The burden of mental illness on the family. Results of observations in four developing countries. *Acta Psychiatrica Scandinavica*, **68**, 186–201.

HARDING, T. W., DE ARANGO, M. V., BALTHAZAR, J., *et al* (1980) Mental disorders in primary health care: a study of their frequency and diagnosis in four developing countries. *Psychological Medicine*, **10**, 231–241.

——, CLIMENT, C. E., DIOP, M., *et al* (1983) The WHO collaborative study on strategies for extending mental health care. II. The development of new research methods. *American Journal of Psychiatry*, **140**, 1474–1480.

HUDELSON, P. M. (1994) *Qualitative Research for Health Programmes*. Geneva: WHO.

ISAAC, M., JANCA, A. & SARTORIUS, N. (1994) *The ICD–10 Symptom Glossary for Mental Disorders*. Geneva: WHO.

JABLENSKY, A., SCHWARZ, R. & TOMOV, T. (1980) WHO collaborative study on impairments and disabilities associated with schizophrenic disorders. A preliminary communication: objectives and methods. In *Epidemiological Research as a Basis for the Organization of Extramural Psychiatry* (eds E. Strömgren *et al*). *Acta Psychiatrica Scandinavica*, **62** (suppl. 286), 152–159.

——, SARTORIUS, N., ERNBERG, G., *et al* (1992) Schizophrenia: manifestations, incidence and course in different cultures: a World Health Organization ten-country study. *Psychological Medicine*, monograph suppl. 201.

JANCA, A., ROBINS, L. N., COTTLER, L. B., *et al* (1992) Clinical observation of assessment using the Composite International Diagnostic Interview (CIDI): an analysis of the CIDI field trials-wave II at the St Louis site. *British Journal of Psychiatry*, **160**, 815–818.

—— & CHANDRASHEKAR, C. R. (1993) *Catalogue of Assessment Instruments Used in the Studies Coordinated by the WHO Mental Health Programme*. Geneva: WHO.

——, USTUN, T. B., EARLY, T. S., *et al* (1993) The ICD–10 Symptom Checklist – a companion to the ICD–10 Classification of Mental and Behavioural Disorders. *Social Psychiatry and Psychiatric Epidemiology*, **28**, 239–242.

——, —— & SARTORIUS, N. (1994*a*) New versions of World Health Organization instruments for the assessment of mental disorders. *Acta Psychiatrica Scandinavica*, **90**, 73–83.

——, ——, VAN DRIMMELEN, J., *et al* (1994*b*) *The ICD–10 Symptom Checklist for Mental Disorders, Version 2.0*. Geneva: WHO.

——, KASTRUP, M. C., KATSCHNIG, H., *et al* (1996*a*) The World Health Organization Short Disability Assessment Schedule (WHO DAS-S). A tool for the assessment of difficulties in selected areas of functioning of patients with mental disorders. *Social Psychiatry and Psychiatric Epidemiology*, **31**, 349–354.

——, MEZZICH, J. E., KASTRUP, M., *et al* (1996*b*) Contextual aspects of mental disorders: a proposal for axis III of the ICD–10 multi-axial system. *Acta Psychiatrica Scandinavica*, **94**, 31–36.

LORANGER, A., HIRSCHFIELD, R., SARTORIUS, N., *et al* (1991) The WHO/ADAMHA international pilot study of personality disorders: background and purpose. *Journal of Personality Disorders*, **5**, 296–306.

——, SARTORIUS, N., ANDREOLI, A., *et al* (1994) The International Personality Disorder Examination (IPDE): the WHO/ADAMHA international pilot study of personality disorders. *Archives of General Psychiatry*, **51**, 215–224.

ROBINS, L. N., WING, J. E., WITTCHEN, H-U., *et al* (1988) The Composite International Diagnostic Interview: an epidemiologic instrument suitable for use in conjunction with different diagnostic systems and in different cultures. *Archives of General Psychiatry*, **45**, 1069–1077.

——, COTTLER, L. B. & BABOR, T. (1990) *CIDI Substance Abuse Module*. St Louis: Department of Psychiatry, Washington University School of Medicine, St Louis, Missouri, USA.

ROOM, R., JANCA, A., BENNETT, L. A., *et al* (1996) WHO cross-cultural applicability research on diagnosis and assessment of substance use disorders: an overview of methods and selected results. *Addiction*, **91**, 1529–1538.

SARTORIUS, N. (1979) Cross-cultural psychiatry. In *Psychiatrie der Gegenwart, Vol. III* (2nd edn) (eds K. P. Kisker, I. E. Meyer, C. Muller & E. Strömgren), pp. 711–737. Berlin: Springer-Verlag.

—— (1989) Recent research activities in WHO's mental health programme. *Psychological Medicine*, **19**, 233–244.

—— (1990) Cultural factors in the etiology of schizophrenia. In *Psychiatry: A World Perspective, Vol. 4. Social Psychiatry Ethics and Law: History of Psychiatry, Psychiatric Education* (eds C. N. Stefanis *et al*), pp. 33–44 (International Congress Series). Amsterdam: Excerpta Medica.

—— (1993) WHO's work on the epidemiology of mental disorders. *Social Psychiatry and Psychiatric Epidemiology*, **28**, 147–155.

—— (1998) SCAN translation. In *Diagnosis and Clinical Measurement in Psychiatry – A Reference Manual for SCAN* (eds J. K. Wing, N. Sartorius & T. B. Ustun), pp. 44–57. Cambridge: Cambridge University Press.

——, JABLENSKY, A., GULBINAT, W., *et al* (1980) WHO collaborative study: assessment of depressive disorders. Preliminary communication. *Psychological Medicine*, **10**, 743–749.

——, DAVIDIAN, H., ERNBERG, G., *et al* (1983) *Depressive Disorders in Different Cultures. Report on the WHO Collaborative Study on Standardized Assessment of Depressive Disorders*. Geneva: WHO.

—— & KUYKEN, W. (1994) Translation of health status instruments. In *Quality of Life Assessment: International Perspectives* (eds J. Orley & W. Kuyken), pp. 3–18. Berlin: Springer-Verlag.

SAUNDERS, J. B. & AASLAND, O. G. (1987) *WHO Collaborative Project on the Identification and Treatment of Persons with Harmful Alcohol Consumption. Report on Phase 1. Development of a Screening Instrument*. Geneva: WHO.

——, AASLAND, O. G., ARUNDSEN, A., *et al* (1993*a*) Alcohol consumption and related problems among primary health care patients. WHO collaborative project on early detection of persons with harmful alcohol consumption. I. *Addiction*, **88**, 339–352.

——, ——, BABOR, T. F., *et al* (1993*b*) Development of the Alcohol Use Disorders Identification Test (AUDIT). WHO collaborative project on early detection of persons with harmful alcohol consumption. II. *Addiction*, **88**, 617–629.

SELL, H. & NAGPAL, R. (1992) *Assessment of Subjective Well-Being. The Subjective Well-Being Inventory (SUBI)*. New Delhi: WHO Regional Office for South-East Asia.

—, THARA, R., PADMAVATI, R., *et al* (1998) *The Burden Assessment Schedule (BAS)*. New Delhi: WHO Regional Office for South-East Asia.

TSIANTIS, J., CALDWELL, B., DRAGONAS, T., *et al* (1991) Development of a WHO child care facility schedule (CCFS): a pilot collaborative study. *Bulletin of the World Health Organization*, **69**, 51–57.

VAN GOOR-LAMBO, G., ORLEY, J., POUSTKA, F., *et al* (1990) Classification of abnormal psychosocial situations: preliminary report of a revision of a WHO scheme. *Journal of Child Psychology and Psychiatry*, **31**, 229–241.

WING, J. K., COOPER, J. E. & SARTORIUS, N. (1974) *Measurement and Classification of Psychiatric Symptoms: An Instruction Manual for the PSE and CATEGO Program*. London: Cambridge University Press.

—, BABOR, T., BRUGHA, T., *et al* (1990) SCAN: Schedules for Clinical Assessment in Neuropsychiatry. *Archives of General Psychiatry*, **47**, 589–593.

—, SARTORIUS, N. & USTUN, T. B. (1998) *Diagnosis and Clinical Measurement in Psychiatry: A Reference Manual for SCAN*. Cambridge: Cambridge University Press.

WITTCHEN, H-U., ROBINS, L. N., COTTLER, L., *et al* (1991) Cross-cultural feasibility, reliability and sources of variance of the Composite International Diagnostic Interview (CIDI) – results of the multicentre WHO/ADAMHA field trials (wave I). *British Journal of Psychiatry*, **159**, 645–653.

WORLD HEALTH ORGANIZATION (WHO) (1973) *Report on the International Pilot Study of Schizophrenia, Vol. I*. Geneva: WHO.

— (1980) *International Classification of Impairments, Disabilities and Handicaps*. Geneva: WHO.

— (1984) *Mental Health Care in Developing Countries: A Critical Appraisal of Research Findings. Report of a WHO Study Group*. Geneva: WHO.

— (1988) *Draft Multiaxial Classification of Child and Adolescent Psychiatric Disorders. Axis V. Associated Abnormal Psychosocial Situations Including Glossary Descriptions of Items and Diagnostic Guidelines*. Geneva: WHO.

— (1990*a*) *WHO Child Care Facility Schedule with User Manual*. Geneva: WHO.

— (1990*b*) *Parent Interview Schedule. Draft for Comments and Field Testing*. Geneva: WHO.

— (1991) *Interview Schedule for Children. Draft for Comments and Field Testing*. Geneva: WHO.

— (1992) *The ICD–10 Classification of Mental and Behavioural Disorders: Clinical Descriptions and Diagnostic Guidelines*. Geneva: WHO.

— (1993*a*) *The Composite International Diagnostic Interview, Core Version 1.1*. Washington, DC: American Psychiatric Association Press.

— (1993*b*) *International Personality Disorder Examination*. Geneva: WHO.

— (1993*c*) *Computerized CIDI (CIDI-Auto)*. Geneva: WHO.

— (1994) Schedules for Clinical Assessment in Neuropsychiatry (SCAN). Washington, DC: American Psychiatric Research.

— (1997*a*) *International Classification of Impairments, Activities and Participation: Beta-1 Draft for Field Trials*. Geneva: WHO.

— (1997*b*) *Multiaxial Presentation of the ICD–10 for Use in Adult Psychiatry*. Cambridge: Cambridge University Press.

WHOQOL Group (1994) The development of the WHO Quality of Life Assessment Instrument (the WHOQOL). In *Quality of Life Assessment: International Perspectives* (eds J. Orley & W. Kuyken), pp. 41–57. Berlin: Springer-Verlag.

13 Properties of the Composite International Diagnostic Interview (CIDI) for measuring mental health outcome

HANS-ULRICH WITTCHEN,
RONALD C. KESSLER and BEDIRHAN ÜSTÜN

History and general characteristics of the CIDI

The World Health Organization (WHO) Composite International Diagnostic Interview (CIDI; WHO, 1990) is a comprehensive, fully standardised diagnostic interview originally developed for use in epidemiological studies by an international group of researchers under the patronage of the US National Institutes of Health and the WHO. Initially based on two predecessors, the National Institute of Mental Health (NIMH) Diagnostic Interview Schedule (DIS; Robins *et al*, 1981) and the Present State Examination (PSE; Wing *et al*, 1974), the CIDI has gone through various revisions and updates and has been considerably expanded. Some of the available versions are official WHO products, namely the WHO CIDI versions 1.0 through to 2.1; others (see below) are modified and supplementary versions developed for use in specific populations or studies, sharing the core features with regard to symptom and diagnostic assessment. The common core of this interview in all revisions is a standardised set of questions designed for the assessment of a wide range of mental disorders according to the symptom and diagnostic criteria of both the DSM and ICD systems (see below). Over the past decade, the scope of these diagnostic modules has been considerably expanded and they now cover a wide range of affective, anxiety, substance, somatoform, eating- and stress-related disorders and conditions. Further, more recent optional additions include assessment modules on age of onset and course of illness, impairments and disabilities, help-seeking behaviours and service utilisation, as well as treatment.

The core of the CIDI comprises fully standardised interview questions with standard probing, coding, training and data analysis procedures for which reliability and validity have been established (for a review see Wittchen, 1994). Analyses and diagnostic decisions are entirely based on computerised algorithms by use of the CIDI standard data entry file, which throughout revisions maintains a high degree of consistency. Although paper-and-pencil versions are available in several languages for subsequent computerised data entry, the more recent versions of the CIDI recommend the use of computer-assisted versions to ease training and administration and to reduce potential sources of interrater discrepancies: these Computer-Assisted Personal Interview (CAPI) versions are the CIDI-Auto (Andrews *et al*, 1993, 1998) and the DIA-X-M-CIDI (Wittchen & Pfister, 1997).

These characteristics ensure that results from different studies are directly comparable, that the interview can be repeatedly administered in a uniform style and that even non-clinical interviewers can administer the CIDI. Because of the comprehensive nature of the instrument, which allows the assessment of up to 75 diagnostic categories in both the DSM and ICD classification systems, its flexible, modular format allows researchers to use only those sections that are relevant to their objectives. Further, users may choose between lifetime and 12-month cross-sectional interview versions.

This chapter briefly reviews the content, structure and options of the 'CIDI toolbox' and describes the main features of the more frequently used modifications. These include the primary care version of the CIDI (CIDI-PMC), developed by the WHO (Üstün & Sartorius, 1995), the University of Michigan CIDI (UM-CIDI; Wittchen & Kessler, 1994), the Munich-CIDI (M-CIDI; Wittchen & Pfister, 1997), as well as the version used in the World Mental Health Survey 2000 (Kessler *et al*, 1999). Particular emphasis will be placed upon those features of the CIDI that are potentially relevant for the measurement of mental health outcomes.

The core of the CIDI (version 2.0)

Characteristics

The core of the CIDI consists of close to 200 questions related to symptoms of mental disorders, frequently arranged in a diagnosis-specific stem–branch structure with many skip options. Some of the core symptom questions are followed up by so-called probe questions by use of a differentiated probe flowchart (Table 13.1). These probe questions aim to determine whether the symptom was severe enough to cause either impairment or professional help seeking, as well as to what degree symptoms may be attributed to either physical diseases or conditions or the effect of substances. The following information can be collected using the chart: whether the symptom was present; whether the respondent talked with a medical doctor or another mental health professional about the symptom; whether the respondent took medication because of the symptom; and whether the symptom has caused significant impairment.

Some of the CIDI's CAPI versions (M-CIDI) further allow the recording of medical doctor's type of diagnoses, beyond the global rating of the standard version. The coding of most symptom and diagnostic questions in the standard core CIDI is strictly categorical (yes/no format), whereas some of the modified versions (UM-CIDI, M-CIDI) also allow for dimensional ratings, for example with regard to distress, impairments and disability.

Another set of questions in many diagnostic sections allows an assessment of the length of an episode for key syndromes (general anxiety disorder and affective disorders), the frequency of the episodes (e.g. affective disorders) as well as the respondent's age at first onset and the most recent occurrence. The CIDI core version is accompanied by a diagnostic program that facilitates the classification of the respondent's symptoms according to DSM–IV (American Psychiatric Association, 1994) or the ICD–10 Criteria for Research (WHO, 1993). Besides reporting diagnoses, the program prints out the times at which criteria were first and last met. The coding options for this are: within the past two weeks, two weeks to one month, one month to six months, six months to one year and more than a year in the past. For the last coding option, the age of the respondent at that time is registered.

Use of CIDI core in mental health outcome and service research

Despite the lack of any dimensional measures, the standard CIDI, similarly to the DIS, has been used for outcome measurement in several ways (Kessler *et al*, 1995, 1999).

First, measures of remission for each diagnosis can be derived by examining whether a specific episode is currently still present. This judgement is based on the recency probes relating to the diagnosis of key syndromes. These recency probes allow the calculation of remission for various periods of time (syndrome present in the past two weeks, six months or year). If remission occurred more than a

TABLE 13.1
Examples of CIDI questions and other information extractable from the CIDI core

Domain	Example	Coding
Questions regarding symptoms with probing	C.7: Have you ever had a lot of trouble with back pain? Doctor diagnosis: ... Other attributions: ...	Probing for doctor and diagnosis, other health professional, interference, relationship physical illness/substances (Codes: probes 1 2 3 4 5)[1]
Series of explicit questions regarding help-seeking and interference	D27: Did you tell a doctor about your fears of ...? 1. Did you tell any other professional about any of them? 2. Did you take medication more than once because of these fears? 3. Did these fears interfere with your life or activities a lot?	NO/YES NO/YES NO/YES NO/YES
Questions on frequency	E41: In your lifetime how many spells like that have you had that lasted two weeks or more?	Number of spells
Questions on onset and recency	E37: When was the first time you had a period of two weeks or more, when you had several of these problems and also felt low, uninterested or depressed? And when was the last time...?	Onset: 1 2 3 4 5 6 Age at onset: ... Recency: 1 2 3 4 5 6[2] Age: ...

1. 1 = no; 2 = yes, but not severe; 3 = yes, but always due to medication, drugs or alcohol; 4 = yes, but always due to physical disorders or conditions; 5 = yes, probably mental health problem.
2. 1 = within past 2 weeks; 2 = within past month; 3 = within past 3 months; 4 = within past 6 months; 5 = within past 6–12 months; 6 = more than 1 year ago.

year previously, it is also possible to indicate at what age the respondent last experienced the problem.

Second, measures of duration can be obtained by specific questions for some syndromes (e.g. depression, mania, generalised anxiety disorder). Some authors have also used the time difference between recency and onset to derive a rather crude measure of duration. This measure merely indicates that the respective syndrome was at least present at the age of onset and at age of recency. It does not necessarily indicate, however, whether it has been present during the interval.

Third, measures of help seeking and impairment can be obtained for many symptoms and syndromes (e.g. anxiety, affective and psychotic disorders) using the probe flowchart. The CIDI allows a determination of whether the person sought professional help from medical doctors or other health professionals, took medication more than once or reported a lot of interference. This information, however, is not specifically dated and refers to lifetime reports. By using the computerised version (CIDI-AUTO) it is also possible to print out this information for each individual symptom for which probe questions were used.

Fourth, measures of change cannot be derived directly from the CIDI core, owing to the lack of any dimensional cross-section items. However, some research groups have used the CIDI in longitudinal studies by simply modifying the questions in the follow-up investigation to cover exclusively the follow-up period. By assessing lifetime information and by focusing, for example, on a one-year time frame in the case of a one-year follow-up investigation, an indirect assessment of changes in diagnostic status can be done. The resulting measures are new diagnoses that occurred in the interval between investigations. By using more sophisticated analytical procedures, changes between subthreshold and threshold conditions based on the number of diagnostic criteria met can also be identified.

In summary, the standard CIDI core version has not been constructed for outcome measurement; thus it is not surprising that only rather limited options are available.

University of Michigan CIDI (UM-CIDI)

Characteristics

This interview is a modified version of the CIDI in which the CIDI diagnostic programs are used for generating DSM–III–R diagnoses. It has been modified to meet the needs of the US National Comorbidity

Survey (Kessler *et al*, 1994), the first national study of mental disorders in the United States and also the first to examine the frequency, form and the implications of comorbidity of mental disorders. The modifications include:

- deletion of some sections of the CIDI, such as the lengthy section on somatoform disorders
- modification of some CIDI questions, such as breaking down long complex questions into separate sub-questions, placing important explanations for words or concepts that are part of the CIDI Interviewer Manual directly into the interview, and adding clarifying probes in places where pilot tests showed that there was confusion in the original CIDI (the probe flowchart questions were also streamlined)
- rearrangement of the order in which CIDI questions are asked to improve comprehension and flow (e.g. many of the stem questions were moved to the beginning of the interview)
- the addition of dimensional ratings for impairment questions as well as questions to assess service utilisation and the time when such services were used for the very first time
- the addition of standard disability questions assessing the number of days the respondent has been partially or entirely disabled by symptoms or syndromes of mental disorders
- the use of visual symptom checklists and review cards to simplify the complex cognitive tasks required of respondents during the interview
- implementation of a lifetime review section for diagnostic stem questions.

Mental health service and outcome measures

Although almost identical to the CIDI core in most respects, the UM-CIDI incorporates a slightly wider range of measures, potentially relevant for mental health service and outcome research (Kessler *et al*, 1998; Alegria *et al*, 2000). For each diagnosis, the UM-CIDI comprises a longer series of help-seeking questions, including separate questions for medical doctors, psychiatrists, other mental health specialists and other professionals. Separate questions are asked for each category about the age at which the respondent first contacted them. Thus lifetime symptom information can be more accurately related to certain episodes.

The standard questions regarding psychosocial impairment as well as some other symptoms were transformed into four-point ratings, with response options ranging from a lot of interference to none.

Furthermore, additional questions were added in most sections to assess the effect of prescribed medication on mental disorders (e.g. anxiety) and remission from episodes (e.g., depression), and to determine the sequence in which psychopathological syndromes occurred. Similar to the CIDI core, the focus is on the lifetime assessment and no current state information is assessed for any of these domains.

Primary Care Version of the CIDI (CIDI-PMC)

Characteristics

The CIDI-PMC was developed in the context of an international WHO multi-centre study in primary care (Üstün & Sartorius, 1995). Designed as a longitudinal study, specific emphasis was placed on modifications of the CIDI core that would allow both comparisons to be made over time and the quantification of change. Because mental disorders in primary care were believed to be frequently atypical, subthreshold conditions, as well as mixed anxiety disorders, modifications were made to allow the derivation of various new DSM–III–R (American Psychiatric Association, 1987) and ICD–10 diagnoses, which were not originally covered in the CIDI core (e.g. a combination of anxiety, depression and neurasthenia, generalised anxiety syndrome). The CIDI-PMC enables the researcher to code both lifetime information and symptoms that are currently present (past four weeks). This allows the calculation of current symptom scores for all major syndromes covered (somatoform and pain, generalised anxiety, depressive syndromes). It is important to note, however, that the CIDI-PMC covers only some of the CIDI diagnostic sections. For example, there are no sections for substance use disorders (except alcohol), hypochondriasis, simple, social phobia and obsessive–compulsive disorder, mania and psychotic as well as eating disorders. It is noteworthy that the CIDI-PMC has not yet been updated for DSM–IV.

Mental health service and outcome measures

In addition to the information gathered by the standard CIDI, the CIDI-PMC allows for:

- the derivation of syndrome and symptom counts, which can be compared over time
- the monitoring of changes in specific symptoms over time
- the evaluation of subthreshold conditions as well as changes between subthreshold and threshold status.

Thus the researcher can directly compare changes in current symptoms between different examinations and monitor changes over time for each of the key syndromes. No corresponding changes were implemented for the CIDI psychosocial impairment questions, because this study used a generic dimensional disability measure, the Disability Assessment Schedule (Üstün & Sartorius, 1995).

Munich CIDI (M-CIDI)

Characteristics

The M-CIDI (Lachner *et al*, 1998; Wittchen *et al*, 1998*a*) was the first DSM–IV CIDI version, and was designed as a much more comprehensive modularised 'toolbox', giving users a high degree of flexibility in terms of choices for diagnostic sections and modules. Still maintaining comparability with the ICD–10 diagnostic criteria of CIDI versions 1.2 and 2.0, various procedural modifications were implemented, such as:

- the use of several respondent lists to reduce the administration time and to take advantage of cognitive probes (comparable to the UM-CIDI)
- the use of dimensional lifetime ratings for psychosocial impairments and disabilities for each diagnosis, instead of the categorical ratings
- the use of specific current (four weeks) psychosocial impairment ratings for each diagnosis, allowing an evaluation of the degree of impairment with regard to work, household, study, leisure activities and interpersonal aspects, as well as standard disability days questions, identical to those used in the UM-CIDI
- the possibility of directly relating the symptom assessed to one specific episode in time, including current syndromes, which allows the determination of several course and severity specifiers for many key syndromes covered
- a separate module to assess lifetime and past-year service utilisation of a wide range of specific providers, in addition to the standard CIDI diagnosis-specific questions (Wittchen *et al*, 1998*b*)
- a mental health treatment module describing for which condition what type of treatment was provided (Wittchen *et al*, 1999*a*).

In addition, three compatible interview versions are available: lifetime assessment (M-CIDI-LT), past 12 months (M-CIDI-12 month) and an interval version (M-CIDI-Int) for flexible time intervals to assess incidence and changes in symptoms over time. Each version permits the computation of current diagnoses and symptom counts (see Table 13.2, pp. 222–223). M-CIDI differs from previous versions in the following respects: coverage of DSM–IV criteria, coverage of a wider spectrum of diagnoses (post-traumatic stress disorder, subtypes of disorders, organic anxiety and depressive disorders) as well as various subthreshold conditions. Because of the greater complexity of the M-CIDI, the use of the CAPI M-CIDI is recommended, known as the DIA-X-M-CIDI, which is available in various languages.

Unlike other CIDI versions, the computerised DIA-X-M-CIDI is constructed in a modular way so that users can choose their optimal configurations in terms of sections that can be skipped completely and the choice of additional scales and instruments that might be of interest for a specific research project. In an initial entry menu, the user is prompted to make choices from the 'toolbox menu'; the computer program then automatically configures the interview accordingly, ensuring that all diagnostically relevant standard questions and sections are still available and given prompts. This change was made in response to the fact that the vast majority of users in the past did not use the full CIDI core, but rather restricted themselves to certain sections, to reduce time and resources.

Mental health service and outcome measures

Both the lifetime and the 12-month versions of the M-CIDI are specifically designed for follow-up studies of mental disorders, as well as to measure a change in status over time. In addition to all the above-mentioned options (diagnoses, age of onset and finish, duration, frequency, impairment and help seeking) the M-CIDI also includes the following features:

- the measurement of 12-month cross-sectional symptom counts, including severity for selected somatoform syndromes, panic, generalised anxiety disorder, social and agoraphobia, post-traumatic stress disorder, expressive and psychotic disorders as well as substance use disorders.
- the assessment of impairments specific to the current disorder, related to those of each disorder, with one generic measure for the peak of illness severity as well as more specific measures (work, household management, leisure time and social interaction) relating to the past four weeks (Wittchen *et al*, 1999*b*)

- a fuller description of illness course, by providing standardised age-at-onset information for symptoms, syndromes and full diagnoses, the determination of peak episodes (when symptoms were at their worst) for many conditions, the recency of each threshold and subthreshold condition, along with information about remission, number and length of episodes and persistence (graphic course patterns for three-month intervals may also be evaluated and computed)
- the addition of a lay person's version of the Brief Psychiatric Rating Scale, to measure the current severity of several psychopathological syndromes.

It is noteworthy that the M-CIDI can be combined with questionnaires that are compatible with the interview. Three scales developed from the M-CIDI methodological studies are available, for screening purposes: the Anxiety Screening Questionnaire (ASQ; Wittchen & Boyer, 1998), the Depression Screening Questionnaire (DSQ; Wittchen *et al*, 2000) and the Stress Screening Questionnaire (SSQ; Wittchen & Pfister, 1997) can be used in an initial screening before starting the M-CIDI interview. This may considerably shorten the average administration time of 65 minutes.

CIDI 2000

Background and characteristics

The WHO is carrying out a landmark international survey on the epidemiology of mental disorders in the year 2000, known as the World Mental Health 2000 (WMH2000) project (Kessler, 1999) (more information on CIDI 2000 and the WMH2000 initiative can be obtained from www.hcp.med.harvard.edu/icpe). Close to 200 000 respondents will be interviewed in general population surveys carried out in over 20 countries throughout the world. The CIDI has been revised for this purpose in a number of ways. Both hard-copy and computer-administered versions of the instrument, CIDI 2000, are available for use by other investigators.

CIDI 2000 elaborates upon the earlier CIDI by incorporating the best of the innovations in earlier versions (the CIDI-PMC, UM-CIDI, and M-CIDI) as well as in the most recent version of the DIS. There are four of these, involving the assessment of course of illness, 12-month persistence and severity, comparative functional impairments, and service use.

Course of illness. Earlier versions of the CIDI, with the exception of the M-CIDI, were weak in their assessment of lifetime course. CIDI

2000 has rectified this problem by including a series of parallel questions for each diagnostic section on illness course. Included here are questions on the number of years between the age of onset and age of recency when the disorder was active, and, for episodic disorders, the number of lifetime episodes. Similar questions in the M-CIDI and DIS were the model for this series of questions.

Twelve-month persistence and severity. Critics of earlier versions of the CIDI complained that it was impossible to determine the clinical significance of recent disorders because no information was included on recent persistence or severity (Regier *et al*, 1998). This problem has been rectified in CIDI 2000 by the inclusion of detailed, disorder-specific data of this sort. The 12-month persistence data assess the number of weeks in the past 12 months when each disorder was active. The severity data consist of structured versions of standard clinical severity measures (e.g. the Hospital Anxiety and Depression scale for generalised anxiety disorder and major depression, and the Liebowitz Social Anxiety Scale for social anxiety disorder).

Functional impairments. A related concern of critics is that earlier versions of the CIDI lacked detailed assessments of role impairments. This information is necessary to evaluate the clinical importance of disorders. CIDI 2000 includes a series of disorder-specific questions in each diagnostic section to evaluate the impact of 12-month disorders on functioning in family, work and social roles. In order to increase the breadth of comparison among the disorders, CIDI 2000 also includes a checklist of chronic physical conditions. The same disorder-specific questions about functional impairment are administered about a series of randomly selected chronic physical disorders for each respondent, making it possible to obtain data on the comparative impacts of mental and physical disorders. CIDI 2000 also includes the WHO Disability Assessment Schedule (WHO-DAS; Üstün & Chatterji, 1998), which asks about recent difficulties in functioning due to any health problem rather than to one particular disorder. By using statistical analysis to predict WHO-DAS scores from information about morbidities and comorbidities among the wide range of mental and physical disorders assessed in the instrument, it will be possible to evaluate the effects of mental disorders in mediating the impact of physical disorders on functioning as well as to evaluate the effects of comorbidity on functioning.

Service use. CIDI 2000 includes an expanded set of questions on help-seeking. Although the vast majority of CIDI surveys carried out since the CIDI was first released in 1990 have included questions on service use, no previous WHO version of the CIDI contained a standardised series of questions about service use or about the help-seeking process. This has limited comparative analyses of the help-seeking process in cross-national comparative studies based on CIDI surveys (Alegria *et al*, 2000; International Consortium of Psychiatric Epidemiology, 2000).

The new services questions included in CIDI 2000 are of several types. There are disorder-specific questions about delays in initial help-seeking after incident episodes of particular disorders. These questions are based on questions included in the UM-CIDI. There are more general questions about patterns of lifetime and 12-month help-seeking for emotional problems and substance use problems that include details regarding sector, number of visits, duration of visits and content of therapies (e.g. names and dosages of medications). Also, there are questions about barriers to seeking care, reasons for not seeking care and reasons for treatment drop-out.

Summary and outlook

The various versions of the CIDI discussed above were not specifically designed for measuring outcome. As a primarily epidemiological diagnostic instrument, along with the operation-alised and explicit criteria of DSM and ICD, the strength of the CIDI lies in its reliability and validity as a diagnostic instrument, and in its ease of administration even by trained non-clinicians. Although measurement of syndrome change is possible with at least some of the CIDI variations, this is not its main purpose. Hence, for the vast majority of researchers interested in outcome and mental health service evaluation more specific interview questions or questionnaires are needed to supplement the CIDI. However, taking the M-CIDI and the CIDI 2000 as examples, this situation seems likely to change.

This chapter has described several useful and unique options in each of the CIDI variants. In particular, the more recent modifications made in the M-CIDI and more comprehensively in the CIDI 2000 constitute considerable expansions and improvements of the rather crude measurements that have been possible with the CIDI core. The WHO advisory group that supervises and coordinates the develop-ment of the CIDI has recently acknowledged the emerging trend to favour cross-sectional and dimensional measures as well as the modular approach (adopted in the CIDI toolbox). The group is currently exploring various options for the further development and refinement of this approach.

References

ALEGRIA, M., KESSLER, R. C., BIJL, R., *et al* (2000). Comparing mental health service use data across countries. In *Unmet Need in Mental Health Service Delivery* (ed. G. Andrews), pp. 97–118. Cambridge: Cambridge University Press.

AMERICAN PSYCHIATRIC ASSOCIATION (1987) *Diagnostic and Statistical Manual of Mental Disorders* (3rd edn, revised) (DSM–III–R). Washington, DC: APA.

—— (1994) *Diagnostic and Statistical Manual of Mental Disorders* (4th edn) (DSM–IV). Washington, DC: APA.

ANDREWS, G., MORRIS-YATES, A., PETERS, L., *et al* (1993) *CIDI-Auto. Administrator's Guide and Reference, Version 1.1.* Sydney: Training and Reference Center for the WHO.

——, ——, ——, *et al* (1998) *CIDI-Auto. Administrator's Guide and Reference, Version 2.0.* Sydney: Training and Reference Center for the WHO.

INTERNATIONAL CONSORTIUM OF PSYCHIATRIC EPIDEMIOLOGY (2000) Cross-national comparisons of the prevalences and correlates of mental disorders: results from the WHO International Consortium of Psychiatric Epidemiology. *Bulletin of the World Health Organization,* **78**, 413–426.

KESSLER, R. C. (1999) The World Health Organization International Consortium in Psychiatric Epidemiology (ICPE): initial work and future directions – the NAPE lecture 1998. *Acta Psychiatrica Scandinavica,* **99**, 2–9.

——, MCGONAGLE, K. A., ZHAO, S., *et al* (1994) Lifetime and 12-month prevalence of DSM–III–R psychiatric disorders in the United States: results from the National Comorbidity Survey. *Archives of General Psychiatry,* **51**, 8–19.

——, SONNEGA, A., BROMET, E., *et al* (1995) Posttraumatic stress disorder in the National Comorbidity Survey. *Archives of General Psychiatry,* **52**, 1048–1060.

——, OLFSON, M. & BERGLUND, P. A. (1998) Patterns and predictors of treatment contact after first onset of psychiatric disorders. *American Journal of Psychiatry,* **155**, 62–69.

——, DUPONT, R. L., BERGLUND, P., *et al* (1999) Impairment in pure and comorbid generalized anxiety disorder and major depression at 12 months in two national surveys. *American Journal of Psychiatry,* **156**, 1663–1678.

LACHNER, G., WITTCHEN, H.-U., PERKONIGG, A., *et al* (1998) Structure, content and reliability of the Munich-Composite International Diagnostic Interview (M-CIDI). Substance use sections. *European Addiction Research,* **4**, 28–41.

REGIER, D. A., KAELBER, C. T., RAE, D. S., *et al* (1998) Limitations of diagnostic criteria and assessment instruments for mental disorders: implications for research and policy. *Archives of General Psychiatry,* **55**, 109–115.

ROBINS, L. N., HELZER, J. E., CROUGHAN, J., *et al* (1981) National Institute of Mental Health Diagnostic Interview Schedule: its history, characteristics and validity. *Archives of General Psychiatry,* **38**, 381–389.

ÜSTÜN, T. B. & SARTORIUS, N. (1995) *Mental Illness in General Health Care. An International Study.* Chichester: Wiley.

—— & CHATTERJI, S. (1998) Editorial. Measuring functioning and disability – a common framework. *International Journal of Methods in Psychiatric Research,* **7**, 79–83.

WING, J. K., COOPER, J. E. & SARTORIUS, N. (1974) *Measurement and Classification of Psychiatric Symptoms.* London: Cambridge University Press.

WITTCHEN, H-U. (1994) Reliability and validity studies of the WHO-Composite International Diagnostic Interview (CIDI): a critical review. *Journal of Psychiatric Research,* **28**, 57–84.

—— & KESSLER, R. C. (1994) *Modification of the CIDI in the National Comorbidity Survey: The Development of the UM-CIDI.* NCS Working Paper 2. Ann Arbor: Institute of Social Research, University of Michigan.

—— & PFISTER, H. (eds) (1997) *DIA-X-Interviews: Manual für Screening-Verfahren und Interview; Interviewheft Längsschnittuntersuchung (DIA-X-Lifetime); Ergänzungsheft (DIA-X-Lifetime);*

Interviewheft Querschnittuntersuchung (DIA-X-12 Monate); Ergänzungsheft (DIA-X-12Monate); PC-Programm zur Durchführung des Interviews (Längs- und Querschnittuntersuchung); Auswertungsprogramm. Frankfurt: Swets & Zeitlinger.

—— & Boyer, P, (1998) Screening for anxiety disorders. Sensitivity and specificity of the Anxiety Screening Questionnaire (ASQ–15). *British Journal of Psychiatry*, **173** (suppl. 34), 10–17.

——, Lachner, G., Wunderlich, U., *et al* (1998a) Test–retest reliability of the computerized DSM–IV version of the Munich-Composite International Diagnostic Interview (M–CIDI). *Social Psychiatry and Psychiatric Epidemiology*, **33**, 568–578.

——, —— & Storz, S. (1998b) Psychische Störungen: Häufigkeit, psychosoziale Beeinträchtigungen und Zusammenhänge mit körperlichen Erkankungen. *Das Gesundheitswesen*, **60** (suppl. 2), 95–100.

——, Üstün, B. & Kessler, R. C. (1999a) Diagnosing mental disorders in the community. A difference that matters? *Psychological Medicine*, **29**, 1021–1027.

——, Müller, N., Pfister, H., *et al* (1999b) Affektive, somatoforme und Angststörungen in Deutschland. Erste Ergebnisse des bundesweiten Zusatzsurveys "Psychische Störungen". *Das Gesundheitswesen*, **61**, 216–222.

——, Höfler, M., & Meister, W. (2000) *Depressionen in der Allgemeinpraxis. Die bundesweite Depressionsstudie.* Stuttgart: Schattauer Verlag.

World Health Organization (1990) *Composite International Diagnostic Interview (CIDI).* Geneva: WHO.

—— (1993) *The ICD–10 Classification of Mental and Behavioural Disorders – Diagnostic Criteria for Research.* Geneva: WHO.

14 Assessment instruments in psychiatry: description and psychometric properties

L. SALVADOR-CARULLA and D. SALAS

Basic concepts

Assessment may be defined as the process of applying a systematic method to describing phenomena or objects. Its degree of systematisation may vary widely, from merely assigning pre-established codes to algorithmic quantification systems. Assessment may be subjective or objective. Subjective assessment is characterised by the description of hypothetical or intangible elements (e.g. quality of life, depression), as opposed to the tangible entities described by the experimental sciences, such as weight or height, that is, objective assessment. In the health sciences, this differentiation is not always very clear, since there is a great deal of individual discretion in the interpretation of complex complementary evidence (e.g. histology, imaging diagnosis, neurophysiology). This means that many quality norms are the same for objective and subjective instruments. Subjective assessment is less precise, and has been under-valued until very recently. The growing demand for intangible parameters – such as satisfaction, support, autonomy, quality of life and level of disability – has determined that the use of these instruments is currently essential in any health care field.

Assessment may also be qualitative or quantitative. Qualitative assessment describes in words rather than numbers the qualities of phenomena through observation, unstructured interviews and a series of qualitative research techniques (Bowling, 1997). On the other hand, quantitative assessment consists of elaborating rules to assign numbers to a given phenomenon, with the aim of quantifying one or more of its attributes. These rules are a codified series of procedures for assigning numbers. When assessing a certain phenomenon, it is important to situate it within a categorical or dimensional model, and in the latter case to delimit whether it is uni- or multi-dimensional.

Assessment instruments comprise a variable number of items. An item is the basic information unit of an assessment instrument, and usually consists of a question – generally a closed question – and an answer, which can be assigned a code. The glossary is an additional list of explanatory notes regarding the precise definition of each item, and how to combine them in categories or dimensions (Strömgren, 1988).

Bases for description and classification of assessment instruments

Bech *et al* (1993) proposed a description of assessment scales based on the scales' objectives and composition:

- assessment area – diagnostic, symptomatic and personality scales and scales for other specific purposes
- type of administration – scales for the patient, the doctor and other health care staff
- retrospective time access – time frame of the assessment
- selection of items – distinguishes among first-generation scales (based on clinical experience) and second-generation scales (derived from the former)
- number of items on the scale
- definition of individual items.

The work of other authors (such as Thompson, 1989*a*; Streiner & Norman, 1996; Badia *et al*, 1999) has led to modifications of Bech's original proposal to permit a more complete description of the different instruments used in mental health. In general terms, the classification is based on instruments' complexity, purpose (condition assessed, population of reference, assessment period, etc.) and construction (structure, composition of its items, and the prevention of potential bias in its completion). These changes in terminology with respect to that used by Bech are detailed below.

Complexity

Assessment instruments may be classified in a series of groupings, according to their complexity. *Descriptive questionnaires* (e.g. socio-demographic questionnaires) may be situated in the first group, as well as symptom inventories (e.g. inventories of adverse effects). The items on these instruments cannot be quantified, so they may be considered merely checklists.

On a second level are the *rating scales*. As their name indicates, their items can be accumulatively scaled, generating overall scores at the end of the assessment. They are composed of individual items, each one describing a well-defined characteristic of the phenomenon being assessed. Their accumulative nature differentiates them from data collection questionnaires and simple symptoms inventories.

On a third level are the *standardised interviews*. These are classified by their objectives (general or specific) and according to the level of training required for their administration. The latter depends on how structured they are as far as formulating the questions and codifying the answers are concerned (the more structured the interview, the less experience interviewers need to administer it). Standardised interviews may be accompanied by a computerised correction system for assigning diagnostic criteria.

Standardised diagnostic systems constitute a fourth level. They provide a codification of nosological entities, with a detailed description of each one of them in a glossary, to make diagnosis easier. Diagnostic systems are called operational when they provide a series of rules for diagnosis based on inclusion criteria (presence of a minimum number of characteristics of the phenomenon for its diagnosis) and exclusion criteria (casting off other characteristics unrelated to the phenomenon). When the exclusion criteria refer to the presence of other syndrome-related entities, the system is considered hierarchical, since it imposes a hierarchical structure on the nosological entities included in the system for their differential diagnosis. If the standardised diagnostic system also allows for the codification of various entities or aspects related in different axes, it is considered a multi-axial system. There are two principal systems of hierarchical and multi-axial operative diagnosis currently in use: the ICD–10 research system (World Health Organization, 1993) and DSM–IV (American Psychiatric Association, 1994). According to some authors, diagnostic systems should not be considered assessment instruments. However, in their construction and use, diagnostic systems fit into the general rules of standardised subjective evaluation (see Muthen *et al*, 1993*a,b*; Room *et al*, 1996).

Composite assessment batteries may be placed on the next level. These are sets of different instruments (e.g. a data collection questionnaire, assessment scales incorporated into a battery, a standardised interview on past symptoms and/or current state, and a computerised system for multiple diagnoses, which allows for diagnostic codification according to different systems). Examples of compound batteries are the Schedules for the Assessment of Neuropsychiatry (SCAN; Pull &

Wittchen, 1991; Vazquez-Barquero, 1993), and the Comprehensive Assessment of Symptoms and History (CASH) battery for assessment of schizophrenia and mood disorders (Andreasen *et al*, 1992).

Clinical information systems comprise a whole array of automated instruments designed for handling databases (Mezzich, 1986).

Purpose of a scale

The purpose of a scale will determine the content of its items and different aspects related to its structure. A scale should always limit itself to the area for which it has been designed, at least until it can be standardised. The purpose is related to the dimension being assessed, the population under study, the assessment period and how the scale is filled out.

Area to be assessed

The different psychosocial scales assess a wide range of areas, such as symptoms (clinical scales), personality, social, family, sexual and vocational functioning or disability. Bech *et al* (1993) make a distinction between two types of clinical scale: diagnostic and symptomatic. This distinction, however, is not precise, since there are symptomatic scales that have been used for diagnosis (and vice versa) after calculating cut-off points by means of a predictive validity study (see under Quality parameters of assessment instruments, below). (The various scales given as examples below are discussed and referenced by Bech *et al*, 1993.)

Objective of the study

It is important to differentiate between general scales (e.g. for evaluating psychiatric 'caseness') and specific scales (e.g. for the evaluation of depression). Specific scales may focus on different stages of levels of a given disease, such as the Hamilton Rating Scale for Depression (HRSD), for the assessment of major depression, and the Newcastle scale, for the assessment of endogenous depression).

Wittchen & Essau (1990) distinguish between scales based on a 'wide' or 'restrictive' concept of mental disorder. The most restrictive instruments value specificity over sensitivity and vice versa (this factor is particularly important in the use of standardised diagnostic systems).

Time frame

According to the stability of the phenomenon under assessment, we can differentiate between *trait scales*, which assess phenomena that are relatively stable over time (e.g. personality tests, locus of control), and *status scales*, which assess the subject's current situation (such as depression or positive and negative symptoms), usually during the previous month, the previous week or few weeks, or during the three days before the assessment ('here and now' scales). The time frame should be detailed in the instructions for administering the scale.

In status scales, the assessment period is what differentiates *detection scales*, for example for identifying psychiatric cases, such as the General Health Questionnaire (GHQ), from *follow-up scales. Non-transitional* follow-up scales, such as the HRSD, assess change based on the difference in the score from one assessment to another; *transitional* follow-up scales, such as the Clinical Global Impression change scale (CGI), assess the degree of improvement or worsening experienced by the patient between the two assessments. When using a follow-up scale, it is important to know its sensitivity to change.

Type of administration

Self-administered scales are designed to be filled out by the subject, or by an informant. Sometimes they include items to calibrate the validity of the answers based on a tendency to dissimulate or simulate (e.g. the Eysenck's Personality Questionnaire, EPQ). Bech *et al* (1993) call this group of instruments "questionnaires"; however, this term is too general.

Interviewer-administered scales (which Bech *et al* termed "observer scales") are filled out by an examiner. Such instruments require different degrees of professional training for their use (this factor is particularly important in designing and administering structured interviews). These scales require a previous standardisation of raters by means of an analysis of their agreement with an examiner of reference (see under Reliability, below). Two extremes in the application of interviewer-administered scales have been pointed out: an *alpha situation* (expert rater who carries out a closed interview and uses a scale with a few well-defined items, and which includes criteria of improvement and health), and a *beta situation* (unskilled rater, who conducts an open-ended interview and uses a scale with many poorly defined items, and without criteria of improvement and health) (Bech *et al*, 1993).

Some clinical assessment instruments are of a mixed type, including one section for reported symptoms and another for symptoms observed during the interview.

Construction of assessment scales

As mentioned above, the item is the basic information unit of an assessment instrument, and generally consists of a closed question and its answer.

Number of items

Scales may be divided into two types: unitary or global scales, composed of a single item (e.g., CGI, Global Assessment Scale, analogue scales of pain or well-being); and multi-item scales. As a general rule, it is agreed that a phenomenon should be assessed with a minimum of six items (Bech *et al*, 1993). Scales generally consist of 10–90 items. Different scales are available in different versions: Goldberg's GHQ in versions with 60, 30, 28, and 12 items; the HRSD in versions with 21 or 17 items (in addition to other scales derived from this test).

Content of the items

Uni-dimensional and multi-dimensional scales are differentiated by their content. On a uni-dimensional scale, more than 80% of the items evaluate a single dimension, in accordance with Israel's model (Israel *et al*, 1983). For example, McGill's Pain Questionnaire evaluates the physical dimension (symptoms related to somatic or medical aspects), the Beck Depression Inventory evaluates psychic dimensions (cognitive aspects) and the Activities of Daily Living Index (ADL) evaluates the social dimension. With multi-dimensional scales (e.g. the GHQ or HRSD), the items assess two or three of these dimensions. With interviewer-administered scales, there is also a distinction made between the items reported by the patient and those observed by the interviewer.

The item bias or its orientation refers to the part of the syndrome that appears best reflected in the scale. This is represented by a percentage of the maximum theoretical score for each category of symptoms (Thompson, 1989*a*). For example, the HRSD has an item bias for the somatic symptoms of depression.

Definitions

The definition of items should be exhaustive and mutually exclusive (Guilford's criteria; see Bech *et al*, 1993). The following aspects should be considered when formulating the questions and alternative answers and when ordering the set of items that compose the scale.

Comprehension. The language and formulation of the questions and answers need to be adapted to the patient's socio-cultural environment. For example, comprehension of the use of linear analogues tends to be better in some cultural environments, while understanding of decimal numeric analogues is better in others. There are different indices for assessing the comprehensibleness of a text (e.g. Flesch's Index for English) (Thompson, 1989*a*). The problem of

comprehension is extremely important in assessing specific populations, such as the mentally retarded. On the other hand, the
translation and adaptation of a scale previously developed in another
language, for another cultural context, should follow a specific
procedure, including the process of back-translation. Recently, more
complex systems have been applied, such as conceptual translation
(see below).

Cultural acceptability. It is fundamental that the items be acceptable
to the subject under evaluation. Social desirability is a type of
potential bias that can alter the validity of the answers given (Wittchen
& Essau, 1990). This should be taken into account when formulating
questions for certain items (this type of bias is important in assessing
attitudes regarding certain illnesses, such as AIDS and mental
retardation, because the subject tends to give the most socially
acceptable answers). It is also necessary to limit the number of items,
to avoid fatigue and to encourage the subject's collaboration (this
problem is evident on questionnaires or batteries with more than
100 items, such as the Minnesota Multiphasic Personality Inventory,
MMPI).

Preventing bias in completion. Acquiescence (the tendency to
answer a question affirmatively) requires that alternate questions
be formulated 'positively' and 'negatively'. However, this may
significantly diminish the patient's comprehension, as well as the
reliability of the answers (e.g. items such as 'It is untrue that
Columbus sailed to America – T/F' may easily confound patients
with low attention span). 'Central tendency error' refers to the
reluctance to choose the extreme alternatives in an item, giving
preference to the central ones. This problem mainly affects verbal
analogue scales with three or five alternatives (e.g., None, Some,
A lot). Another type of bias is related to the tendency to answer
more with the alternatives situated to the right or to the left, and
this bias increases when one of the two extremes always contains
the 'desirable' alternatives. This can be avoided by alternating
which side the positive alternatives are on.

When an interviewer-administered scale is designed, different types
of specific biases should be kept in mind. The 'halo effect' refers to
the tendency to make a judgement at the beginning of the interview
(e.g. heuristic diagnosis), which influences how the following items
are filled out. This can happen when completing the HRSD, which
groups items directly related with depression and severity at the
beginning of the interview. The halo effect is important in the
assessment of comorbidity with those instruments that use a single
evaluator (Buchanan & Carpenter, 1994). 'Logical error' occurs in
all those items that are apparently related and scored in a similar

way (thus, it may be assumed that a patient with a high score on 'suicidal ideation' will also have a high score on 'hopelessness'). 'Proximity error' leads the rater to score adjoining items in a similar way. Another source of error is 'terminology variance', and is due to the attribution of different meanings to the same term. This problem may have a marked effect on clinical scales, given the different interpretations of a term according to an evaluator's psycho-pathological orientation or background knowledge. This bias can be avoided by including an appendix with a glossary, as is done with the Brief Psychiatric Rating Scale (BPRS).

Selection, analysis and ordering of the items

Meehl & Golden (1982) described a series of principles or steps in the construction of a symptoms assessment scale:

1   Select the items based on their clinical relevance and validity.
2   Select the items based on their internal correlation when they are applied to a mixed group of patients (one which includes patients with and without the assessed symptom).
3   Select items with different hierarchical weights (describing different aspects of the phenomenon assessed); that is, they should not be redundant.
4   All things being equal, select items with the greatest potential for consensus.
5   Check the results of the group of items selected based on different external criteria (age, gender, etc.), in order to assess their transferability.
6   When steps 3, 4 and 5 cannot be carried out, repeat the analysis with modified items regarding definition or content.

Items can also be selected based on their usefulness. This is assessed in accordance with three criteria (Thompson, 1989*b*):

- *calibration* – sufficient frequency of replies on an individual item in the population being tested in order to guarantee its inclusion in the scale (arbitrarily this can be fixed at 10%)
- *ascending monotonicity* – significant correlation of each item with the global assessment
- *dispersion* – low dispersion with regard to the line of regression of the above correlation.

There are various models for the psychometric analysis of items (Garcia-Cueto, 1993; Martinez-Arias, 1995). Classical test theory (CTT) is a psychometric model that describes the influence of measurement errors on the scores observed for an individual. The true score for a given variable is defined as that which really corresponds to an individual. However, when something is measured with any instrument, a measurement error is always made, which gives rise to a difference between the true (theoretical) score and the observed score. The CTT is based on a mathematically acceptable definition of the true score that is conceptually usable and makes certain basic suppositions which relate the true score to measurement error.

Item response theory (IRT), or latent trait theory, attempts to specify the relationship between a subject's 'observable' score in a test, and the 'latent traits' which it is assumed lie behind these scores. The models are uni- or multi-dimensional, depending on the set of latent traits necessary to explain the behaviour under study. Although the IRT considers two more parameters to be kept in mind when studying the psychometric characteristics of a test, namely getting the right answer by chance and by false positives, both are complementary for the analysis and construction of a test. The process of constructing an assessment scale composed of binary items may begin with the use of total–item correlation indices of the classic test model, followed by an analysis of its latent structure using Rasch's model[1]. Thus it is possible to establish the relationship between observable scores and latent traits by means of manifest answers and the latent dimension (Andersen *et al*, 1989).

Generalisability theory (GT) uses a set of techniques for studying the degree to which a series of measures from a group of subjects can be generalised (i.e. extended to a different group of subjects). GT takes into account the multiple factors that can produce variations in subjects' scores by means of applying a multivariate design. This makes it possible to estimate the variance attributable to each one of them, as well as their interactions. By diversifying the measurement conditions, it increases the representativeness (generalisability) of the results. It also facilitates the design of measurement procedures in which the confounding factors are represented (Muñiz, 1992).

---

[1] In the Rasch model the sample is split into two groups, one comprising individuals with predominantly low answers, the other those with predominantly high answers. For each group, a set of item parameters expressing the likelihood that the items will produce high answers is calculated. If the item parameters for the two groups are in close agreement, the items and individuals can be characterised on their own. This characteristic makes it meaningful to regard the individual's parameters as a measure of the phenomenon described in the rating scale (Rasch, 1980; Lund, 1989).

Factor analysis enables investigators to check the uni- or multi-dimensional structure of an instrument. It is more generally applied to instruments that have already been constructed or to new versions of them, rather than to the construction of new instruments, and so it is discussed in more detail below, under 'Consistency'.

System of answers codification

Dichotomous categorical scales comprise a series of questions with two possible answers: yes/no or true/false. Examples are personality tests such as the EPQ and the MMPI.

Analogue scales can be differentiated, on the basis of the analogue system used for the answer, into five different types.

First, on a linear analogue scale ranking, say of pain or well-being, is done on a line 7–10 cm long.

Not at all sad	As sad as I have ever been

Second, on analogue numerical scales ranking is similar to that of analogue scales except that numbers are used (from 0 to 7 or 10). With thermometric unitary scales, the numbers are arranged vertically. These may be graded from 0 to 100, as is done on the General Assessment of Functioning scale (GAF). Sometimes, visual and numerical analogues are combined to increase comprehension.

Not at all sad 0 1 2 3 4 5 6 7 8 9 As sad as I have ever been

Third, on graphic scales ranking is by means of drawings, as is done on the Face scale for the assessment of well-being. Some authors consider graphic scales to be linear.

Fourth, on verbal analogue scales ranking is done using previously calibrated verbal categories (e.g. by means of Guttman's escalation system), such as:

No more than usual	Somewhat less than usual	Somewhat more than usual	Much more than usual

Generally, the response options range between three and seven. Likert considered five to be the optimal number of alternatives. Goldberg preferred to use four options to avoid central tendency bias. It is generally agreed that with more than six options the level of reliability diminishes significantly. Severity scales use more options than detection scales (e.g. the CGI has seven, while the GHQ has four). These scales are also called Likert scales, in honour of the man who introduced them 60 years ago

(Bech *et al*, 1986). However, a specific scoring system bears the same name, so this usage can be confusing.

Fifth, categorical analogue scales comprise a series of scales which combine numeric and verbal ranking (e.g. the CGI and GAF) (Bech *et al*, 1986). They are also known as discretised analogues scales (DISCAN).

1	2	3	4	5	6	7	8	9
	No more than usual		Somewhat less than usual		Somewhat more than usual		Much more than usual	

Scoring the items

The scoring system can vary substantially from one scale to another and even within the same scale, in the case of verbal analogue scales.

Unitary scales of severity (non-transitional) tend to have a maximum score of 8 or 10 when dealing with verbal analogues or other combined forms (DISCAN). The GAF can be scored up to 99, but it really presents 10 degrees of response in decimals.

Unitary global scales of a transitional type are generally bipolar, allowing for a positive or negative score (from greater worsening to greater improvement):

$-3/-2/-1/0/1/2/3$

For technical reasons, they can also be scored from 1 to 7, although the scale's polarity may not be adequately reflected in this approach.

$1/2/3/4/5/6/7$

Multi-item verbal scales allow for different numerical assignations. Thus, Goldberg's GHQ permits three different scorings: two are based on the system originally proposed by Likert in the 1930s, and the other was proposed by Goldberg himself. The HRSD and the Scales for the Assessment of Positive and Negative Symptoms are scored in accordance with a system (proposed by Hamilton) that differentiates between the options of absent (0), doubtful (1) and different degrees of intensity (from 2 to 4 or 5).

Goldberg	0–0–2–2
Likert I	0–1–2–3
Likert II	0–0–1–2
Hamilton	0–1–2–3–4

Quality parameters of assessment instruments

There are four basic parameters for assessing the quality of an assessment instrument: its feasibility; its consistency or 'structural validity'; its reliability; and its validity. For follow-up scales, a fifth should be added: sensitivity to change. Other parameters to consider are construction, adequacy, redundancy and transcultural applicability. Unfortunately, there is no consensus on a definition of these terms in epidemiology; their meaning varies from common use, varies among different areas of study and even varies between authors within the same area. Furthermore, different dimensions may be assigned to more than one parameter. Several guidelines for assessing the quality of assessment instruments have been published, particularly in quality-of-life research (Burke, 1998; Marquis, 1998). Badia *et al* (1999) use an 11-item checklist that produces a global rating for assessing the level of an instrument's development (the GRAQoL index). An 'Assessment instrument quality checklist' is given as an appendix to this chapter.

Adequacy

Adequacy addresses the suitability of a particular instrument to the purpose of a specific assessment procedure (i.e. in routine clinical practice, in research or in outcome management). Adequacy is not related to the intrinsic properties of the scale, but to its applicability to a defined purpose for a distinct condition in a specific environment. Thus, adequacy should be valued separately from other quality parameters.

Construction

Several aspects of the instrument's construction should be taken into consideration for appraising its overall quality. It is important to assess whether the purpose of the scale is clearly defined, whether there is an accompanying glossary and an instruction manual that clarify the completion process, the time frame as well as the rater's requirements.

Feasibility

Feasibility has become a relevant issue owing to the increasing importance of routine outcome measures in health assessment (Salvador-Carulla, 1999). There is no consensus on how feasibility should be defined and measured. Slade *et al* (1999) have suggested a definition in the context of routine outcome assessment.

Andrews *et al* (1994) identified three dimensions of feasibility: applicability, acceptability, and practicality. The 'applicability' of a measure was defined as the degree to which it addresses dimensions of importance to the consumer, is useful for service providers in formulating and conducting decisions, and allows for the aggregation of data in a meaningful way to meet the purposes of service management. (This aspect, defined as 'relevance' by Slade *et al* (1999), may be framed as: 'Is the description meaningful to recipients, such as health authorities, managers, staff, patients/families?') The acceptability of a measure describes the ease with which a consumer or clinician can use a particular measure (i.e. user-friendliness). Practicality relates to implementation, training requirements, and complexity of scoring, reporting and interpreting the data.

Efficiency may be regarded as the fourth dimension of feasibility. It could be defined as the relationship between an instrument's practicality and the costs incurred by using it.

Consistency (structural validity or internal reliability)

Consistency comprises the psychometric solidity of a scale, its internal structure, the level to which its different items are interrelated and the possibility of adding them up to obtain overall scores. It has been defined as that "property which defines the level of agreement or conformity of a set of measurements among themselves" (Hernandez-Aguado *et al*, 1990). Some authors include consistency within the category of reliability (Thompson, 1989*b*; McDowell & Newell, 1996) or validity (Badia *et al*, 1999). To avoid such confusion, we distinguish here between the *internal consistency* and the *external reliability* of a test.

Some statistical methods, such as factor analysis, provide data both on the internal structure of a scale and on its relationship to external models. This is the case with the Scales for the Assessment of Positive and Negative Symptoms of schizophrenia, a factor analysis of which can serve to validate, revise or even refute the models on which the construction of the instrument itself is based (Liddle, 1987; Buchanan & Carpenter, 1994).

Many of the aspects related to consistency have been mentioned above in the context of selecting items or the hierarchy of their order. *Homogeneity* indicates the degree of agreement among the items on a scale, which determines whether they can accumulate and generate an overall score. It can be obtained by studying the correlation of the items with the total (split-half or Cronbach's alpha correlation), by factor analysis or by using Rasch's statistical objectivity models (Rasch, 1980). The split-half estimates the degree of homogeneity as the correlation between two equivalent halves of the scale (e.g. items from the first half versus items from the second half, or odd-numbered items versus even ones). Cronbach's alpha coefficient indicates the degree to which different items exhibit a positive correlation (internal consistency above 0.7 is considered adequate; Bech *et al*, 1993). Another test for calculating internal consistency, which is less often used, is the Kuder–Richardson test. Homogeneity based on factor analysis (acceptability of the global score as the sum of that obtained on each item) is confirmed if a uni-dimensional structure is obtained; that is, all the items show a positive load on the first factor (Thompson, 1989*b*).

In addition to exploratory factor techniques, such as principal-component analysis and principal-factor analysis, the structure of a scale can be assessed using other techniques, such as non-metric multi-dimensional scaling or structural equation analysis (Buchanan & Carpenter, 1994). Rasch's uni-dimensional model considers a scale to be homogeneous when all of its items contribute independently to the total information contained in the scale. In latent trait theory, the nexus between manifest (clinical) answers and their latent (theoretical) dimension is defined by the requirement that the answers can be combined by adding them until a total score is reached (Andersen *et al*, 1989). Rasch's model also makes it possible to study the internal hierarchy of a scale, classifying its homogeneous items in a hierarchy ranging from the most inclusive (those which measure the dimension's most severe symptoms).

The reproducibility coefficient indicates to what degree the scale reflects all of the subject's response patterns regarding the parameter measured. This concept is linked to the content validity (see below).

Transferability refers to the degree to which the scale can be applied to different population groups which present the evaluated phenomenon, independent of their age, gender or other relevant external criteria (Bech *et al*, 1993).

Reliability (external reliability)

Reliability indicates the degree to which the results of a test are reproducible. This depends on the stability of the test's measures, in spite of changes in different external parameters (i.e. that are not inherent in the test). It has been defined as the proportion of variance in a measurement that is not error variance, excluding errors related to consistency (attributable to the internal structure of the instrument). The study of external reliability will provide information about the reproducibility of the test's results in different situations.

A study on the reliability of a diagnostic test should include at least an analysis of the level of agreement obtained when the same sample is assessed under the same conditions by two different raters (interrater reliability). This has also been termed interobserver reliability. The importance of having evaluators with similar experience, as far as their training and use of the assessment instrument being analysed are concerned, has been pointed out. Andersen *et al* (1989) indicate other factors that differentiate between interobserver and intraobserver reliability, such as their attitudes about assessment scales and therapeutic preferences.

A measure of stability is obtained when the same sample is assessed by the same rater in different situations (test–retest reliability or intraobserver reliability). In some situations (e.g. child psychiatry or mental handicap), data are obtained from informants, making it necessary to analyse the agreement of the data obtained with the test using the same sample and the same evaluator, but collecting the data from two different informants (inter-informant reliability). The procedure for obtaining such information has been extensively reviewed by Costello (1994).

The statistical index used for evaluating concordance depends on the characteristics of the variables to be assessed. The use of Kendall's concordance coefficient (Siegel, 1966) in various studies is open to discussion. In the case of dichotomous or binary variables, item-by-item concordance can be analysed using the percentage agreement and unweighted kappa (Kramer & Feinstein, 1981). The kappa concordance coefficient reveals the level of agreement obtained, once concordance that was produced by chance has been eliminated. This makes it more reliable than a simple percentage agreement. However, the same kappa value can result from different response patterns. Therefore, it is also expedient to record the frequency of each item's appearance and its agreement percentage (Costello, 1994), as well as the confidence interval. Feinstein (1985) proposes the scheme shown in Table 14.1 for analysing kappa results.

In the case of ordinal variables, analysis of item-by-item concordance can be conducted using the weighted agreement percentage and the weighted kappa. These are considered better than their unweighted analogues, since they give a more realistic measure of the level of agreement. This is achieved by weighting disagreement according to the number of degrees separating the score assigned by one evaluator from that assigned by another. Thus, the assigned weight can be '0' for complete agreement, '1' when there is one degree of difference, '2' when there are two, and so on (Kramer & Feinstein, 1981).

The method for analysing the concordance of a test's overall score is controversial. Usually correlation coefficients are used to determine the degree of agreement. These coefficients should not be used to analyse concordance between two evaluations: the tendency can be perfect, with a correlation coefficient of 1 (Feinstein, 1985). In

TABLE 14.1
Feinstein's (1985) categorisation of kappa results

Kappa value	Level of agreement
<0	Poor
0–0.20	Low
0.21–0.40	Fair
0.41–0.60	Moderate
0.61–0.80	Strong
0.81–1.0	Almost perfect

continuous variables, the intraclass correlation coefficient (ICC) can be used (Bartko & Carpenter, 1976). Bech *et al* (1993) also proposed the use of the ICC to assess test–retest reliability when the data are collected by different evaluators, although this is a debatable application. There is currently no general agreement on the sample size required for reliability studies of scales (Bech *et al*, 1993).

Validity

Validity indicates what proportion of the information collected is relevant to the formulated question, and is defined by the degree to which an instrument measures what it is supposed to measure. It is considered present when the measurement predicts a criterion (criterion validity), or consistently fits a series of related constructs within the context of an accepted theory (construct validity) if there is no external criterion that serves as a 'gold standard' (Thiemann *et al*, 1987). There are several forms of validity, with the further complication that some authors use the same term to refer to different concepts. The six principal forms of validity can be distributed into two axes: one revolving around the presence or absence of a 'gold standard' for the dimension assessed (criterion validity versus construct validity), and the other focusing on whether mathematical techniques are used in their calculation (descriptive validity versus statistical validity). Thus, a certain type of validity can be considered of the criterion or the construct type, depending on the dimension assessed. Concurrent validity of a scale for service assessment forms part of criterion validity, whereas the concurrent validity for a quality-of-life scale, for which there is no 'gold standard', should be considered as part of its construct validity. Likewise, estimation of discriminant validity or convergent validity may be merely descriptive, or may involve the use of statistical procedures.

The absence of a conceptual framework has led to a notable degree of confusion in the definition and classification of different forms of validity. For example, concurrent and predictive validity are types of criterion validity according to some authors (Strang *et al*, 1989; Martinez-Arias, 1995); others consider them types of construct validity (Thompson, 1989*a*). In fact, the majority of psychological attributes and mental processes are intangible parameters, which cannot be measured directly (unlike, say, height or weight); therefore, they should be considered hypothetical constructs. However, it is accepted that many psychiatric constructs are close to a 'gold standard' (e.g. somatic symptoms of depression, anhedonia), while others cannot be compared with external criteria (e.g. quality of life, social integration).

Bearing in mind these considerations and exceptions, the principal types of validity of an assessment instrument are discussed under separate headings below.

Simple validity (face validity)

This is a type of descriptive criterion validity, and reflects what experts consider significant measures. There may be a certain amount of confusion between this concept and that of applicability. However, the latter refers to the judgement of a wide-ranging group of users (e.g. health care managers and clinicians) of the instrument or of the information derived from it, whereas the assessment of face validity is limited to the expert's opinion.

Content validity

This defines the degree to which the set of items on a test adequately represents the domain assessed, that is, the level of representativeness of the items of the set of components under assessment (Martinez-Arias, 1995). In reality, this concept does not differ much from that of consistency, so that they may be considered synonymous. According to Thompson (1989*a*), this type of validity is descriptive, and cannot be analysed using statistical techniques.

Discriminant validity

This refers to the degree to which an instrument measures those features belonging to one domain and not to others, as well as the degree to which the features of different domains are not included within the domain examined by the instrument (inclusion and exclusion discriminant validity). Discriminant validity may be assessed either descriptively or with statistical procedures.

Convergent validity

This refers to the assessment of a certain feature of a domain using two different methods (e.g. the assessment of depression using an assessment scale and a biological test). This term has also been used to denote the use of two assessment instruments, each covering a different dimension, in order to find a third (e.g. the use of clinical and functioning scales to study the validity of a quality-of-life scale).

Concurrent validity

This provides a measure of the association between the scores for different items and the overall scores for other reference scales with an equivalent purpose and content. It is generally limited to the study of inter-score correlation. Czobor *et al* (1991) suggested the use of canonical component analysis, a method which is an extension of factor analysis for two groups of variables. Although some authors have considered this type of validity as a form of construct validity, it actually constitutes one of the strategies used to assess the validity of a test in the absence of a 'gold standard'.

Predictive validity

Predictive validity refers to the probability that a scale will give a correct judgement of the observed phenomenon. The use of Bayes' analysis makes it possible to determine the predictive validity of a test, its utility and its comparability, based on an analysis of the distribution of 'cases' and 'non-cases' in a given population, as well as its relationship with the results obtained on the test under study (positive or negative). A 2×2 contingency table expresses this relationship in terms of true positives (TP), true negatives (TN), false positives (FP), and false negatives (FN). Table 14.2 defines the predictive validity coefficients obtained from the contingency table. Sensitivity (x) corresponds to the TP rate, and is defined by the rate of correct positive results on the test in relation to the total of true cases in the population assessed (TP/TP + FN). Specificity (y) corresponds to the rate of TN on the test among all of the non-cases (TN/TN + FP). Other measures related to the above are the FP rate ($1 - y$), the FN rate ($1 - x$) and Youden's index ($x + y - 1$).

Positive predictive value (PPV) corresponds to the quotient of TP results with regard to the total of positives (TP/TP + FP); negative predictive value (NPV) corresponds to the total of TN with regard to the total of negatives (TN/TN + FN). It is important to bear in mind

TABLE 14.2
Bayes' analysis and parameters of predictive validity
(modified from Baldessarini et al, 1988)

(A) Prevalence: 50% $(P = 0.5)$
Criterion reference (i.e. diagnosis – Dx)

		Present (P)	Absent (1 – P)
Test result	(+)	TP (a)	FP (b)
	(–)	FN (c)	TN (d)

Parameter	Definition	Computation	Symbol
Sensitivity	TP/All Dx	$a/(a + c)$	x
Specificity	TN/All no Dx	$d/(b + d)$	y
False positive rate	FP/All no Dx	$b/(b + d)$	$1 - y$
False negative rate	FN/All Dx	$c/(a + c)$	$1 - x$
Efficiency	TP+TN/All subjects	$(a + d)/n$	Ef
Positive predictive value	TP/TP + FP	$a/(a + b)$	PPV
Negative predictive value	TN/TN + FN	$d/(c + d)$	NPV
Error ratio	False results/TP	$(b + c)/a$	ER
Prevalence	All Dx/All subjects	$(a + c)/n$	P
'Well rate'	All no Dx/All subjects	$(b + d)/n$	$1 - P$
Youden Index		$x + y - 1$	YI
Odds ratio (pre-test)		$P/(1 - P)$	OR

(B) Prevalence rate different than 50% $(P \neq 0.5)$
Criterion reference (i.e. diagnosis – Dx)

		Present (P)	Absent (1 – P)
Test result	(+)	$(P)(x)$	$(1 - P)(1 - y)$
	(–)	$(P)(1 - x)$	$(1 - P)(y)$

Parameter	Computation	Symbol
Positive predictive value	$[(P)(x)+(1 - P)(1 - y)]$	PPV
Negative predictive value	$[(1 - P)(y)]/[(1 - P)(y) + (P)(1 - x)]$	NPV

the prevalence of the reference criteria in the population assessed, since prevalence rates above or below 50% will alter the PPV and NPV rates. Baldessarini *et al* (1988) provided a clear example of the influences of these variations.

Other parameters obtainable by applying Bayes' theorem are positive and negative predictive power, the misclassification rate, efficiency (cases not detected by the test in relation to the total number of cases), bias (quotient between those assessed who were considered positive or negative) and the odds ratio (Table 14.2).

These coefficients make it possible to adjust the cut-off point, according to the objective of the study. If the purpose is to conduct a two-phase sampling study, we should look for the cut-off point that enables us to enrol the maximum number of cases, even though some of them may be FP (acceptable specificity with optimal sensitivity). If, on the contrary, we aim to learn the probable morbidity of a population with a test score, we should select that cut-off point that enables us to rule out the highest number of non-cases, although this could mean the loss of some FN (acceptable sensitivity with optimal specificity).

Alternatively, a test's ideal cut-off point can be calculated with receiver operating characteristics (ROC) analysis. This technique was developed in the 1960s to assess radar controllers' capacity to discriminate between signals. First, a graphic representation of the TP (sensitivity) and FP (specificity) rates is obtained for each cut-off point; calculation of the area beneath the resulting curve then indicates the test's discriminatory capacity throughout the spectrum of morbidity. When discriminatory capacity is equal to that obtained randomly, the result is a diagonal line whose lower area is 0.5 (sensitivity equal to the FP rate). Although an ideal test would produce 100% TP before admitting a single FN, so that the area below the curve obtained would be 1.0, in practice the area below the curve oscillates between 0.5 and 1.0. This makes it possible to produce a graphic representation of different tests' discriminatory capacities for the same dimension – with the best one being that which corresponds to the curve farthest away from the diagonal (cf. Thompson, 1989*b*).

Those tests for which the standard TP deviations are very different from the FN deviations are called 'asymmetric' or 'eccentric'. In such cases, it may be necessary to use two cut-off points in order to differentiate between the 'positive' and 'negative' subjects. Somoza (1996) proposed a new definition of sensitivity and specificity that takes into account the existence of asymmetric assessment instruments, showing their properties by applying an ROC analysis.

Meta-analysis is a set of techniques used to quantify the information contained in similar studies. It is intended to produce more precise estimates of the effect being studied, and to assess consistency between different studies analysing the same variables in order to combine their results; therefore, one of its principal uses is for the assessment of diagnostic examinations. In this sense, techniques for meta-analysis of scales are being used to assess the precision of a diagnostic test and its ideal cut-off point. The different studies that assess the discriminant capacity of a test tend to present discordant results as far as the FP and FN rates are concerned, due mainly to the use of different cut-off points and of samples from different populations. This technique uses the results presented in different studies that use ROC analysis to determine such an ideal cut-off point: it is a matter of combining the results of these studies by presenting a summary ROC curve. Different authors have described the methodology used in this kind of meta-analysis (Littenberg & Moses, 1993; Midgette *et al*, 1993; Moses *et al*, 1993).

External redundancy

Generally, redundancy or overlapping of the items on a scale is assessed only while the scale itself is being constructed (internal redundancy). However, it is also important to investigate the possible redundancy of the items and overall scores with other, similar scales (external redundancy). This parameter is not equivalent to the association obtained in concurrent validity; for example, in multi-variate cases it is possible to find near-zero redundancy even though there may be a perfect fit between the two tests (Czobor *et al*, 1991). The use of equivalent scales with redundant items in similar populations does not increase the amount of information obtained; however, it does raise the possibility of completion errors (due to fatigue, transcription mistakes, etc.), increase type I and type II statistical errors, and diminish the cost-utility of administering the tests (Thiemann *et al*, 1987; Czobor *et al*, 1991). According to Wollenberg (1977), redundancy analysis can be considered an extension of factor analysis for two groups of separate variables. Factors are taken from a group of variables (e.g. test A) that explain the variance in another group of variables (e.g. test B). The derivation of linear criterion variates makes it possible to assess the importance of each variate in the redundancy relationship between two instruments (Johansson, 1981).

Thiemann *et al* (1987) expressed the opinion that, in a way, redundancy is somewhat equivalent to the instrument's inter-test reliability. In fact, redundancy has sometimes been assessed according to the kappa agreement of the items (Fenton & McGlashan, 1992; Kibel *et al*, 1993).

Sensitivity to change

Sensitivity to change can be examined in correlation studies and by analysing the principal components at the baseline and after the assessment period (e.g. after treatment), comparing the factor structures at both points. For calculating sensitivity to change, it is useful to compare ratings with a transitional global measure (e.g. using the CGI to evaluate a well-being scale's sensitivity to change). In this case, a covariance analysis can be conducted on the score obtained after treatment, taking the baseline score as a covariable, regarding the factor of change in the severity determined by the variation in the other scale (Salvador-Carulla *et al*, 1996).

Selection of an assessment instrument

The appropriate selection of a subjective assessment instrument is essential for any clinical research in psychiatry. In light of this, the limited number of methodological reviews of this specific area is surprising. Bech *et al* (1993) mention a series of key aspects to consider in a clinical trial:

1 Identify the purpose – why is it necessary to use an assessment scale in the study?
2 Identify the problem – what is being assessed?
3 Identify its importance – what is the relevance of scales in relation to the hypothesis being investigated?
4 Efficiency evaluation – what is the utility of the information obtained by means of the instrument in relation to the cost of its use?

The last aspect is overlooked with excessive frequency in clinical research. In this case, cost–utility evaluation considers the need for training and preparation before the scale can be used, taking into account the necessary time and requirements for statistical analysis. It is also important to evaluate whether the additional information to be obtained justifies the higher costs and the time employed in both scoring the tests and analysing the data. The possibility of increased bias with the addition of a supplementary instrument to an assessment battery should also be considered, whether due to interviewee fatigue or an increase in measurement or type I or II errors when using redundant scales, such as jointly administering the BPRS and the Scale for the Assessment of Negative Symptoms (Thiemann *et al*, 1987; Czobor *et al*, 1991).

Criteria for the transcultural use of assessment instruments

The use of the same questionnaire in different cultures involves a series of exceedingly complex methodological problems, two of the most important being equivalence levels and translation systems.

Levels of transcultural equivalence

The possibility of international use is a major aspect in the selection of assessment instruments. It involves a considerable number of problems, to the point that some authors feel it necessary to tackle this aspect in the construction of the questionnaire itself. This is really not very feasible, so other alternatives must be sought.

Flaherty *et al* (1988) proposed five levels of transcultural equivalence:

1   *Content equivalence.* The content of each item on the instrument is relevant to the phenomenon in each culture.
2   *Syntax equivalence.* The meaning of each item is identical in each culture after its translation into the idiomatic language (written and oral) of each culture. There are a number of sources of variation, here (words, colloquialisms, register).
3   *Technical equivalence.* The assessment method (e.g. pencil and paper, interview) is comparable in each culture with regard to the data produced.
4   *Criterion equivalence.* The interpretation of the measurement of the variable remains the same when compared with the norm for each culture studied.
5   *Conceptual equivalence.* The instrument measures the same theoretical construct in each culture. Sometimes the translation of a word can be very close to the original, while being extremely different on a conceptual level in the two languages.

Translation systems

The most widely used system is that of the back-translation (see also Chapter 12). This differs from direct translation in that after a first translation by one or more translators, the instrument is 'retranslated' by another translator or team. The 'retranslated' version can then be compared with the original. This system, however, is not ideal, and its results are often poor as far as conceptual equivalence is concerned (Brislin, 1970). In mental health studies, investigators have tried to complement this system with techniques that enable them to turn a merely linguistic translation into a cultural one. Among these, some of the most striking are pre-test techniques (based on the congruence of the answers obtained) and different forms of translating committees. The translation of the SCAN into Spanish is a good example of the systematisation of these processes in what has been called a conceptual translation (Vazquez-Barquero, 1993; Room *et al*, 1996). A conceptual translation is one in which the essence of the experience being assessed is clearly reflected in the version in a second language. Concept equivalence takes precedence over syntax. The preparation of such a version is considerably more complicated than the methods discussed above. First, a literal translation is prepared, on the basis of which two independent teams make conceptual translations. Next, these translations are verified to detect problematic terms and concepts, and a consensus is arrived at in accordance with the target environment's cultural reality. This version is then back-translated, and finally the head of the project evaluates the conceptual similarity of each item.

Other tests for transcultural evaluation

There is no consensus regarding the psychometric tests required for an assessment instrument to be used in different cultures. Some authors consider that an instrument should go through the entire analytical process once again. However, this tends to be too expensive. There is, though, certainly a need to reassess reliability (Wittchen *et al*, 1991) and validity (above all in the case of screening instruments in which a cut-off point for detection has been established). The need for an exhaustive analysis of internal consistency is questionable.

Conclusions

The use of psychiatric assessment scales is well established in different areas, from clinical epidemiology to pharmacology (the purpose for which many clinical follow-up scales were originally developed). However, given their number, diversity and the fact that new ones are being developed all the time, computerised, systematic inventories are now more important than ever for the orientation of clinicians and investigators. One guide for their classification could be based on the following parameters: complexity, purpose and design. An evaluation of each instrument's quality could be based on a series of parameters related to its adequacy, construction, feasibility, consistency, reliability, validity and sensitivity to change. Lastly, it is necessary to consider cost-effectiveness or efficiency aspects in the selection of an instrument, as well as its relationship to other instruments used in the study (redundancy). Adequate adaptation and standardisation should be performed in every different cultural setting.

Appendix: Assessment instrument quality checklist (AIQCL) (beta version)

Name and acronym (if translation, note original versions, as well):

Objective of the instrument:

Purpose for which the rater intends to use the instrument:

Dimensions to be evaluated:

Score the following items based on all available literature and your previous experience with the instrument. Use the information obtained in every section to score the overall ratings (do not rate sections which are not applicable for this particular instrument):

Adequacy

Overall rating: 1. Poor   2. Fair   3. Good   4. Excellent

Is the instrument relevant to the purpose for which the rater intends to use it?
   1. Not at all   2. Insufficient   3. Acceptable   4. Excellent

Is instrument's complexity appropriate to the purpose for which the rater intends to use it?
   1. Not at all   2. Insufficient   3. Acceptable   4. Excellent

Does the instrument cover the dimensions to be assessed?
   1. Not at all   2. Insufficient   3. Acceptable   4. Excellent

If not, can it be 'batterised' (administered jointly with other instruments in order to assess different dimensions of the same phenomenon)?
   1. Not at all   2. Insufficient   3. Acceptable   4. Excellent

Is there information available on the instrument's standardisation in the specific cultural/group environment in which it is to be used?
   1. Not at all   2. Insufficient   3. Acceptable   4. Excellent

Construction

Overall rating: 1. Poor   2. Fair   3. Good   4. Excellent

Is the instrument's objective defined explicitly?
   1. Not at all   2. Insufficient   3. Acceptable   4. Excellent

Is there a glossary? *(With the exception of very simple instruments)*
   1. Not at all   2. Insufficient   3. Acceptable   4. Excellent

Is there an instruction manual or any equivalent within the test that clearly specifies instructions for filling it out, the time frame, and rater requirements?
   1. Not at all   2. Insufficient   3. Acceptable   4. Excellent

Feasibility

Overall rating: 1. Poor   2. Fair   3. Good   4. Excellent

Is the description given in the questionnaire meaningful for its recipients (e.g. investigators, health care professionals, users, managers)? *(applicability)*
   1. Not at all   2. Insufficient   3. Acceptable   4. Excellent

Is the instrument user-friendly in terms of its comprehensibility, ease of filling out, completion time? *(acceptability)*
   1. Not at all   2. Insufficient   3. Acceptable   4. Excellent

Is the instrument's data coding and data handling practical? (*practicality*)
  1. Not at all   2. Insufficient   3. Acceptable   4. Excellent

What is the usefulness of the information obtained in relation to its costs (completion time and personnel) (*efficiency*)
  1. Not at all   2. Insufficient   3. Acceptable   4. Excellent

Consistency

Overall rating: 1. Poor   2. Fair   3. Good   4. Excellent

Has the consistency analysis been carried out on a sufficient number of subjects?
  1. Not at all   2. Insufficient   3. Acceptable   4. Excellent

If the instrument generates global ratings, has its internal consistency been analysed?
  1. Not at all   2. Insufficient   3. Acceptable   4. Excellent

If so, name the statistical test(s) used:

Has its factor structure been analysed?
  1. Not at all   2. Insufficient   3. Acceptable   4. Excellent

Reliability

Overall rating: 1. Poor   2. Fair   3. Good   4. Excellent

Has the reliability analysis been carried out on a sufficient number of subjects?
  1. Not at all   2. Insufficient   3. Acceptable   4. Excellent

Has test–retest reliability been analysed?
  1. Not at all   2. Insufficient   3. Acceptable   4. Excellent

If applicable, has interrater reliability been analysed?
  1. Not at all   2. Insufficient   3. Acceptable   4. Excellent

If applicable, has inter-informant reliability been analysed?
  1. Not at all   2. Insufficient   3. Acceptable   4. Excellent

Validity

Overall rating: 1. Poor   2. Fair   3. Good   4. Excellent

Has the validity analysis been carried out on a sufficient number of subjects?
  1. Not at all   2. Insufficient   3. Acceptable   4. Excellent

Are the results obtained significant and relevant to the expert rater? (*simple validity*)
  1. Not at all   2. Insufficient   3. Acceptable   4. Excellent

To what extent does the questionnaire describe the different characteristics of the phenomenon to be observed, in the expert rater's opinion? (*content validity*)
  1. Not at all   2. Insufficient   3. Acceptable   4. Excellent

If applicable, to what extent are similar characteristics included in the same group, and divergent ones in different groups? (*precision/discriminant validity*)

    1. Not at all   2. Insufficient   3. Acceptable   4. Excellent

If applicable, is information on convergent validity available?

    1. Not at all   2. Insufficient   3. Acceptable   4. Excellent

If applicable (i.e. instrument of reference available), is information on concurrent validity available?

    1. Not at all   2. Insufficient   3. Acceptable   4. Excellent

If applicable, is information on predictive validity available?

    1. Not at all   2. Insufficient   3. Acceptable   4. Excellent

If so, name the statistical test(s) used:

If applicable, is information on factorial or dimensional validity available? (*Use of exploratory factor analysis should be considered insufficient, unless the data are based on extensive coinciding literature, in which case it should be rated acceptable.*)

    1. Not at all   2. Insufficient   3. Acceptable   4. Excellent

Sensitivity to change

Overall rating: 1. Poor   2. Fair   3. Good   4. Excellent

If it is a follow-up questionnaire, what is the quality of available information on sensitivity to change?

    1. Not at all   2. Insufficient   3. Acceptable   4. Excellent

Redundancy avoidance

Overall rating: 1. Poor   2. Fair   3. Good   4. Excellent

If the questionnaire is being used within a battery of instruments, what is the quality of available information on redundancy?

    1. Not at all   2. Insufficient   3. Acceptable   4. Excellent

Generalisability

Overall rating: 1. Poor   2. Fair   3. Good   4. Excellent

To what extent has the usefulness of the instrument been analysed using different populations and settings?

    1. Not at all   2. Insufficient   3. Acceptable   4. Excellent

To what extent do data on the instrument's psychometric properties proceed from studies other than the original?

    1. Not at all   2. Insufficient   3. Acceptable   4. Excellent

Transcultural equivalence

Overall rating: 1. Poor   2. Fair   3. Good   4. Excellent

What is the quality of the available data on the instrument's transcultural standardisation? *(Unless the instrument has been validated in more than three different major languages/cultures, it should not be rated excellent.)*

    1. Not at all   2. Insufficient   3. Acceptable   4. Excellent

Adequacy:
AIQCindex:%

$$\text{AIQC index} = \frac{\text{Addition of all applicable overal ratings}}{\text{Maximum score among applicable sections}} \times 100$$

Acknowledgements

This work was supported in part by grants CICYT PM-96/0109 (Interministerial Commission of Science and Technology, Ministry of Education), and FIS 99/0035-01 (Health Research Fund, Ministry of Health).

References

AMERICAN PSYCHIATRIC ASSOCIATION (1994) *Diagnostic and Statistical Manual of Mental Disorders* (4th edn) (DSM–IV). Washington, DC: APA.

ANDERSEN, J., LARSEN, J. K., SCHULTZ, V., *et al* (1989) The Brief Psychiatric Rating Scale: dimension of schizophrenia – reliability and construct validity. *Psychopathology*, **22**, 168–176.

ANDREASEN, N. C., FLAUM, M. & ARNDT, S. (1992) The Comprehensive Assessment of Symptoms and History (CASH): an instrument for assessing diagnosis and psychopathology. *Archives of General Psychiatry*, **49**, 615–623.

ANDREWS, G., PETERS, L. & TEESON, M. (1994) *Measurement of Consumer Outcome in Mental Health: A Report to the National Mental Health Information Strategies Committee*. Sydney: Clinical Research Unit for Anxiety Disorders.

BADIA, X., SALAMERO, M. & ALONSO, J. (1999). *La medida de la salud: Guía de escalas de medición en español* (2nd edn). Barcelona: Edimac.

BALDESSARINI, R. J., FINKLESTEIN, S. & ARANA, G. W. (1988) Predictive power of diagnostic tests. In *Psychobiology and Psychopharmacology* (ed. F. Flasch), pp. 175–189. New York: Norton.

BARTKO, J. J. & CARPENTER, W. T. (1976) On the methods and theory of reliability. *Journal of Nervous and Mental Diseases*, **163**, 307–317.

BECH, P., KASTRUP, M. & RAFAELSEN, O. J. (1986) Mini compendium of rating scales for states of anxiety, depression, mania, schizophrenia with corresponding DSM–III syndromes. *Acta Psychiatrica Scandinavica*, **73** (suppl. 326), 1–37.

——, MALT, U. F., DENCKER, S. J., *et al* (eds) (1993) Scales for assessment of diagnosis and severity of mental disorders. *Acta Psychiatrica Scandinavica*, **87** (suppl. 372), 1–87.

BOWLING, A. (1997) *Research Methods in Health: Investigating Health and Health Services*. Buckingham: Open University Press.

BRISLIN, R. W. (1970) Back-translation for cross-cultural research. *Journal of Cross-cultural Psychology*, **1**, 185–216.

BUCHANAN, R. W. & CARPENTER, W. T. (1994) Domains of psychopathology. An approach to the reduction of heterogeneity in schizophrenia. *Journal of Nervous and Mental Diseases,* **182**, 193–204.

BURKE, L. B. (1998) Quality of life evaluation: the FDA experience. *Quality of Life Newsletter,* March, 8–9.

COSTELLO, C. G. (1994) Advantages of the symptom approach to schizophrenia. In *Symptoms of Schizophrenia* (ed. C. G. Costello), pp. 1–26. New York: Wiley.

CZOBOR, P., BITTER, I. & VOLAVKA, J. (1991) Relationship between the Brief Psychiatric Rating Scale and the Scale for the Assessment of Negative Symptoms: a study of their correlation and redundancy. *Psychiatry Research,* **36**, 129–139.

FEINSTEIN, A. R. (1985) *Clinical Epidemiology.* Philadelphia: W. B. Saunders.

FENTON, W. & MCGLASHAN, T. H. (1992) Testing systems for assessment of negative symptoms in schizophrenia. *Archives of General Psychiatry,* **49**, 179–184.

FLAHERTY, J. A., GAVIRIA, F. M., PATHAK, D., *et al* (1988) Developing instruments for cross-cultural psychiatric research. *Journal of Nervous and Mental Diseases,* **176**, 257–263.

GARCIA-CUETO, E. (1993) *Introducción a la psicometría.* Madrid: Siglo XXI.

HERNANDEZ-AGUADO, I., PORTA, M., MIRALLES, M., *et al* (1990) La cuantificación de la variabilidad en las observaciones clínicas. *Medicina Clínica,* **95**, 424–429.

ISRAEL, L., KOZAREVIC, D. & SARTORIUS, N. (1983) *Source Book for the Geriatric Assessment: I. Evaluation in Gerontology.* Basel: Karger/WHO.

JOHANSSON, J. K. (1981) An extension of Wollenberg's redundancy analysis. *Psychometrika,* **46**, 95–103.

KIBEL, D. A., LAFFONT, I. & LIDDLE, P. F. (1993) The composition of the negative syndrome of chronic schizophrenia. *British Journal of Psychiatry,* **162**, 744–750.

KRAMER, M. S. & FEINSTEIN, A. R. (1981) Clinical biostatistics: LIV. The biostatistics of concordance. *Clinical and Pharmacological Therapy,* **29**, 111–123.

LIDDLE, P. F. (1987) Schizophrenic syndromes, cognitive performance and neurological dysfunction. *Psychological Medicine,* **17**, 49–57.

LITTENBERG, B. & MOSES, L. E. (1993) Estimating diagnostic accuracy from multiple conflicting reports: a new meta-analytic method. *Medical Decision Making,* **13**, 313–321.

LUND, J. (1989) Measuring behaviour disorder in mental handicap, *British Journal of Psychiatry,* **155**, 379–383.

MARQUIS, P. (1998) Strategies for interpreting quality of life questionnaires. *Quality of Life Newsletter,* March (special issue), 3–4.

MARTINEZ-ARIAS, R. (1995) *Psicometria: Teoria de los tests psicológicos y educativos.* Madrid: Editorial Síntesis.

MCDOWELL, I. & NEWELL, C. (1996) *Measuring Health: A Guide to Rating Scales and Questionnaires.* New York: Oxford University Press.

MEEHL, P. & GOLDEN, R. R. (1982) Taxonometric methods. In *Handbook of Research Methodology in Clinical Psychology* (eds P. C. Kendall & J. N. Butcher), pp. 127–181. New York: Wiley.

MEZZICH, J. E. (ed.) (1986) *Clinical Care and Information Systems in Psychiatry.* Washington, DC: American Psychiatric Press.

MIDGETTE, A. S., STUKEL, T. A. & LITTENBERG, B. (1993) A meta-analytic method for summarizing diagnostic test performances: reveiver-operating-characteristic – summary point stimates. *Medical Decision Making,* **13**, 253–257.

MOSES, L. E., SHAPIRO, D. & LITTENBERG, B. (1993) Combining independent studies of a diagnostic test into a summary ROC curve: data-analytic approaches and some additional considerations. *Statistics in Medicine,* **12**, 1293–1316.

MUÑIZ, J. (1992) *Teoría clásica de los test.* Madrid: Ediciones Pirámide.

MUTHEN, B. O., HASIN, D. & WISNICKI, K. (1993a) Factor analysis of ICD–10 symptom items in the 1988 National Health Interview Survey on Alcohol Dependence. *Addiction,* **88**, 1071–1077.

——, GRANT, B. & HASIN, D. (1993*b*) The dimensionality of alcohol abuse and dependence: factor analysis of DSM–III–R and proposed DSM–IV criteria in the 1988 National Health Interview Survey. *Addiction*, **88**, 1079–1090.

PULL, C. B. & WITTCHEN, H-U. (1991) The CIDI, SCAN, and IPDE: structured diagnostic interviews for ICD–10 and DSM–III–R. *European Psychiatry*, **6**, 227–285.

RASCH, G. (1960) *Studies in Mathematical Psychology. I. Probabilistic Models for Some Intelligence and Attaintment Tests*. Copenhagen: Danmarks Paedagogiske Institut.

—— (1980) *Probabilistic Models for Some Intelligence and Attainment Tests*. Chicago: University of Chicago Press.

ROOM, R., JANCA, A., BENNET, L. A., *et al* (1996) WHO cross-cultural applicability research on diagnosis and assessment of substance use disorders: an overview of methods and selected results. *Addiction*, **91**, 199–220.

SALVADOR-CARULLA, L. (1999) Routine outcome assessment in mental health research. *Current Opinion in Psychiatry*, **12**, 207–210.

——, HUETE, T., HERNAN, M. A., *et al* (1996) Validación del indice de bienestar general en pacientes con depresión mayor. In *Avances en trastornos afectivos* (eds M. Gutierrez, J. Ezcurra & P. Pichot), pp. 289–306. Barcelona: Ediciones en Neurociencias.

SIEGEL, S. (1966) *Non-parametric Statistics for Behavioral Sciences*. New York: McGraw-Hill.

SLADE, M., THORNICROFT, G. & GLOVER, G. (1999) The feasibility of routine outcome measurement. *Social Psychiatry and Psychiatric Epidemiology*, **34**, 243–249.

SOMOZA, E. (1996) Eccentric diagnostic tests: redefining sensitivity and specificity. *Medical Decision Making*, **16**, 15–23.

STRANG, J., BRADLEY, B. & STOCKWELL, T. (1989) Assessment of drug and alcohol use. In *The Instruments of Psychiatric Research* (ed. C. Thompson), pp. 211–232. Chichester: Wiley.

STREINER, D. L. & NORMAN, G. R. (1996) *Health Measurement Scales: A Practical Guide to Their Development and Use* (2nd edn). New York: Oxford University Press.

STRÖMGREN, E. (1988) The lexicon and issues in the relation of psychiatric concepts and terms. In *International Classification in Psychiatry* (eds J. E. Mezzich & M. von Cranach), pp. 175–179. Cambridge: Cambridge University Press.

THIEMANN, S., CSERNANSKY, J. G. & BERGER, P. (1987) Rating scales in research: the case of negative symptoms. *Psychiatry Research*, **20**, 47–55.

THOMPSON, C. (1989*a*) Introduction. In *The Instruments of Psychiatric Research* (ed. C. Thompson), pp. 1–17. Chichester: Wiley.

—— (1989*b*) Affective disorders. In *The Instruments of Psychiatric Research* (ed. C. Thompson), pp 87–126. Chichester: Wiley.

VAZQUEZ-BARQUERO, J. L. (ed.) (1993) *SCAN. Cuestionarios para la evaluación clínica en psiquiatría*. Madrid: Meditor.

WITTCHEN, H-U. & ESSAU, C. A. (1990) Assessment of symptoms and psychosocial disabilities in primary care. In *Psychological Disorders in General Medical Settings* (eds N. Sartorius, D. Goldberg, G. de Girolamo, *et al*), pp. 111–136. Toronto: Hogrefe & Huber.

——, Robins, L. N., Cottler, L. B., *et al* (1991) Cross-cultural feasibility, reliability and sources of variance of the Composite International Diagnostic Interview (CIDI). *British Journal of Psychiatry*, **159**, 645–653.

WOLLENBERG, A. L. (1977) Redundancy analysis: an alternative for canonical correlation analysis. *Psychometrika*, **42**, 207–219.

WORLD HEALTH ORGANIZATION (1993) *The ICD–10 Classification of Mental and Behavioural Disorders – Diagnostic Criteria for Research*. Geneva: WHO.

15 Graphical models for the multi-dimensional assessment of outcome

**ANNIBALE BIGGERI, GIULIA BISOFFI,
PAOLA RUCCI, MIRELLA RUGGERI
and MICHELE TANSELLA**

The need for comprehensive models to assess outcome

The impression of reductionism may overwhelm clinicians when they read most literature on the outcome of psychiatric care. What clinicians consider *reductionism* often corresponds to an attempt by researchers to *simplify* the enormous complexity of psychiatry. This attitude has had a major role also in the choice of the indicators of outcome; in fact, morbidity and mortality rates or data on service use have almost exclusively been the indicators of choice for outcome studies, although their limits in reflecting the real outcome of psychiatric care have often been emphasised (Jenkins, 1990; Mirin & Namerow, 1991; Attkisson *et al*, 1992; Ruggeri & Tansella, 1995, 1996; Tansella & Ruggeri, 1996; Everitt & Landau, 1998). The result of this tendency has been to enlarge the gap between research and clinical practice and favour the widespread use of treatments whose efficacy has never been proven. Indicators of outcome should instead fit the needs and the complexity of routine clinical practice; psychiatric services, on their side, should be flexible in their organisation and able to modify their treatment strategies on the basis of the feedback from outcome studies.

As mentioned in Chapter 4, it is now clear that in order to be valid and useful in clinical practice, outcome studies should first of all be comprehensive and combine optimal measures of both the 'service level' (Tansella, 1989) and the 'patient level' (Ruggeri & Tansella, 1996). At the service level, process variables seem still to give useful information on the outcome of care, provided they are integrated with other indicators. At the patient level, indicators should explore an intervention's effect on clinical variables (the severity and course of symptoms), social variables (social functioning, social support, quality of life) and the users' views of that intervention (needs, burden, satisfaction). Moreover, the assessment should take simultaneously into account various points of view, or axes. In fact, in psychiatric settings, professionals, paraprofessionals, patients and relatives are all involved in care and should be considered legitimate judges of an intervention's effectiveness, albeit from differing perspectives (Mayer & Rosenblatt, 1974; Dowds & Fontana, 1977; Garrard *et al*, 1988; Gunkel & Priebe, 1993; Andrews *et al*, 1986).

Thus, *multi-dimensionality* and *multi-axiality* are key components of the assessment of outcome; a fundamental requirement is also to perform outcome studies in 'real services', according to a longitudinal design. An advantage of such a design is that it provides a complete cross-sectional and follow-up picture without preliminary (and, in the light of current knowledge, dubious) assumptions about the relevance of one indicator, or perspective. A drawback is that it takes simultaneously into account so many variables that their mutual interaction may be obscured without appropriate data analysis; moreover, the common statistical techniques are unsatisfactory for this purpose. To deal with this complexity, and gain insight into the phenomena investigated, integrated methods of data representation and analysis are needed.

The aims of this chapter are to introduce an integrated statistical method to the study of the relationships between variables, based on graphical modelling, and to show its practical application on a data-set from a project on the outcome of community psychiatric care that is currently being conducted in South-Verona and that is based on a multi-dimensional and multi-axial assessment model (Ruggeri *et al*, 1998*a,b*).

Statistical methods of analysing complex sets of data

Regression models

The approach to the study of the association between outcome (response) variables and one or more predictors (covariates) is based on multiple regression models. The need for mathematical and statistical modelling emerged when the researcher had to manage several quantitative and qualitative predictors and stratified analysis was not possible because there were insufficient data.

Most epidemiological variables are categorical or measured on an ordinal scale. Great effort has therefore been devoted over the last

20 years to finding suitable techniques for analysing non-continuous data. In particular, the logistic regression model for dichotomous outcomes (dead/alive; ill/healthy, etc.) became very popular and alternative techniques, such as discriminant analysis, which relies on strong distributional assumptions on the set of predictors, were virtually abandoned (Greenland, 1987). The reasons for this can be traced to the straightforward interpretation of the regression coefficients: in the logistic model they are log odds ratios and, depending on study design, can be read as the logarithm of relative risks, a sensible measure of association between outcome and predictors. In contrast, other regression models for discrete data based on trigonometric transformations of the response variable led to uninterpretable parameters. Parallel to this trend, covariance selection models were refined for continuous data (Dempster, 1972).

When an association is found between two variables, it is good practice to check whether it is a spurious or indirect relationship. This is especially required in case-control and cohort studies, where the distribution of the set of predictors (i.e. of putative risk factors) and of the responses is conditioned by the study design and associations between variables cannot be properly interpreted as causal relationships because the assumption of random assignment does not hold. When potential confounders of the true association between two variables are too many or are mostly unknown, log–linear and regression models are needed to control for their effect. Graphical modelling (Whittaker, 1990; Edwards, 1995; Cox & Wermuth, 1996; Lauritzen, 1996) takes advantage of these techniques by integrating them within a common framework. The idea behind it is that "any kind of relationship should be analysed as a *conditional* relationship" (Kreiner, 1996); that is, a relationship between two variables exists if and only if it does not disappear when one controls for the effect of antecedent or intervening variables. Graphical modelling extends the regression models to more than one response and more than one group of covariates, in such a way that purely explanatory and intermediate variables can be modelled simultaneously. While we limit our illustration to continuous Gaussian data, the method discussed is quite general and allows continuous, categorical and a mixture of quantitative and qualitative variables.

We can imagine three sets of variables: *A* contains the responses, *B* the intermediate variables that affect the responses and *C* the explanatory variables that could affect both *A* and *B*. At least three issues can be addressed:

- we may wish to evaluate the effect of each predictor (not considering its status as explanatory or intermediate) on each response, having fixed all the other variables in the model

- we may wish to evaluate the pattern of associations among explanatory variables and their effect on the intermediate variables
- we may wish to study the reciprocal influence of the responses.

This chapter aims to show how graphical models can help in analysing complex patterns of association among variables like those emerging in a comprehensive assessment of outcome and to address the above-mentioned issues.

Graphical models and log–linear models

The idea of representing graphically a statistical model and causal relationships between variables is an old one. Readers may be familiar with path analysis, which gained some popularity in psychological research (Fienberg, 1980). Log–linear models were used to analyse contingency tables cross-classifying the subjects by several discrete variables. They model the expected frequencies of the table as a log–linear function of parameters that are interpretable as log odds (main effects), log odds ratios (first-order interactions), log ratios of odds ratios (second-order interactions) and so on. The associations between the discrete variables are then modelled in terms of odds ratios. These associations can vary according to the presence or absence of other variables in the model: this phenomenon is known as 'Simpson's paradox'. The true association between two variables is obtained by adjusting for confounding variables and their interactions under a given causal model.

The parameters of interest are therefore adjusted odds ratios obtained from a model with all the relevant relationships correctly specified. Let us suppose, for example, that we wish to analyse a 2 × 2 × 2 contingency table obtained by classifying the subjects enrolled in a cross-sectional study according to: their score (low/high) for psychopathology, using, say, the Brief Psychiatric Rating Scale (BPRS); marital status (married/unmarried); and education (low/high). The log–linear model that specifies the relationships among all three variables is the following, where the three variables are respectively indicated as X, Y, Z:

$$\log m(ijk) = 1 + \lambda(X) + \lambda(Y) + \lambda(Z) + \lambda(XY) + \lambda(XZ) + \lambda(YZ)$$

where $m(ijk)$ denotes the expected frequency for the cell (ijk) of the table. The main effects parameters $\lambda(X)$, $\lambda(Y)$, $\lambda(Z)$ are log odds, and they are different from 0 if the distribution of values between the categories of the respective variable is asymmetrical. The first-order interaction terms, such as $\lambda(XY)$, are log odds ratios and denote an association between the variables. We can distinguish *crude* or *marginal* log odds ratios of the simpler model, e.g.

$$\log m(ijk) = 1 + l(X) + l(Y) + l(XY),$$

from the log odds ratios of the previous models which are adjusted for the third variable (Z). Log odds ratios have the same meaning of correlation coefficients. The *adjusted* log odds ratios can be interpreted as partial correlation coefficients.

Restricting our attention to the relationship between a high score on the BPRS and marital status, $\lambda(XY)$, the crude odds ratio is not useful in making a causal inference since it may depend on an unbalanced distribution of education (Z) in the actual sample being analysed. The adjusted odds ratios, in contrast, reflect the association XY given the third variable Z. To analyse the pattern of associations correctly, we need to take into account all the relevant variables. In the case of continuous variables, this means that we have to consider the matrix of partial correlation coefficients.

Finally, it should be noted that no second-order interaction terms, $\lambda(XYZ)$, have been considered; their interpretation is effect modification – for example, the effect of marital status on psychopathology is modified by education. While these interactions can easily be included in a log–linear model, there is no counterpart in multivariate Gaussian models for continuous data.

For each multivariate regression model, such as log–linear models, we can draw a unique graph, which is a schematic representation of the conditional independence relationships between several variables. It consists of vertices and edges. Each vertex represents one variable; it is drawn as a circle if the variable is on a continuous scale, or as a point if it is discrete. Any edge between a pair of vertices denotes the presence of an association between the two variables, given all the other variables in the graph.

Two variables are said to be *conditionally independent* if there is no direct association between them and therefore there is no edge connecting the two respective vertices in the graph. This does not mean that the two variables are *marginally* independent. In this case the two vertices would be connected by an indirect path, involving other vertices.

The partial correlation matrix is used to obtain the conditional association graph for continuous variables. For any pair of variables, a 0 partial correlation coefficient means conditional independence and lack of a direct edge between the corresponding vertices in the graph. The statistical analysis aims to model the partial correlation matrix or its inverse. The estimated association graph is drawn from estimated partial correlation matrices (an example is given below). With discrete variables, adjusted odds ratios substitute for the correlation coefficient; an odds ratio equal to 1 denotes an absence of association. With mixed data, the partial correlation matrix is calculated separately for each level of the categorical variables.

The usefulness of graphical models is even more evident when we consider *directed graphs*. In these graphs an arrow between vertices (variables) denotes associations that can be interpreted directionally (causally). Variables can be hierarchically ordered as responses (dependent) and potentially explanatory (independent) or inter-mediate/intervening variables on the basis of previous knowledge. A trivial example of hierarchy is when variables are temporally ordered, as in longitudinal studies, where subsequent assessments are scheduled. In this case associations between variables measured at different times should be statistically evaluated, 'conditionally to' (taking into account) all the associations among previous and concomitant ones.

We finally introduce *graphical chain models*. These are especially suited to the analysis of complex sets of variables, some of which are responses, some predictors and some intermediate. The study of the undirected associations between such variables is conducted within each set, and directed causal association is then assessed conditionally to all the associations among predictors and intermediate variables, step by step.

We do not discuss methods of estimation and fitting of graphical models in this chapter. Maximum-likelihood estimates and likelihood ratios to compare nested models are used in the example given in the next section. For discrete data the maximum-likelihood equations follow from Poisson or multinomial sampling and for continuous data from the multivariate Gaussian sampling (see Lauritzen & Wermuth, 1989, for mixed data). Formerly, in the statistical literature, log–linear modelling for discrete data and covariance selection models for continuous data were widely used. The novelty of the graphical approach resides in the treatment of mixed data and on the modelling strategy using conditional independence. Directed and chain graphs extend the capability of such models to cover a wide range of substantive research hypotheses.

An application of the conditional independence model to the multi-dimensional assessment of outcome

The South-Verona Outcome Project

The South-Verona Outcome Project is an attempt to standardise information that clinicians collect and record, in periodical reviews of cases in treatment, in their everyday clinical practice and to employ for service evaluation the same professionals involved in the clinical work (Ruggeri *et al*, 1998*a,b*). Most of the assessments are actually completed, after a short period of training, by the clinicians themselves, while other assessments are made by the patients, with the help of research workers. Standardised assessments include global functioning, psychopathology, social disability, needs for care, quality of life, and satisfaction with services. They take place twice a year: from April to June (wave A) and from October to December (wave B). During these periods both first-ever patients and patients already in contact with the service are assessed at the first or, at latest, the second time they are seen. In wave A, the assessment is made only by the key professional (in most cases a psychiatrist or a psychologist) and includes the Global Assessment of Functioning Scale (GAF; Endicott *et al*, 1976), the BPRS expanded version (Lukoff *et al*, 1986), eight items from the Disability Assessment Scale (DAS-II; World Health Organization, 1988), and the Camberwell Assessment of Needs (CAN; Slade *et al*, 1999). In wave B the assessment is made by both the key professional (again the GAF, BPRS and DAS-II, plus) and the patients, who are requested to complete the Lancashire Quality of Life Profile (LQL; Oliver, 1991) and the Verona Service Satisfaction Scale (VSSS; Ruggeri & Dall'Agnola, 1993; Ruggeri *et al*, 1994). Socio-demographic characteristics, psychiatric history of the patients and service utilisation are routinely recorded in the South-Verona psychiatric case register (PCR). All these data are entered into the clinical records and are available to clinicians.

The project started in 1994 and about 80% of the patients in contact with the service in that year were assessed in both waves. Costs calculated using service utilisation data were attached to each service contact recorded on the PCR, and individual total direct costs referring to the period between every assessment were calculated for each patient using the registry data and a dedicated software package (Amaddeo *et al*, 1997, 1998).

A graph drawn from a subset of variables from the South-Verona Outcome Project

We use only six variables from South-Verona assessments obtained in wave B 1994 (B94) and wave B 1996 (B96): mean GAF and DAS-II scores from wave B94, mean GAF, DAS-II and VSSS scores from wave B96, and individual daily total direct costs in the interval between the two waves. The GAF, DAS-II and VSSS B96 scores can be considered response variables, the total daily costs referred to the period between B94 and B96 can be considered a process indicator, while GAF B94 and DAS-II

B94 can be considered explanatory variables. Here a distinction was made *a priori* among the variables considered.

The aim in using a graphical model in the present data-set was threefold: to assess the influence of explanatory and process variables on the set of response variables; to assess the influence of explanatory variables on the process indicators; and to analyse the relationships between response variables. We represent the relationships among the six variables (baseline GAF and DAS-II, total costs, outcome GAF and DAS-II, VSSS) in the chain graph shown as Fig. 15.1. The analysis proceeds as follows:

Step 1. Relationships in the first box are calculated. The empirical (observed) Pearson's correlation coefficient between the two variables GAF B94 and DAS-II B94 is −0.743 (the more social disability, the less is the global functioning for a given patient). It is evident that the two variables are not marginally independent. Sometimes, as the variables in the first box are fixed by design, this step is omitted.

Step 2. Relationships between the pseudo-response 'total costs of psychiatric care' (actually a process indicator) and the two predictors, GAF and DAS-II B94, are considered. This is simply a multiple regression analysis of the logarithm of total costs against baseline GAF and DAS-II (Table 15.1). The magnitude of social disability (DAS-II B94) affects the individual total direct costs.

Step 3. Relationships between the variables in the third box and dependencies between the variables in the third box on the variables in the first and second boxes are calculated. The empirical (observed) partial correlation matrix for the six variables considered, GAF and DAS-II B94 (baseline), total costs (process) and GAF, DAS-II and VSSS B96 (outcome), is shown in Table 15.2 together with the fitted partial correlation matrix. It is evident, on inspecting the matrix, that outcome DAS-II B96 is independent of baseline GAF B94 ($r = -0.007$) and of total costs ($r = 0.077$), keeping the other variables constant, while outcome GAF B96 is independent from baseline DAS-II B94 ($r = -0.071$), again keeping constant the other variables.

We point out that the entries in the matrix are the partial correlation coefficients given all the other variables; for example,

TABLE 15.1
Multiple regression analysis of log(total direct cost) against GAF and DAS-II scores at wave B, 1994 (data derived from the South-Verona case register)

	Coefficient	SE	t	P	95% CI
GAF	−0.0174162	0.0116736	−1.492	0.138	−0.0404552 to 0.0056229
DAS-II	0.8022713	0.2283642	3.513	0.001	0.351569 to 1.252974
Constant	2.02836	0.8553907	2.371	0.019	0.3401502 to 3.71657

TABLE 15.2
Empirical (observed) and fitted partial correlation matrices

	GAF B94	DAS-II B94	GAF B96	DAS-II B96	VSSS B96	Costs
Empirical, discrete, linear and partial correlation parameters						
GAF B94	1.000					
DAS-II B94	−0.613	1.000				
GAF B96	0.173	−0.071	1.000			
DAS-II B96	−0.007	0.154	−0.498	1.000		
VSSS	−0.010	−0.014	0.149	−0.078	1.000	
Costs	−0.072	0.202	−0.109	0.077	0.020	1.000
Fitted discrete, linear and partial correlation parameters						
GAF B94	1.000					
DAS-II B94	−0.617	1.000				
GAF B96	0.201	0.000	1.000			
DAS-II B96	0.000	0.196	−0.521	1.000		
VSSS	0.000	0.000	0.193	0.000	1.000	
Costs	−0.062	0.223	−0.153	0.000	0.000	1.000
Fitted concentration matrix (inverse partial correlation matrix)						
GAF B94	0.010					
DAS-II B94	0.121	3.947				
GAF B96	−0.002	0.000	0.010			
DAS-II B96	0.000	−0.620	0.081	2.524		
VSSS	0.000	0.000	−0.040	0.000	4.430	
Costs	0.004	−0.278	0.009	0.000	0.000	0.396

Partial correlation coefficients equal to zero denote conditional independence.

−0.613 is the correlation coefficient between GAF B94 and DAS-II B94, given all the other variables, including those in the later boxes. The ordering among the variables (baseline – process – outcome) renders this coefficient irrelevant to the analysis, because it is illogical to assume that any correlation between baseline variables must be adjusted for the outcome variables. In contrast, with the outcome variables, the ordering is of great relevance, for example the partial correlation coefficient −0.498 between outcome GAF B96 and outcome DAS-II B96, given all the other variables, is directly interpretable as these variables are all in the previous boxes. The meaning of this coefficient is that there is a residual association between the two variables, after taking into account the associations induced by the common regressors.

The modelling strategy consists in setting to zero the appropriate entries of the partial correlation matrix. Table 15.2 also shows the fitted partial concentration matrix. The model has a good fit ($P = 0.88$) and the regression coefficients of interest are obtained from the concentration matrix (i.e. the inverse of the fitted partial correlation matrix); for example, the regression coefficient of Xj on Xi,

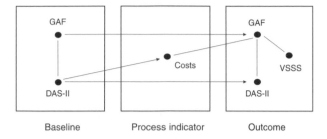

Fig. 15.1. *Chain graph showing the relationships between variables from the South-Verona Outcome Project (n = 178). Points denote variables, lines between variables denote direct associations, arrows denote causal relationships. The lack of a line between variables indicates conditional independence*

given all the other predictive variables in the graph, is $\beta_{j|i} = -\sigma_{ij}/\sigma_{jj}$, where σ_{ij} denotes the ij-th element of the concentration matrix (see Whittaker, 1990, chapter 5, for details). In our example, the regression coefficient between the outcome GAF B96 and the baseline GAF B94 is 0.20 (95% confidence interval (CI) 0.10 to 0.30) (since the coresponding concentrations in Table 15.2 are –0.002 and 0.010) and that between GAF B96 and total costs is –0.023 (95% CI –0.04 to –0.006); for the outcome variable DAS-II B96, only the correlation with DAS-II B94 is statistically significant, with a coefficient of 0.246 (95% CI 0.12 to 0.37); and finally no explanatory variables directly predict VSSS.

The results highlight the gain in precision with this approach: the standard errors of the estimates are systematically lower than those that would be obtained by separate multiple regressions. Moreover, they are more efficient since irrelevant associations between variables are dropped.

When dealing with continuous variables, it is assumed that a multivariate Gaussian distribution will apply. An important consequence of this would be the absence of non-linearity and second-order interactions among variables. This assumption is usually addressed when building up a regression model by checking: first, whether there is an important non-linear effect of the covariate of interest; and second, whether the effect of a covariate is modified by another covariate. By regressing each variable in turn on any other plus the respective quadratic term, we have, in our example data, a total of 30 (6 × 5) tests; and by regressing each variable against each pair of covariates, plus their interaction term, we have a total of 60 tests (6 × the number of combinations of 2 out of 5). To avoid the problem of multiple comparisons, a graphical assessment has been suggested by Cox & Wermuth (1994).

In the event that an evaluation suggests some inadequacies of the model, the analysis should be replicated either after having transformed (e.g. by taking logarithms) or after having categorised some variables, and the results of these different strategies should be presented and discussed. It is also important to perform a sensitivity analysis, for example replicating the results using Box–Cox transformed data or after deleting some outlying or influential observations.

Findings from our analysis can be summarised as follows:

- disability and global functioning are strongly correlated and the baseline conditions recorded in 1994 are strongly predictive of the corresponding conditions at the 1996 reassessment;
- service utilisation measurements (process indicators), namely individual total direct costs, are directly dependent on baseline status; they are only weakly associated with the outcomes considered, with higher costs predicting lower global functioning at the 1996 reassessment;
- service satisfaction is predicted by explanatory variables only indirectly, through outcome global functioning status.

These preliminary findings are promising and already show the ability of the model to encapsulate a complex set of variables without splitting the analysis into a series of independent tasks.

Conclusions

Bridging the gap between reductionism and over-complexity in evaluating mental health service outcomes is a challenge in psychiatric epidemiology research. Certainly this work will require both a large-scale application of comprehensive models of outcome assessment and, consequently, the capacity to manage large sets of data and understand complex relationships between variables. A necessary step in epidemiological research in this area is to accept that we are in a hypothesis-generating, not a hypothesis-testing, phase. The implication is that we have to proceed as far as possible without restrictive *a priori* assumptions regarding the data.

The multi-dimensional and multi-axial model that we propose for the assessment of outcome, and its application to a naturalistic and longitudinal design that makes use of the information that clinicians collect and record in their everyday clinical practice, seems a good compromise between practicality and comprehensiveness. Graphical modelling and the strategy based on conditional independence on which it relies represent a powerful tool in dealing with the complexities involved in assessing outcome. Moreover, they provide a sound statistical ground for both generating and testing hypotheses, because of the possibility they offer of interpreting the undirected (non-causal) and directed (causal) relationships between variables.

Acknowledgements

This study was supported by the Fondazione Cassa di Risparmio di Verona Vicenza Belluno e Ancona, Progetto Sanità 1996–1997, through a grant for 'The role of social factors on onset, course and outcome of mental disorders: an epidemiological approach', to Professor Michele Tansella.

References

AMADDEO, F., BEECHAM, J., BONIZZATO, P., *et al* (1997) The use of a case register to evaluate the costs of psychiatric care. *Acta Psychiatrica Scandinavica*, **95**, 189–198.

——, ——, ——, *et al* (1998) The cost of community-based psychiatric care for first-ever patients. A case register study. *Psychological Medicine*, **28**, 173–183.

ANDREWS, S., LEAVY, A., DeCHILLO, N., *et al* (1986) Patient–therapist mismatch: we would rather switch than fight. *Hospital and Community Psychiatry*, **37**, 918–922.

ATTKISSON, C., COOK, J., KARNO, M., *et al* (1992) Clinical services research. *Schizophrenia Bulletin*, **18**, 627–668.

COX, D. R. & WERMUTH, N. (1994) Tests of linearity, multivariate normality and the adequacy of linear score. *Applied Staistics*, **43**, 347–355.

—— & —— (1996) *Multivariate Dependencies. Models, Analysis and Interpretation*. London: Chapman & Hall.

DEMPSTER, D. P. (1972) Covariance selection models. *Biometrics*, **28**, 157–175.

DOWDS, B. & FONTANA, A. (1977) Patients' and therapists' expectations and evaluations of hospital treatment. *Comprehensive Psychiatry*, **18**, 295–300.

EDWARDS, D. (1995) *Introduction to Graphical Modelling*. New York: Springer-Verlag.

ENDICOTT, J., SPITZER, R. L., FLEISS, J. L., *et al* (1976) The Global Assessment Scale. A procedure for measuring overall severity of psychiatric disturbance. *Archives of General Psychiatry*, **33**, 766–771.

EVERITT, B. S. & LANDAU, S. (1998) The use of multivariate statistical methods in psychiatry. *Statistical Methods in Medical Research*, **7**, 253–277.

FIENBERG, S. E. (1980) *The Analysis of Cross-Classified Categorical Data*. Cambridge, MA: MIT Press.

GARRARD, J., HAUSMAN, W., MANSFIELD, E., *et al* (1988) Educational priorities in mental health professions: do educators and consumers agree? *Medical Education*, **22**, 60–66.

GREENLAND, S. (1987) *Evolution of Epidemiologic Ideas*. Chestnut Hill: Epidemiology Research Inc.

GUNKEL, S. & PRIEBE, S. (1993) Different perspectives of short-term changes in the rehabilitation of schizophrenic patients. *Comprehensive Psychiatry*, **34**, 352–359.

JENKINS, R. (1990) Toward a system of outcome indicators for mental health care. *British Journal of Psychiatry*, **157**, 500–514.

KREINER, S. (1996) An informal introduction to graphical modelling. In *Mental Health Service Evaluation* (eds H. C. Knudsen & G. Thornicroft), pp. 156–175. Cambridge: Cambridge University Press.

LAURITZEN, S. L. (1996) *Graphical Models*. Oxford: Oxford Science Publications.

—— & Wermuth, N. (1989) Graphical models for associations between variables, some of which are qualitative and some quantitative, *Annals of Statistics*, **17**, 31–54.

LUKOFF, D., NUECHTERLEIN, K. & VENTURA, J. (1986) Manual for expanded Brief Psychiatric Rating Scale (BPRS). *Schizophrenia Bulletin*, **4**, 594–602.

MAYER, J. & ROSENBLATT, A. (1974) Clash in perspective between mental patients and staff. *American Journal of Orthopsychiatry*, **44**, 432–441.

MIRIN, S. M. & NAMEROW, M. J. (1991) Why study treatment outcome? *Hospital and Community Psychiatry*, **42**, 1007–1013.

OLIVER, J. P. (1991) The social care directive: development of a quality of life profile for use in community services for the mentally ill. *Social Work and Social Science Review*, **3**, 4–45.

RUGGERI, M. (1994) Patients' and relatives' satisfaction with psychiatric services: the state of the art of its measurement. *Social Psychiatry and Psychiatric Epidemiology*, **28**, 212–227.

—— & DALL'AGNOLA, R. (1993) The development and use of the Verona Expectations for Care Scale (VECS) and the Verona Service Satisfaction Scale (VSSS) for measuring expectations and satisfaction with community-based psychiatric services in patients, relatives and professionals. *Psychological Medicine*, **23**, 511–523.

—— & TANSELLA, M. (1995) Evaluating outcome in mental health care. *Current Opinion in Psychiatry*, **8**, 116–121.

—— & —— (1996) Individual patient outcomes. In *Mental Health Service Evaluation* (eds H. C. Knudsen & G. Thornicroft), pp. 281–295. Cambridge: Cambridge University Press.

——, DALL'AGNOLA, R., AGOSTINI, C., *et al* (1994) Acceptability, sensitivity and content validity of VECS and VSSS in measuring expectations and satisfaction in psychiatric patients and their relatives. *Social Psychiatry and Psychiatric Epidemiology*, **29**, 265–276.

——, BIGGERI, A., RUCCI, P., *et al* (1998*a*) Multivariate analysis of outcome of mental health care using graphical chain models. The South-Verona Outcome Project 1. *Psychological Medicine*, **28**, 1421–1431.

——, RIANI, M., RUCCI, P., *et al* (1998*b*) Multidimensional assessment of outcome in psychiatry: the use of graphical display. The South-Verona Outcome Project 2. *International Journal of Methods in Psychiatric Research*, **7**, 187–199.

SLADE, M., THORNICROFT, G., LOFTUS, L., *et al* (1999) *CAN: Camberwell Assessment of Need*. London: Gaskell.

TANSELLA, M. (1989) Evaluating community psychiatric services. In *The Scope of Epidemiological Psychiatry* (eds P. Williams, C. Wilkinson & K. Rawnsley), pp. 386–403. London: Routledge.

—— & RUGGERI, M. (1996) Monitoring and evaluating a community-based mental health service: the epidemiological approach. In *The Scientific Basis of Health Services* (eds R. Smith & M. Peckham), pp. 160–169. London: British Medical Journal Publishing Group.

—— (1999) Evaluating community psychiatric services. In *The Scope of Epidemiological Psychiatry* (eds P. Williams, C. Wilkinson & K. Kawnsley), pp. 386–403. London: Routledge.

WHITTAKER, J. (1990) *Graphical Models*. Chichester: Wiley.

WORLD HEALTH ORGANIZATION (1988) *WHO Psychiatric Disability Assessment Schedule* (WHO/DAS). Geneva: WHO.

16 Assessing needs for mental health services

SONIA JOHNSON, GRAHAM THORNICROFT, MICHAEL PHELAN and MICHAEL SLADE

If mental health services aim to meet needs at the levels of both the individual patient and the whole population, then three key issues emerge: how can needs be defined, who should assess them and how can this information be best used? This chapter addresses these issues in three stages: by presenting definitions of need, by reviewing methods of assessing individual needs for treatment and by outlining how needs for services at the population level can be measured.

Needs: the problem of definition

There is at present no consensus on how needs should be defined (Holloway, 1994) or who should define them (Ellis, 1993; Slade, 1994). The *Oxford English Dictionary* offers "necessity, requirement and essential" and, in a different sense, "destitution, distress, indigence, poverty or want". These clusters of meanings overlap in so far as they define 'need' as a vital element that is lacking, and this chapter uses this sense as its point of departure. Need will therefore be used here to refer to essentials of life that are not present. The fact that a need is present does not mean that it can be met. For example, some needs may remain unmet because other problems take priority, because an effective method is not available locally, or because the person in need refuses treatment.

In psychological terms, Maslow (1968) has set out a hierarchy of five levels reflecting, in sequence, needs for physiological functioning, safety, love, self-esteem and self-actualisation. Similarly, in a philosophical analysis of the field, Liss (1990) has distinguished four elements of need. The first is the 'ill health' approach, which equates

271

need with a deficiency in health that requires medical care. In this model the required intervention is simply the provision of the absent treatment. For Mallman & Marcus (1980), for example, need is "an objective requirement to avoid a state of illness" (p. 165). Second, Liss describes the 'supply notion', where the existence of a need presumes that an acceptable and effective treatment exists to offer remedy, and this is referred to by Stevens & Gabbay (1991) as "the ability to benefit in some way from health care". Third, the 'normative notion' of need proposes that need is a matter of opinion, and therefore a needs assessment has to be put in the context of the beliefs of those involved, often referred to as 'felt' or 'perceived' needs, to distinguish them from needs that are considered to have a more objective basis. The view that "need is seen as a shortfall compared with a state of being which is generally acceptable" exemplifies this approach (Davies & Challis, 1986, p. 562). Fourth, the 'instrumental view' of need is that health is required to reach a certain state or defined goal. For example, Tracy (1986) described a need as "a lack of a specific resource which is useful for or required by the purpose of [a living system]" (p. 212). In this view, the accuracy of the needs assessment and the effectiveness of the treatment intervention can therefore be gauged by the extent to which the instrumental goal is achieved. Need in this sense can be distinguished from demand (expressed wish) and supply (utilisation).

Need, demand and supply are related to each other (Stevens & Gabbay, 1991). A demand for care exists when an individual expresses a wish to receive it. In an alternative formulation, demand is what people would be willing to pay for in a market or might wish to use in a system of free health care (Stevens & Raftery, 1994). Supply includes interventions, agents and settings, whether or not they are used in any particular case. Care coordination entails providing such a pattern of service after initial assessment and then updating the assessment regularly to assess outcomes and to modify the care if needs remain unmet. Overprovision occurs when provision exceeds need, while need in excess of provision is unmet need. A need may exist, as defined by a professional, even if the intervention is refused by a patient. At the same time, a proper needs assessment process should not lead to the imposition of expert solutions upon patients. A professionally defined need may remain unmet and have to be replaced by one acceptable to the patient.

Another approach to defining need has been proposed by health economists. Their contributions include, first, the proposal that need refers to both the capacity to benefit from an intervention and the amount of expenditure required to reduce the capacity to benefit to zero; it is therefore a product of benefit and cost-effectiveness (Culyer

& Wagstaff, 1992). Second, health economists have proposed that diagnosis-related groups are notably irrelevant for mental health services (McCrone & Strathdee, 1994). Third, empirical data should guide operational needs definitions (Beecham *et al*, 1991).

In the particular case of mental health services, needs have been described in terms of the gaps between the service needs of patients and of populations and the services actually provided. Lehtinen *et al* (1990) interpret needs as reflecting an inadequate level of service for the severity of the problem: patients with severe disorders who receive primary rather than specialised psychiatric care would therefore be rated as having unmet need. Similarly, for Shapiro *et al* (1985), unmet needs are defined as the combination of definite morbidity and lack of mental health service utilisation. A third view is that needs represent an insufficient supply of particular treatment interventions, and this approach is embodied in the three individual needs assessment instruments now described.

Needs at the individual level

Patients who suffer from severe mental illness have a range of needs that go far beyond the purely medical, as described in the National Institute of Mental Health's document *Toward a Model Plan for a Comprehensive Community-Based Mental Health System* (1987). The issue of how best to make an individual assessment of need has taxed both researchers and clinicians, not least because their requirements differ. An ideal assessment tool for use in a routine clinical setting would be one that is brief, is easily learned, takes little time to administer, does not require the use of personnel in addition to the usual clinical team, is valid and reliable in different settings and, above all, can be used as an integral part of routine clinical work. MacDonald (1991) suggests that such a scale should also be sensitive to change, the potential interrater and test–rater reliability should be high, and it should logically inform clinical management (Hillier *et al*, 1991; Thornicroft & Bebbington, 1996). The decision about which scale to use depends on whether the approach is to focus on particular diagnostic or care groups, on the balance to be struck between economy of time and inclusiveness of the ratings, and on the range of areas of clinical and social functioning to be assessed.

Camberwell Assessment of Need (CAN)

A clinically orientated and relatively brief instrument is the Camberwell Assessment of Need (CAN), which has been published by the

PRiSM team at the Institute of Psychiatry (Phelan *et al*, 1995; Slade *et al*, 1999). It is intended both for research and for clinical use, especially in relation to the requirements of the NHS and Community Care Act 1990 to undertake needs assessments of people with severe mental health problems. It includes both patient and staff views, considers a comprehensive range of health and social needs, and assesses needs separately from interventions.

The principles that have guided the development of the CAN are that needs are universal, that many psychiatric patients have multiple needs, that needs assessment should be an integral part of clinical practice and that the process should involve ratings by both staff and patients. In the construction of the scale, the authors aimed to ensure that it had adequate psychometric properties, could be completed within 30 minutes, was comprehensive, was usable by wide range of staff, could record help from informal carers and staff, and would be suitable for both research and clinical use.

The 22 areas assessed are basic needs (accommodation, food and occupation), health needs (physical health, psychotic and neurotic symptoms, drugs and alcohol, safety to self and others), social needs (company, intimate relationships and sexual expression), everyday functioning (household skills, self-care and child care, basic education, budgeting) and service receipt (information, telephone, transport and welfare benefits). The psychometric properties of the scale have now been established in terms of both validity (face, consensual, content, criterion and construct) and reliability (Phelan *et al*, 1995) and the results are acceptable (Table 16.1). It was striking that in a survey of severely disabled psychiatric patients in south London, the mean number of problems identified by staff was 7.5 (95% confidence interval, 6.7 to 8.4) and by patients was 7.9 (6.8 to 8.9). When examined in detail, however, the degree of agreement by staff and patients for individual items was rather poor, so that the hypothesis that staff and patients would rate problems similarly was rejected (Slade *et al*, 1996).

TABLE 16.1
Camberwell Assessment of Needs: summary of reliability scores

	r	*Significance level*
Interrater		
Staff	0.99	$P < 0.001$
Patient	0.98	$P < 0.001$
Test–retest		
Staff	0.78	$P < 0.001$
Patient	0.71	$P < 0.001$

The CAN has now been used in a variety of published research studies (e.g. Leese *et al*, 1998; Wiersma *et al*, 1998; Boardman *et al*, 1999). A brief version, the Camberwell Assessment of Need Short Appraisal (CANSAS), is now also available (Slade *et al*, 1999). This takes only around 10 minutes to complete, and involves rating level of need in each of the 22 areas listed above as no need, met need or unmet need. Unlike the fuller version of the instrument, amount and appropriateness of help currently received are not rated, so that it is less useful than the original for individual care planning, but is suitable for purposes such as assessing outcomes in mental health services research or examining the profile of needs among clients of a particular service or on the caseloads of individual professionals. The original CAN is intended for use with adults with severe mental illnesses, but versions are now also available or being developed for people with learning disabilities, children and older people, and translations have been made into at least 11 languages (Slade & McCrone, 2001).

MRC Needs for Care Assessment

The Medical Research Council (MRC) Needs for Care schedule (Brewin, 1992) is based on the following formal definitions:

- a need is present when a patient's functioning (social disablement) falls below or threatens to fall below some minimum specified level, and this is due to a remediable, or potentially remediable, cause
- a need is met if it has attracted some at least partly effective item of care, and if no other items of care of greater potential effectiveness exist
- a need is unmet when it has attracted an only partly effective or no item of care and when other items of care of greater potential effectiveness exist.

In this schedule, 'needs for care' have been defined as requirements for specific activities or interventions that have the potential to ameliorate disabling symptoms or problems in social functioning. In contrast, 'needs for services' reflect institutional requirements and are defined as needs for specific agents or agencies to deliver those interventions (Brewin *et al*, 1987). Mangen & Brewin (1991) outline a procedure for deriving estimates of needs for services from individuals' needs for specific items of care. Substantial data have now been presented on individual needs assessments using this instrument (Brewin *et al*, 1988, 1990; Lesage *et al*, 1991; Pryce *et al*, 1993; Van Haaster *et al*,

1994), along with a detailed critique of this approach (Hogg & Marshall, 1992; Brewin & Wing, 1993).

Cardinal Needs Schedule

A third approach to individual needs assessment is that of Marshall (1994), who has developed the Cardinal Needs Schedule. This is a modification of the MRC Needs for Care approach, intended to be briefer and simpler than the original in terms of both data collection and rating, and to provide a more structured procedure for incorporating users' and carers' views. 'Cardinal problems' are identified through the application of three criteria:

- the 'cooperation criterion' (the patient is willing to accept help for the problem)
- the 'carer stress criterion' (the problem causes considerable anxiety, frustration or inconvenience to people caring for the patient)
- the 'severity criterion' (the problem endangers the health or safety of the patient or the safety of other people).

Information is collected using the Manchester Scale for mental state assessment, the REHAB scale and specially developed additional schedules including a Client Opinion Interview and a Carer Stress Interview. The rating procedure has been computerised. Marshall *et al* (1995) report data on the practicality and psychometric properties of the instrument; the procedure apparently is indeed substantially shorter than the MRC Needs for Care Assessment, and the interrater and test–retest reliability are good in most areas, although only moderate in a few.

Population-based needs assessment

The ideal method for the development of comprehensive and appropriate local services is the use of a standardised method such as those discussed above for individual assessment of the needs of all those identified as mentally ill within the catchment area. Services should then be developed so that they fit the aggregated needs of this population as closely as possible. However, direct data on service needs are often absent or of very poor quality, so that local planners need methods of estimating the extent of local needs for services from widely available demographic and service use data.

A number of proxies for more comprehensive needs assessment have been developed, each with its own limitations (Shapiro *et al*, 1985). First, local need may be estimated on the basis of epidemiological studies that provide figures for the national prevalence of the disorders that may bring individuals into contact with the psychiatric services. Second, data about national and international patterns of service utilisation and provision may be extrapolated to give expected levels of service use by the local population. Third, current local services may be compared with expert views on desirable levels of services. Fourth, the validity of these various types of estimate may be increased by using a deprivation-weighted approach. Estimates of service need may be adjusted on the basis of knowledge about relationships of psychiatric disorders to age, sex, ethnic group, marital status, economic status and other social variables. Finally, the geographical distribution of mental health facilities should also be considered: services should be accessible to all, and their availability in parts of the catchment area where need is likely to be highest should be a particular consideration.

Each of these methods is summarised below, and illustrations of how population need may be estimated for a catchment area are provided by Johnson *et al* (1996).

Estimating local needs from epidemiological data

Taking the first of the approaches, a simple estimate of local morbidity may be derived from epidemiological studies of the prevalence of psychiatric disorders carried out elsewhere. The strength of prevalence data from community surveys is that they allow estimates to be made of the total levels of need existing in the population. However, this method does not identify the types of services likely to be required to meet these needs. This is problematic for disorders such as depression or anxiety, where most symptomatic individuals will not require referral to specialist mental health services. Such community prevalence data are more useful for schizophrenia and other psychoses, as it is reasonable to assume that the majority of people with such illnesses will require some form of long-term contact with secondary services. A consensus on the range of interventions that are effective in, and should be available for, each disorder, and on the proportion of people with each disorder who are likely to benefit from each type of intervention, would allow much more accurate extrapolation from patterns of psychiatric disorder to needs for services and treatments.

Service use as a proxy for service need

The work of Goldberg & Huxley (1980, 1992) may be used as a basis for comparing local service use with national and international data on service utilisation. For example, their calculations suggest that in an average area, 2.4% of the adult population are expected to have contact with specialist mental health services in any one year and 0.6% will be admitted to a psychiatric hospital. Other sources of data on service use include statistics on admissions collected nationally, such as the Hospital Episode Statistics in the UK, and data from local case registers, which have the advantage that they are likely to provide more accurate data than national statistics, particularly for out-patient and community services (Glover, 1991).

Service utilisation data of this kind may be used to calculate the levels of service use that would be expected for a local catchment area. This does not, of course, allow a normative assessment of the services that an area *should* ideally have. However, service planners may find it useful to have some idea of whether current numbers of contacts with particular components of their local services are large or small compared with patterns elsewhere.

Comparing local services with desirable levels of service provision

There is considerable debate about optimal numbers of psychiatric treatment and care places required to meet local needs (Wing, 1971, 1989; Thornicroft & Strathdee, 1994). In the UK, a Royal College of Psychiatrists working party estimated an acute requirement of 44 beds per 100 000 population (Hirsch, 1988). Strathdee & Thornicroft (1992) have set out targets for service provision based on epidemiological findings regarding the prevalence of psychiatric disorder and on a Delphi method of summarising expert opinion. The targets assume that, as far as possible, services should be community based, with community residential and day places taking the place of institutional care. Wing (1992) has made a similar set of estimates of targets for general adult residential services. These estimates are shown in Table 16.2: they provide a basis for comparing actual local service provision with desirable numbers of places of various types.

A deprivation-weighted approach to estimating population needs

The approaches delineated so far do not provide a way of taking into account the particular socio-demographic characteristics of the local catchment area. This is unsatisfactory, as the evidence for a close

TABLE 16.2
Estimated need for general adult residential provision per 250 000 population
(Wing, 1992; Strathdee & Thornicroft, 1992)

Type of accommodation	Wing (1992)		Strathdee & Thornicroft (1992)	
	Midpoint	Range	Midpoint	Range
Staff awake at night				
Acute and crisis care	100	50–150	95	50–150
Intensive-care unit	10	5–15	8	5–10
Regional secure unit and special hospital	4	1–10	5	1–10
Hostel wards	50	25–75		
Other staffed housing	75	40–110	95	40–150
High-staffed hostel				30–120
Day-staffed hostel	50	25–75	75	30–120
Group homes (visited)	45	20–70	64	48–80
Respite facilities		3	0–5	
No specialist staff				
Supported bed-sits	30	–		
Direct access	30	–		
Adult placement schemes			8	0–35
Total per 250 000	394	226–585	357	174–540

association between social and demographic factors and measured rates of psychiatric disorder is strong. For example, in the UK, the Jarman combined index of social deprivation has been shown to be highly correlated with psychiatric admission rates (Jarman, 1983, 1984; Hirsch, 1988; Thornicroft, 1991; Thornicroft *et al*, 1993), making the Jarman index a potentially useful tool in predicting expected rates of psychiatric service use.

The Mental Illness Needs Index (MINI) has been developed by Glover *et al* (1998) specifically as a tool for estimating likely local needs for mental health service care. It is available in computerised form and is based on local levels of social isolation, poverty, unemployment, permanent sickness and temporary and insecure housing. Glover *et al* (1998) describe a study in which the MINI appeared to be more closely associated with psychiatric admission rates than the Jarman score. Thus a method for making weighted estimates of likely local needs for services may be derived by combining indices such as the MINI or Jarman score with the estimates of the range of places needed in a catchment area shown in Table 16.2. Such a method assumes that more deprived places will require a number of places at the higher end of these ranges, and vice versa.

An illustration of this approach is Ramsay *et al*'s (1997) examination of mental health service provision across London. This work is based on the MINI, combined with expert estimates of the ranges within which are likely to fall the numbers of hospital and residential places required in a catchment area. Actual levels of service provision in each London borough are compared with estimated need, providing some indications of areas and types of provision where there may be shortfalls, although the authors draw attention to a number of reasons for caution in the interpretation of these findings.

Taking overall social deprivation into account is a helpful beginning in making epidemiologically based estimates of needs for services. Such estimates will be improved by taking into account a number of local factors with specific implications for needs for mental health services. Ethnicity is particularly important: ethnic minority populations have been found to have different patterns of service use from others in their communities, and both the effects of local minority populations on numbers of places required and their particular needs for culturally and linguistically appropriate services should be taken into account (King *et al*, 1994; Fernando, 1996; Bhui, 1997). Any groups of recently arrived refugees living locally are likely to be experiencing high levels both of deprivation and of post-traumatic disorders. The extent of the local homeless population should also be considered, as the homeless have high rates of psychiatric disorder and may not be reached by conventional psychiatric services (Marshall, 1989; Timms & Fry, 1989; Scott, 1993).

Assessment through reports of key informants

A further approach used in local needs assessment is to elicit reports by individual or group interview or by questionnaire from key local informants regarding their views about whether local services meet local people's needs. These key informants may include service users, carers, clinicians and service managers. The DISC framework developed by Smith (1998) provides a method for structuring such a needs assessment exercise and is intended to be used in service development. An extensive range of service functions that should be available to meet the needs of a local catchment area are identified using this tool. Thus this procedure allows identification of perceived gaps and shortfalls in local service provision, although it does not lead directly to a quantitative estimate of how much service provision is required to meet local needs.

Service needs from a geographical perspective

Meeting needs across a catchment area requires both the provision of adequate numbers of places in a range of forms of care *and* their location such that they are accessible to those who need them. Not only the overall characteristics but also the detailed geography of a catchment area thus needs to be considered. Sectorisation is now regarded in many European countries as an essential pre-requisite to the development of effective community services (Johnson & Thornicroft, 1993). Such a division of larger catchment areas into smaller geographically defined sectors, with services for each area located centrally within it, is an important principle in ensuring that services are accessible to people throughout the catchment area. It is also important for service planners to examine public transport routes to ensure local bases can be reached reasonably quickly from each part of each sector. A further important principle in considering the geography of the catchment area is that particular attention should be paid to service provision in those areas where the greatest levels of needs may be expected, as in areas where there is severe poverty or where homeless people tend to congregate.

Conclusions

There is now widespread agreement on the principle that the needs of the local population with mental illness should guide the development and provision of community mental health services. No consensus exists as yet on how to define such needs, at either an individual or a population level. However, some methodologies are now available both for needs assessment at an individual level and for estimating the likely aggregate needs of populations. While these methods are still at an early stage of development, their wider application in service planning and provision promises to promote the development of services that are more appropriate for mentally ill individuals. They also make available a means of assessing the current extent of unmet needs and the degree to which services may currently lack resources required to meet the needs of their catchment area populations.

References

BEECHAM, J., KNAPP, M. & FENYO, A. (1991) Costs, needs and outcomes. *Schizophrenia Bulletin*, **17**, 427–439.

BHUI, K. (1997) London's ethnic minorities and the provision of mental health services. In *London's Mental Health* (eds S. Johnson, R. Ramsay, G. Thornicroft *et al*), pp. 143–166. London: King's Fund.

BOARDMAN, A. P., HODGSON, R. E., LEWIS, M., *et al* (1999) North Staffordshire Community Beds Study: longitudinal evaluation of psychiatric in-patient units attached to community mental health centres. I: Methods, outcome and patient satisfaction. *British Journal of Psychiatry*, **175**, 70–78.

BREWIN C. R. (1992) Measuring individual needs for care and services. In *Measuring Mental Health Needs* (eds G. Thornicroft, C. R. Brewin & J. Wing), pp. 220–236. London: Gaskell.

——, WING, J. K., MANGEN, S. R., *et al* (1987) Principles and practice of measuring needs in the long-term mentally ill: the MRC Needs for Care Assessment. *Psychological Medicine*, **17**, 971–981.

——, WING, J. K., MANGEN, S. R., *et al* (1988) Needs for care among the long-term mentally ill: a report from the Camberwell High Contact Survey. *Psychological Medicine*, **18**, 457–468.

——, VELTRO, F., WING, J. K.., *et al* (1990) The assessment of psychiatric disability in the community: a comparison of clinical, staff, and family interviews. *British Journal of Psychiatry*, **157**, 671–674.

—— & WING, J. K. (1993) The MRC Needs for Care Assessment: progress and controversies. *Psychological Medicine*, **23**, 837–841.

CULYER, A. & WAGSTAFF, A. (1992) *Need, Equity and Equality in Health and Health Care.* York: Centre for Health Economics, Health Economics Consortium, University of York.

DAVIES, B. & CHALLIS, D. (1986) *Matching Resources to Needs in Community Care.* London: Gower.

ELLIS, K. (1993) *Squaring the Circle: User and Carer Participation in Needs Assessment.* York: Joseph Rowntree Foundation.

FERNANDO, S. (1996) *Mental Health in a Multi-ethnic Society.* London: Routledge.

GLOVER, G. (1991) The official data available on mental health. In *Indicators for Mental Health in the Population* (eds R. Jenkins & S. Griffiths), pp. 18–24. London: HMSO.

——, ROBIN, E., EMAMI, J., *et al* (1998) A needs index for mental health care. *Social Psychiatry and Psychiatric Epidemiology*, **33**, 89–96.

GOLDBERG, D. & HUXLEY, P. (1980) *Mental Illness in the Community.* London: Tavistock.

—— & —— (1992) *Common Mental Disorders: A Bio-Social Model.* London: Routledge.

HILLIER, W., ZAUDIG, M. & MOBOUR, W. (1991) Development of diagnostic checklists for use in routine clinical care. *Archives of General Psychiatry*, **47**, 782–784.

HIRSCH, S. (1988) *Psychiatric Beds and Resources: Factors Influencing Bed Use and Service Planning.* London: Gaskell.

HOGG, L. & MARSHALL, M. (1992) Can we measure need in the homeless mentally ill? Using the MRC Needs for Care Assessment in hostels for the homeless. *Psychological Medicine*, **22**, 1027–1034.

HOLLOWAY, F. (1994) Need in community psychiatry: a consensus is required. *Psychiatric Bulletin*, **19**, 321–323.

JARMAN, B. (1983) Identification of underprivileged areas. *British Medical Journal*, **286**, 1705–1709.

—— (1984) Underprivileged areas: validation and distribution of scores. *British Medical Journal*, **289**, 1587–1592.

JOHNSON, S. & THORNICROFT, G. (1993) The sectorisation of psychiatric services in England and Wales. *Social Psychiatry and Psychiatric Epidemiology*, **28**, 45–47.

——, THORNICROFT, G. & STRATHDEE, G. (1996) Population-based assessment of needs for services. In *Commissioning Mental Health Services* (eds G. Strathdee & G. Thornicroft), pp. 37–52. London: HMSO.

KING, M., COKER, E., LEAVEY, G., *et al* (1994) Incidence of psychotic illness in London: a comparison of ethnic groups. *British Medical Journal*, **309**, 1115–1119.

LEESE, M., JOHNSON, S., SLADE, M., *et al* (1998) The user perspective on needs and satisfaction with mental health services: the PRiSM Psychosis Study (8). *British Journal of Psychiatry*, **173**, 409–415.

LEHTINEN, V., JOUKAMAA, M., JYRKINEN, E., *et al* (1990) Need for mental health services of the adult population in Finland. Results from the Mini Finland Health Survey. *Acta Psychiatrica Scandinavica*, **81**, 426–431.

LESAGE, A. D., MIGNOLLI, G., FACCINCANI, C., *et al* (1991) Standardised assessment of the needs for care in a cohort of patients with schizophrenic psychoses. In *Community-Based Psychiatry: Long-Term Patterns of Care in South Verona* (ed M. Tansella). *Psychological Medicine*, monograph suppl. 19, pp. 27–33.

LISS, P. (1990) *Health Care Need: Meaning and Measurement.* Linkoping: Studies in Arts and Science.

MACDONALD, A. (1991) How can we measure mental health? In *Indicators for Mental Health in the Population* (eds R. Jenkins & S. Griffiths), pp. 25–29. London: HMSO.

MALLMAN, C. A. & MARCUS, S. (1980) Logical clarifications in the study of needs. In *Human Needs* (ed. K. Lederer), pp. 163–185. Cambridge, MA: Oelgeschlager, Gunn & Hain.

MANGEN, S. & BREWIN, C. R. (1991) The measurement of need. In *Social Psychiatry: Theory, Methodology and Practice* (ed. P. E. Bebbington), pp. 163–181. New Brunswick: Transaction Press.

MARSHALL, M. (1989) Collected and neglected: are Oxford hostels filling up with disabled psychiatric patients? *British Medical Journal*, **299**, 706–709.

—— (1994) How should we measure need? *Philosophy, Psychiatry and Psychology*, **1**, 27–36.

——, HOGG, L. I., GATH, D. H., *et al* (1995) The Cardinal Needs Schedule: a modified version of the MRC Needs for Care Assessment Schedule. *Psychological Medicine*, **25**, 605–617.

MASLOW, A. (1968) *Towards a Psychology of Being* (2nd edn). New York: D. van Nostrand.

MCCRONE, P. & STRATHDEE, G. (1994) Needs not diagnosis: towards a more rational approach to community mental health resourcing in Great Britain. *International Journal of Social Psychiatry*, **40**, 79–86.

MCGOVERN, D. & COPE, R. (1991) Second generation of Afro-Caribbeans and young Whites with a first admission diagnosis of schizophrenia. *Social Psychiatry and Psychiatric Epidemiology*, **26**, 95–99.

NATIONAL INSTITUTE OF MENTAL HEALTH (1987) *Toward a Model Plan for a Comprehensive Community-Based Mental Health System.* Washington, DC: NIMH.

PHELAN, M., SLADE, M., THORNICROFT, G., *et al* (1995) The Camberwell Assessment of Need (CAN): the validity and reliability of an instrument to assess the needs of people with severe mental illness. *British Journal of Psychiatry*, **167**, 589–595.

PRYCE, I., GRIFFITHS, R., GENTRY, R., *et al* (1993) How important is the assessment of social skills in current long-stay psychiatric in-patients? *British Journal of Psychiatry*, **163**, 498–502.

RAMSAY, R., THORNICROFT, G., JOHNSON, S., *et al* (1997) Levels of in-patient and residential provision throughout London. In *London's Mental Health* (eds S. Johnson, R. Ramsay, G. Thornicroft, *et al*), pp. 193–219. London: King's Fund.

SCOTT, J. (1993) Homelessness and mental illness. *British Journal of Psychiatry*, **162**, 314–324.

SHAPIRO, S., SKINNER, E. A., KRAMER, M., *et al* (1985) Measuring need for mental health services in a general population. *Medical Care*, **23**, 1033–1043.

SLADE, M. (1994) Needs assessment: who needs to assess? *British Journal of Psychiatry*, **165**, 287–292.

—— & MCCRONE, P. (2001) The Camberwell Assessment of Need. In *Measuring Mental Health Needs* (2nd edn) (eds G. Thornicroft, C. R. Brewin & J. Wing). London: Gaskell (in press).

——, PHELAN, M., THORNICROFT, G., *et al* (1996) The Camberwell Assessment of Need: comparison of assessments by staff and patients of the needs of the severely mentally ill. *Social Psychiatry and Psychiatric Epidemiology*, **31**, 109–113.

——, Thornicroft, G., Loftus, L., *et al* (1999) *The Camberwell Assessment of Need*. London: Gaskell.

Smith, H. (1998) Needs assessment in mental health services: the DISC framework. *Journal of Public Health Medicine*, **20**, 154–160.

Stevens, A. & Gabbay, J. (1991) Needs assessment needs assessment. *Health Trends*, **23**, 20–23.

—— & Raftery, J. (1994) Introduction. In *Health Care Needs Assessment* (eds A. Stevens & J. Raftery), pp. 11–30. Oxford: Radcliffe Medical Press.

Strathdee, G. & Thornicroft, G. (1992) Community sectors for needs-led mental health services. In *Measuring Mental Health Needs* (eds G. Thornicroft, C. R. Brewin & J. Wing), pp. 140–162. London: Gaskell.

Thornicroft, G. (1991) Social deprivation and rates of treated mental disorder: developing statistical models to predict psychiatric service utilisation. *British Journal of Psychiatry*, **158**, 475–484.

——, Bisoffi, G., De Salvia, G., *et al* (1993) Urban–rural differences in the associations between social deprivation and psychiatric service utilisation in schizophrenia and all diagnoses: a case register study in northern Italy. *Psychological Medicine*, **23**, 487–496.

—— & Strathdee, G. (1994) How many psychiatric beds? *British Medical Journal*, **309**, 970–971.

—— & Bebbington, P. (1996) Quantitative methods in the evaluation of community mental health services. In *Modern Community Psychiatry* (ed. W. Breakey), pp. 120–138. Cambridge: Cambridge University Press.

Timms, P. & Fry, A. (1989) Homelessness and mental illness. *Health Trends*, **21**, 70–71.

Tracy, L. (1986) Toward an improved need theory: in response to legitimate criticism. *Behavioural Science*, **31**, 205–218.

Van Haaster, I., Lesage, A., Cyr, M., *et al* (1994) Problems and needs for care of patients suffering from severe mental illness. *Social Psychiatry and Psychiatric Epidemiology*, **29**, 141–148.

Warr, R., Jackson, P. & Banks, M. H. (1988) Unemployment and mental health: some British studies. *Journal of Social Issues*, **44**, 47–68.

Wiersma, D., Nienhuis, F., Giel, R., *et al* (1998) Stability and change in needs of patients with schizophrenic disorders. *Social Psychiatry and Psychiatric Epidemiology*, **33**, 49–56.

Wing, J. (1971) How many psychiatric beds? *Psychological Medicine*, **1**, 189–190.

—— (ed.) (1989) *Health Services Planning and Research. Contributions from Psychiatric Case Registers*. London: Gaskell.

—— (1992) *Epidemiologically-Based Needs Assessments. Review of Research on Psychiatric Disorders*. London: Department of Health.

17 Outcome measures for the treatment of depression in primary care

WILLIAM E. NARROW
and DARREL A. REGIER

Major depression is among the most disabling and costly of illnesses, yet its burden is often unrecognised. In the USA, where individuals may visit specialists such as psychiatrists and psychologists without first having seen a general practitioner, historically, the primary-care sector of the health system has nevertheless played a large role in both the mental and physical health care of depressed patients. This role has recently been amplified by the managed-care industry, with its emphasis on restricted access to speciality care. This chapter reviews state-of-the-art research on the treatment of depression in primary care, with special attention to the assessment of outcomes.

Epidemiology, service use and costs of depression in primary care

Prevalence of disorder and disability

Major depression is common in primary care, with a point prevalence estimated at 5–10% (Katon & Schulberg, 1992), compared with an estimate of 2.2% (Regier, 1988) in the general population. Associated with this prevalence is a high level of disability. The Medical Outcomes Study (MOS) demonstrated that physical functioning and well-being scores on the 36-item Short Forms scale (SF–36 – see below) for patients with major depression were comparable to, and in some cases significantly worse than, scores for patients with chronic medical conditions. Mental functioning and well-being scores were consistently and significantly worse for the depressed MOS patients than for the medically ill patients (Hays *et al*, 1995). Another longitudinal observational study compared depressed primary-care patients during their 'worst-functioning' assessment interval with non-depressed subjects (Rost *et al*, 1998). The investigators found 3.5–4 times higher scores on SF–36 role limitation–physical scale among depressed primary-care patients, over 9 times higher scores on the role limitations–emotional scale, and 8–10 times more disability days in the past month. In the six months before the assessment, 45–55% had suicidal ideation. These findings point to a high degree of individual suffering and potentially enormous costs to society in terms of lost productivity.

Despite the prevalence and disability of depression, the disorder often goes unrecognised and untreated in primary care. The MOS found that only 46–51% of depressed patients who visited medical clinicians had their depression detected, compared with 78–87% of depressed patients who visited mental health specialists (Wells *et al*, 1989). Higher rates of recognition in primary care, up to 65%, have been reported when the diagnosis of depression was strictly defined to those patients given a structured diagnostic interview, and when clinicians were asked directly about the presence of psychological distress, rather than relying on chart notations. The patients with recognised depression appear to have more severe illness and greater disability than those with unrecognised depression. These patients are also more likely to receive antidepressant treatment (Simon & Von Korff, 1995).

Among those patients whose depression is recognised and treated, the prescribed treatment is often inadequate. General practitioners tend to prescribe inadequate dosages and duration of medication, with infrequent follow-up visits and lack of adjustment of the dose according to patient response. Referrals to speciality care are often not made when needed (Katon *et al*, 1990, 1992; Lin *et al*, 1997; van der Feltz-Cornelis *et al*, 1997). Patient adherence to antidepressant treatment is reasonably high in the first month, with over half of patients taking the prescribed medication. However, there is considerable drop-off in this by four and six months. There is evidence that adherence rates are higher with the newer, non-tricyclic antidepressants (Katon *et al*, 1992; Simon *et al*, 1993, 1995*a*; Lin *et al*, 1995). Adherence to treatment regimens for chronic physical illnesses is a particular problem when comorbid depression is present (Katon, 1996).

Service use

Two large studies have documented the level of mental health service use among Americans with diagnosable major depression. The

National Institute of Mental Health's Epidemiologic Catchment Area (ECA) Program showed that over one year, about 54% of persons with active unipolar major depression used at least one mental health or addiction service, with 45% using the health sector – 27.8% used the speciality sector and 25.3% used the general medical sector for their mental health problems (Regier *et al*, 1993). There were large differences in the average number of mental health visits per treated person per year among the two sectors: 17.5 visits in the speciality sector and 4.2 visits in the general medical sector (Narrow *et al*, 1993).

The National Comorbidity Survey (NCS), done in the early 1990s, 7–10 years after the ECA Program, showed somewhat different results for service use. Among persons with major depression, 36.4% used any mental health service and 27.7% used services in the health sector, with 21.2% using speciality services and 12.1% using general medical services (Kessler *et al*, 1999). It is difficult to explain the lower rate of service use in the general medical settings in the NCS than in the ECA. It may be due to a true decrease in use from the time when the ECA was conducted. Alternatively, methodological differences may account for the disparity. Among the latter possibilities are different respondent recall periods for service use, with the ECA collecting data in three waves, six months apart, and the NCS collecting one wave of data with a one-year service-use recall. Recall for less frequent events, such as general medical visits for depression, may have been enhanced with the longitudinal data collection of the ECA. Average visit frequency was about one visit less per year than in the ECA – 3.4 per treated person per year in the speciality sector and 16.5 per person per year in the general medical sector (Kessler *et al*, 1999).

People with depression are overrepresented among high users of general medical services for physical health reasons (Kessler *et al*, 1987; Katon, 1996; Lefevre *et al*, 1999; Pearson *et al*, 1999). For example, distressed high users were found to have high prevalences of chronic medical problems and illness-related disability. In addition, 24% were found to have current major depression, 17% were found to have current dysthymia and 68% had a lifetime history of major depression (Katon *et al*, 1990).

Costs of care

People with major depression tend to be high users of general medical and mental health services, with attendant high costs to the general medical sector. Simon *et al* (1995*b*) examined age- and sex-matched samples of Health Maintenance Organization (HMO) primary-care attenders with and without depression as diagnosed by their general practitioner. They found that depressed patients had significantly higher annual health care costs – $4246 compared with $2371 for non-depressed patients. The depressed patients had higher costs for each component of care, including in-patient and out-patient care, drugs and laboratory tests, and similar results were found regardless of whether the depression was treated with antidepressant medication. Indeed, among those treated, speciality treatment of the depression accounted for less than 25% of the difference in total costs of care, with about half of the difference accounted for by non-specific increases in out-patient service use. Twofold differences in costs persisted for at least 12 months after the initiation of treatment.

Similar results were found by Unützer *et al* (1997) in a large cohort of older adults. In this study, costs were about 50% higher for patients with significant depressive symptoms, as measured by the Center for Epidemiologic Studies Depression (CESD) scale, than for patients without such symptoms. Again, costs were uniformly increased across all health care components, and speciality care accounted for a very small portion (about 1%) of total costs. It remains to be determined whether the costs of adequately treating depression will be offset by reduced medical costs and improved work productivity (Simon & Katzelnick, 1997; Schulberg *et al*, 1998).

Randomised trials of treatment effectiveness

Based on the foundation presented above, efforts to improve the care of depressed patients in primary care have had several goals – increased recognition and treatment by general practitioners, increased rates of appropriate treatment, increased patient adherence to treatment recommendations, reduction of depressive symptoms and disorder, reduction of disability, increased positive functioning and quality of life, reduced costs of non-mental health medical care, and overall cost-effectiveness. This is a diverse set of goals that encompasses change in outcomes on at least three levels: provider, patient and expenditures. In this chapter we focus on patient-level outcomes assessments. First, recent state-of-the-art research studies in the United States that have examined these issues are briefly described. A description of the outcome measures used in these studies follows. All of these studies had as a goal the use of proven efficacious treatments in actual primary-care practice settings, and so have moved beyond the more tightly controlled efficacy trials to 'real life' effectiveness trials.

The aims of the Collaborative Care intervention trial (Katon *et al*, 1995) were to determine whether the treatment of depression in primary care could be improved to the level of the treatment recommendations of the Agency for Health Care Policy and Research (AHCPR), whether this treatment improved short-term patient outcomes, and whether it was acceptable to the patients and the general practitioners. Patients from general practices in a large HMO who had screening scores of 0.75 or more on the 20-item Symptom Check-List (SCL) were randomised. The intervention arm ($n = 77$) consisted of collaborative depression treatment by one of two on-site psychiatrists along with the general practitioner, who had received didactic training in depression and its treatment. Antidepressant medication along with patient education were the main treatments in the intervention group, although referrals to psychotherapy could be made. The control arm ($n = 76$) was usual care by the general practitioner.

Katon *et al* (1996) subsequently adapted the Collaborative Care model to incorporate non-psychiatrist providers and behavioural (i.e. non-medication) treatment in similar primary-care settings as above. The study aims were similar to those of the previous study, that is, achieving AHCPR guideline-level care, acceptability and improved outcomes. In this study, the intervention ($n = 108$) consisted of a highly structured programme given by an on-site, doctorally trained psychologist involving brief, cognitively orientated psychotherapy, adherence counselling and a relapse-prevention programme. The study psychiatrist acted as a consultant and provided medication recommendations to the general practitioner based on a weekly progress report. The control group ($n = 109$) received care as usual from their general practitioner.

Schulberg *et al* (1996) aimed to test guideline-concordant treatments, including psychotherapy, within a framework of effectiveness research (see also Coulehan *et al*, 1997). They chose patients from four ambulatory health centres, screened for depression with the CESD scale, and confirmed with the Diagnostic Interview Schedule (DIS) and the Hamilton Rating Scale for Depression (HRSD). There were two intervention arms. One intervention group, of 93 patients, received interpersonal psychotherapy from a trained psychologist or psychiatrist in 16 weekly sessions. The second intervention group, of 91 patients, received nortriptyline from an internist (physician specialising in internal medicine) or family practitioners trained in pharmacotherapy through didactic sessions and a manual. The control group of 92 patients received usual care from their general practitioners.

The Partners in Care Study (Wells *et al*, 1999) has been described as the second generation of the Patient Outcomes Research Team (PORT) initiative of the AHCPR. The main goals of Partners in Care are to examine the outcomes of the treatment of depression in terms of patient health and satisfaction, health care and social costs, and the quality and cost-effectiveness of care. The two experimental interventions were basic quality improvement with enhanced medication management and quality improvement with enhanced psychotherapy. These interventions were compared with usual care. Primary-care clinics from seven geographically diverse managed-care organisations were randomised into one of the two intervention groups or the usual-care group. Patients were screened with the Composite International Diagnostic Interview (CIDI) stem questions for major depression and dysthymia. A total of 913 patients were placed in an intervention group and 443 received care as usual.

Patient-level outcome measures used in treatment-effectiveness research on depression in primary care

The outcome measures used for these studies are listed in Table 17.1. For simplicity, these are grouped into five categories: symptoms, functioning/disability, adherence, satisfaction with care and health service use. This chapter concentrates on the measures in the first two categories, which generally have standard measures that have been used extensively and reported in peer-reviewed journals.

Depressive symptoms

The HRSD (Hamilton, 1960, 1967) is frequently used to measure severity of depression as an outcome of treatment. The scale comprises 17 items to assess severity and four additional non-scored items to be used for diagnostic rather than severity purposes (Zitman *et al*, 1990). The items are heavily focused on somatic symptoms: depressed mood, guilt, suicide, insomnia (three items), work and interests, retardation, agitation, psychic anxiety, somatic anxiety, gastrointestinal symptoms, general somatic symptoms, loss of libido, hypochondriasis, loss of insight and loss of weight. Items are scored on a scale of 0–2 or 0–4, although operationalised scoring criteria specific to each item are not consistently provided. The scale is administered in an interview format, and use of collateral information in developing the ratings for a patient was encouraged by the developer of the scale. The interview time frame is the last few days or week. Raters must be trained in the use of the scale and must have clinical experience. To increase its reliability, Hamilton recommended using two raters for each interview and summing the ratings (Hamilton, 1967). The HRSD takes about 30 minutes to administer.

TABLE 17.1

Outcome measures from four US studies of depression treatment in primary care

Study	Symptoms	Functioning/ disability	Adherence	Satisfaction with care	Health service use
Katon *et al* (1995)	SCL–90 depression scale; IDS; NEO Personality Inventory neuroticism scale; CDS; screen for side-effects of medication		Dosage check; took medication for 25 of last 30 days; HMO records for dose and duration	Satisfaction with care; perceived helpfulness of antidepressants	
Katon *et al* (1996)	As above, plus (short-form) DSM checklist		As above, plus self-report adherence		
Schulberg *et al* (1996), Coulehan *et al* (1997)	BDI; HRSD–17; DUSOI	SF–36; GAS			
Wells *et al* (1999)	CESD; CIDI screener for depressive disorder (omitting dysthymia stem)	SF–12 physical and mental health summary scales; current employment	Prescribed medicines used in previous month; medication used for over 1 month in previous 6 months; appropriate use of antidepressants based on guideline dose criteria		Health service use in past 6 months; total medical visits; medical visits for emotional problems; mental health speciality visits; use of individual, individual, family, or group therapy by specialist

SCL, Symptom Checklist; IDS, Inventory for Depressive Symptomatology; CDS, Chronic Disease Score; BDI, Beck Depression Inventory; HRSD, Hamilton Rating Scale for Depression; DUSOI Duke University Severity of Illness Checklist; SF, Short Forms; GAS, Global Assessment Scale; CESD, Center for Epidemiologic Studies Depression Scale; CIDI, Composite International Diagnostic Interview.

In addition to Hamilton's original version of the scale, a different but frequently used version is the ECDEU version (Guy, 1976). Developed for the NIMH Early Clinical Drug Evaluation Unit (ECDEU) programme, this version is more structured and, unlike the original scale, provides anchor points for scoring each item (Nordgren, 1995). It also adds three items to the scale – helplessness, hopelessness and worthlessness – making it a 24-item scale.

Because of concerns about the reliability of individual HRSD items (Cicchetti & Prusoff, 1983; Rehm & O'Hara, 1985), a semistructured interview guide was developed based on the ECDEU version of the instrument (Williams, 1988). This instrument, called the SIGH–D, gives initial and follow-up questions for each of the 21 items of the scale, and allows the interviewer to develop further questions as needed. This method has improved the test–retest reliability of most of the individual items, without lengthening the time of administration (Williams, 1988). A fully structured version of the HRSD, called the SI–HRSD, was developed for use in the MOS (Potts *et al*, 1990). Although this version apparently has lower item-level test–retest reliabilities than the SIGH–D, it has been successfully administered by non-clinicians, and can be given over the telephone. It also uses a past-month time frame. A 14-item version of the SI–HRSD was recommended by the developers of the scale.

The proliferation of 'versions' of the Hamilton scale necessitates careful investigation by the researcher or clinician when choosing the proper instrument. Likewise, when reporting results, the exact version of the scale used, and any modifications, must be reported, to facilitate comparisons with other scales.

The Beck Depression Inventory (BDI) is a 21-item rating scale that is also widely used in the assessment of depressive symptoms. Like the Hamilton scale, there are several versions in current use; unlike the Hamilton, many were developed by the author of the original scale. The original BDI (Beck *et al*, 1961) was developed to be administered by a trained interviewer and assesses symptoms on a current time frame ('right now').

A subsequent version (Beck *et al*, 1979) was released in which items were clarified to allow self-administration and easier scoring, alternative ways of asking the same question were eliminated and double-negative statements were avoided. The time frame used in this revision is 'past week'. The items included are: mood, pessimism, sense of failure, lack of satisfaction, guilt feelings, sense of punishment, self-dislike, self-accusations, suicidal wishes, crying, irritability, social withdrawal, indecisiveness, distortion of body image, work inhibition, sleep disturbance, fatigability, loss of appetite, weight loss, somatic preoccupation and loss of libido. Items are rated on a scale of 0–3 and total scores can range from 0 to 63 (Beck & Steer, 1984.) The scale takes "a few minutes to complete and score" (Nordgren, 1995).

The BDI and the HRSD have many obvious differences, including mode of administration, cost of administration (e.g. training interviewers and avoiding 'interviewer drift' in a study using the HRSD), length of administration and item coverage. All of these factors must enter into a decision on choice of instrument. Studies comparing the two instruments have been inconclusive. Some (Moran & Lambert, 1983; Richter *et al*, 1997) have concluded that the BDI is overreactive in detecting change in response to therapeutic intervention, therefore running the risk of false positives. Others have concluded that the HRSD may be over-reactive (Edwards *et al*, 1984; Lambert *et al*, 1986). One study that directly compared the two instruments with the same patients over time found satisfactory and significant correlations between the total scores for two-thirds of the patients, and poor correlations for the remaining one-third. The authors found no obvious differences in personality or severity of illness that distinguished the latter group (Bailey & Coppen, 1976).

The Inventory for Depressive Symptomatology (IDS; Rush *et al*, 1986, 1996) has both self-report (IDS–SR) and clinician-rated versions (IDS–C). The original scale had 28 items; two were subsequently added to cover atypical symptoms. While not as frequently used as the HRSD or the BDI, both versions of the scale have satisfactory psychometric properties, correlate well with ratings from the HRSD and BDI and, unlike the HRSD and BDI, cover the full range of DSM–IV depression criteria. Items are scored on a 0–3 scale. Factor analysis revealed three dimensions for each scale: cognitive/mood, anxiety/arousal, and vegetative (Rush *et al*, 1996.)

The revised 90-item SCL (SCL–90–R; Derogatis *et al*, 1976; Derogatis & Cleary, 1977; Derogatis, 1983) evolved from an older instrument, the Hopkins Symptom Checklist (Derogatis *et al*, 1974), as a self-report measure of psychopathology. Each of the 90 items is rated on a five-point scale of distress, from 'not at all' to 'extremely'. The SCL–90–R is scored on nine primary symptom dimensions and three global indices of psychopathology. The primary symptom dimensions are somatisation, obsessive–compulsive, interpersonal sensitivity, depression, anxiety, hostility, phobic anxiety, paranoid ideation, and psychoticism. The global indices are the global severity index, the positive symptom distress index, and the positive symptom total. The depression symptom dimension is composed of 13 items, reflecting a broad range of depressive symptoms, including dysphoric mood and affect, withdrawal, lack of motivation, loss of vitality, hopeless feelings, suicidal ideation and other cognitive and somatic symptoms. The depression symptom dimension has an internal consistency coefficient of 0.90 (Derogatis *et al*, 1976).

The SCL–90–R has been criticised for inadequate factor structure and poor discriminant validity, with several investigators finding much of the covariation in symptom dimensions being accounted for by a single global distress factor. In particular, the depression dimension has been found to be highly correlated with the anxiety dimension, raising doubts as to their distinguishability (Morgan *et al*, 1998). However, recent studies have shown that when homogeneous samples of persons with depression or anxiety are used, separate anxiety and depression dimensions can be distinguished (Cox *et al*, 1993; Morgan *et al*, 1998). This finding reinforces the extent to which anxiety and depressive symptoms coexist in unselected patient samples.

The CESD (Radloff, 1977; Radloff & Locke, 1986) was developed at the National Institute of Mental Health for use in epidemiological studies of the presence and severity of depressive symptoms in general populations. It is a 20-item scale, with 16 items assessing symptoms in the negative direction (e.g. "I felt sad") and four items assessing symptoms in the positive direction (e.g. "I enjoyed life"). The latter items were included to discourage tendencies towards a response set as well as to assess positive affect. The items cover a range of depressive symptoms, including depressed mood, feelings of guilt and worthlessness, feelings of helplessness and hopelessness, psychomotor retardation, loss of appetite and sleep disturbance. Items are rated on a 0–3 scale, and the positive items are reversed before scoring, so the highest possible score is 60. The conventional cut-off score signifying significant depressive symptoms is 16 or above. The CESD is a self-report scale, and can be self-administered or interviewer administered.

The Composite International Diagnostic Interview (CIDI; Robins *et al*, 1988; World Health Organization, 1997) is a fully structured diagnostic interview that is suitable for administration by trained lay interviewers. It is available in paper-and-pencil and computer-assisted versions. Responses are scored by computer algorithms to provide psychiatric diagnoses according to either DSM–IV or ICD–10 criteria. The diagnostic sections of the CIDI include phobic and other anxiety disorders, depressive and dysthymic disorders, manic and bipolar affective disorders, schizophrenia and other psychotic disorders, eating disorders, substance use disorders, obsessive–compulsive and post-traumatic stress disorders, dementia, amnesic and other cognitive disorders, and somatoform and dissociative disorders. Diagnoses can be provided in several time frames, including lifetime, one year and one month. Because the CIDI is a modularised instrument, the diagnostic sections of interest can be selected for administration in lieu of the entire interview. The reliability and validity of the CIDI are good for depression and most other diagnoses (Andrews & Peters, 1998).

The NEO Personality Inventory (Costa & McCrae, 1992) measures personality dimensions according to the five-factor model (FFM) of personality (Digman, 1990). The scale originally measured three personality domains: neuroticism, extraversion and openness to experience (hence 'NEO'). Conscientiousness and agreeableness were added in later versions to fit the FFM. The various versions of the inventory were rigorously developed through factor analysis. Test–retest reliability and internal consistency are very good (Costa & McCrae, 1988). The most current version is referred to as the NEO–PI–R. It is a copyrighted inventory containing 240 items with three additional validity items. Each of the five domains contains 'facet scales'. Within the neuroticism domain, these are anxiety, hostility, depression, self-consciousness, impulsiveness and vulnerability (Costa & McCrae, 1988). The entire inventory can be completed in 45 minutes or less, and there are versions for self-administration and administration by a rater who knows the subject well. The inventory has been used successfully in depressed patient populations (Bagby *et al*, 1998, 1999).

Physical symptoms

The Chronic Disease Score (CDS; Von Korff *et al*, 1992) was developed from the population-based computerised prescription system of the Group Health Cooperative of Puget Sound to measure chronic disease status. The scoring system was developed with the following principles in mind: the score should increase with the number of chronic diseases under treatment; the score should increase with increasing complexity of the medication regimen used to treat a specific chronic disease; potentially life-threatening or progressive diseases should be scored higher than benign or stable diseases; medication regimens used in the score should target diseases, not symptoms (e.g. analgesics and sedatives should not be counted). Seventeen diseases were chosen for inclusion, each with one or more medication classes and accompanying scoring rules. For example, high cholesterol was given a score of 1 if antilipaemics were used, diabetes was given a score of 2 if either insulin or oral hypoglycaemics were used. For heart disease, three medication classes were identified and the patient was scored as 3 if one class was used, 4 if two classes were used, or 5 if all three classes were used.

The CDS was found to be correlated with physician ratings of disease severity and it was predictive of hospital admissions and mortality in the following year. There was a modest association with self-reported health status and disability, and the score was not associated with depression or anxiety. Finally, the CDS showed high year-to-year stability in a population sample. For studies with suitable record systems, techniques such as the CDS and related measurements such as the Illness Scale (Mossey & Roos, 1987), which uses insurance claims data, can be used effectively at minimal cost.

The Duke University Severity of Illness Checklist (DUSOI; Parkerson *et al*, 1993) was developed as a generic measure of severity of illness and comorbidity. It is available in paper form and computerised versions (Parkerson *et al*, 1994) and can be completed after a face-to-face medical encounter or from a review of medical records. Training is provided in the form of a four-page users' manual. The checklist comprises a listing of all diagnoses and health problems that are active at the time of the interview or in the previous week. For each diagnosis or health problem, four 'severity parameters' are listed. These are symptom level, complications, prognosis without treatment, and treatability (i.e. need for treatment and expected response to treatment). Each parameter is then rated on a five-point scale. Three main scores can be obtained from the resulting data: the DUSOI diagnosis severity of illness score, which ranges from 1 to 100; the DUSOI overall severity of illness score, which is a weighted sum of all diagnosis severities for a given patient; and the DUSOI comorbidity severity of illness, which is computed in the same way as the overall score but without the index diagnosis score. Less than two minutes are required to complete the computerised version (Parkerson *et al*, 1994.)

One of the main advantages of the DUSOI is its clinical relevance – scores are computed from a clinician's impression, whether the clinician completes the instrument directly, or the chart is audited. Interrater reliability has been moderate to excellent (Parkerson *et al*, 1994; Shiels *et al*, 1997), despite the reliance of the scale on individual judgements and uncertainties in the treatability and prognosis of many conditions. It has been suggested that reliability of the DUSOI may be improved by a more detailed training manual and more explicit criteria for rating severity within parameters (Shiels *et al*, 1997).

Functioning and disability

Probably the most widely used global functioning measures are the Global Assessment Scale (GAS; Endicott *et al*, 1976) and its modification, the Global Assessment of Functioning Scale (GAF; American Psychiatric Association, 1987). The GAS is itself based on an older instrument called the Health–Sickness Rating Scale (Luborsky, 1962), which was developed as a means for clinicians to judge mental health or illness along a single dimension on a 100-point scale. The GAS retains the 100-point continuum of mental illness to mental health, ranging from a score of 1 for the hypothetically sickest individual, to 100 for the hypothetically healthiest individual. The scale is sub-divided into 10-point intervals, and each interval carries a description that includes representative symptoms and impairments in func-tioning. Diagnostic characterisations are avoided in the descriptions. The developers of the scale intended the two highest intervals (81–90 and 91–100) for "those unusually fortunate individuals who not only are without significant psychopathology but also exhibit many positive traits often referred to as 'positive mental health'" (Endicott *et al*, 1976). They wrote that most out-patients would be scored between 31 and 70, and most in-patients between 1 and 40. GAS ratings are based on the individual's lowest functioning level in the preceding week. In order to determine a specific rating within the chosen interval, the two adjacent intervals are examined to determine whether the individual is closer to one or the other. All sources of information can be considered in making the rating. The interrater reliability and validity of the GAS are satisfactory in a research context with proper training in the scale's use (Endicott *et al*, 1976).

Unlike the GAS, the MOS Short Forms measure health profiles across a number of dimensions. Derived from the full-length MOS scale (245 items), two currently popular Short Forms contain 36 items (SF–36; Ware & Sherbourne, 1992) and 12 items (SF–12; Ware *et al*, 1996). The SF–36 was designed to replace older 18- and 20-item Short Forms (Stewart *et al*, 1988), which had problems in comprehensive-ness, content validity and floor effects (Ware & Sherbourne, 1992). The SF–36 measures eight health concepts: physical functioning (10 items), role limitations due to physical problems (4 items), bodily pain (2 items), general health perceptions (5 items), social function-ing (2 items), general mental health (5 items), role limitations due to emotional problems (3 items) and vitality (4 items). An additional item, not used in any of the scales, assesses the respondent's perception of change in his or her health status in the past year. Most questions refer to the past four weeks, and response options vary from question to question, from yes/no responses to six-level Likert-type scales. The SF–36 can be self-administered or admin-istered by telephone or personal interview, although different forms and instructions are used for each method. The scale can be administered in 5–10 minutes (Ware & Sherbourne, 1992).

Data from the MOS were used to assess the psychometric properties of the SF–36 scales that were embedded in the full 245-item MOS assessment. With few exceptions, the SF–36 items met acceptable levels for data completeness, scaling assumptions and scale internal consistency. Floor effects were reduced compared with the SF–20, but remained substantial for the two role disability scales. Ceiling effects were substantial for the role disability scales and the social functioning scale. The investigators of this study emphasised that only the physical functioning scale met minimum standards of internal consistency on an individual patient level, with confidence intervals being unacceptably large for the other scales, so further research is needed before the SF–36 can be used for individual patient assessment and the evaluation of individual treatment effects (McHorney *et al*, 1994).

Further research has identified two summary measures in the SF–36: the Physical Component Summary (PCS), comprising the physical functioning, role limitations – physical, bodily pain, and general health perceptions scales; and the Mental Component Summary (MCS), comprising the social functioning, general mental health, role limitations – emotional, and vitality scales (Ware *et al*, 1996). Research on the SF–36 has shown that physical and mental health factors accounted for 80–85% of the reliable variance in the eight scales. Further, the PCS and the MCS were able to detect hypothesised differences in nearly all tests based on physical and mental criteria, respectively (Ware *et al*, 1996).

The SF–12 was developed in response to the need for even shorter measures than the SF–36 for use in large-scale surveys and monitoring efforts (Ware *et al*, 1996). Items were chosen by applying separate forward step-regression analyses to the SF–36 PCS and MCS. Ten items were found to reproduce more than 90% of the variance in the PCS and MCS, and two additional items were added to represent all eight SF–36 scales. The SF–12 takes two minutes or less to self-administer. Reliability and validity coefficients were acceptable for the SF–12, although predictably somewhat lower than for the SF–36 (Ware *et al*, 1996).

Conclusions

The Global Burden of Disease project estimated that unipolar major depression was the fourth leading cause of disability-adjusted life years (DALYs) in 1990 (Murray & Lopez, 1996*a*) and is projected to be the second leading cause of DALYs by the year 2020 (Murray & Lopez, 1996*b*). Although the scientific basis for primary prevention programmes is increasing, the early identification and treatment of existing depression remains the most effective method of reducing the burden of illness. The primary-care sector has played an important treatment role in the past and will continue to do so in the future, for several reasons. From the patient's perspective, the stigma of mental illness or the costs and inconvenience of obtaining speciality mental health services may make treatment in primary care more attractive. The uneven geographical distribution of speciality mental health services in the United States means that some patients have no access to such services, particularly in isolated and rural areas, and primary-care services may be the only treatment option. Managed-care organisations may also encourage the treatment of depression in primary care, particularly if the case is of mild severity, in order to control costs.

Maximising the effectiveness of the treatment of depression in primary care is critical for the reasons mentioned above, and because of the problems in recognition and treatment adequacy that are known to exist when depressed patients visit their general practitioner.

The patient-level outcome measures described in this chapter are only a part of the picture. Further work is being done in the development of better methods for outcomes assessment at all levels of the treatment process. For example, work on the World Health Organization Disability Assessment Schedule (WHO/DAS–II; World Health Organization, 1999), which is tied to the WHO International Classification of Functioning and Disability (ICIDH–2; Üstün *et al*, 1995), promises to provide a standardised research tool for disability assessment, much as the DIS and CIDI did for the ICD and DSM diagnostic systems. The development and refinement of treatment guidelines for depression provide an anchor for measuring the adequacy of usual treatment and enhanced interventions. The issues of the cost-effectiveness and cost offsets of treating depression are being closely studied (Revicki *et al*, 1998; Von Korff *et al*, 1998). Finally, there is much to be learned from international collaborations, since there are many common issues among different countries and health systems (Üstün & Sartorius, 1995).

References

AMERICAN PSYCHIATRIC ASSOCIATION (1987) *Diagnostic and Statistical Manual of Mental Disorders* (3rd edn, revised) (DSM–III–R). Washington, DC: APA.

ANDREWS, G. & PETERS, L. (1998) The psychometric properties of the Composite International Diagnostic Interview. *Social Psychiatry and Psychiatric Epidemiology*, **33**, 80–88.

BAGBY, R. M., RECTOR, N. A., BINDSEIL, K., *et al* (1998) Self-report ratings and informants' ratings of personalities of depressed outpatients. *American Journal of Psychiatry*, **155**, 437–438.

——, LEVITAN, R. D., KENNEDY, S. H., *et al* (1999) Selective alteration of personality in response to noradrenergic and serotonergic antidepressant medication in depressed sample: evidence of non-specificity. *Psychiatry Research*, **86**, 211–216.

BAILEY, J. & COPPEN, A. (1976) A comparison between the Hamilton Rating Scale and the Beck Inventory in the measurement of depression. *British Journal of Psychiatry*, **128**, 486–489.

BECK, A. T., WARD, C. H., MENDELSON, M., *et al* (1961) An inventory for measuring depression. *Archives of General Psychiatry*, **4**, 561–571.

——, RUSH, A. J., SHAW, B. F., *et al* (1979) *Cognitive Therapy of Depression*. New York: Guilford Press.

—— & STEER, R. A. (1984) Internal consistencies of the original and revised Beck Depression Inventory. *Journal of Clinical Psychology*, **40**, 1365–1367.

CICCHETTI, D. V. & PRUSOFF, B. A. (1983) Reliability of depression and associated clinical symptoms. *Archives of General Psychiatry*, **40**, 987–990.

COSTA, P. T. & MCCRAE, R. R. (1988) Personality in adulthood: a six-year longitudinal study of self-reports and spouse ratings on the NEO Personality Inventory. *Journal of Personality and Social Psychology*, **54**, 853–863.

—— & —— (1992) *Revised NEO Personality Inventory (NEO–PI–R) and NEO Five-Factor Inventory (NEO–FFI) professional manual*. Odessa, FL: Psychological Assessment Resources.

COULEHAN, J. L., SCHULBERG, H. C., BLOCK, M. R., *et al* (1997) Treating depressed primary care patients improves their physical, mental, and social functioning. *Archives of Internal Medicine*, **157**, 1113–1120.

COX, B. J., SWINSON, R. P., KUCH, K., *et al* (1993) Self-report differentiation of anxiety and depression in an anxiety disorders sample. *Psychological Assessment*, **5**, 484–486.

DEROGATIS, L. R. (1983) *SCL–90–R Administration, Scoring, and Procedures Manual – II*. Towson, MD: Clinical Psychometric Research.

——, LIPMAN, R. S., RICKELS, K., *et al* (1974) The Hopkins Symptom Checklist (HSCL): a self-report symptom inventory. *Behavioral Science*, **19**, 1–15.

——, RICKELS, K. & ROCK, A. F. (1976) The SCL–90 and the MMPI: a step in the validation of a new self-report scale. *British Journal of Psychiatry*, **128**, 280–289.

—— & CLEARY, P. A. (1977) Factorial invariance across gender for the primary symptom dimensions of the SCL–90. *British Journal of Social and Clinical Psychology*, **16**, 347–356.

DIGMAN, J. M. (1990) Personality structure: emergence of the five-factor model. *Annual Review of Psychology*, **41**, 417–440.

ENDICOTT, J., SPITZER, R. L., FLEISS, J. L., *et al* (1976) The Global Assessment Scale: a procedure for measuring overall severity of psychiatric disturbance. *Archives of General Psychiatry*, **33**, 766–771.

EDWARDS, B. C., LAMBERT, M. J., MORAN, P. W., *et al* (1984) A meta-analytic comparison of the Beck Depression Inventory and the Hamilton Rating Scale for Depression as measures of treatment outcome. *British Journal of Clinical Psychology*, **23**, 93–99.

GUY, W. (ed.) (1976) *ECDEU Assessment Manual for Psychopharmacology*. DHHS Publication Number ADM 76–336. Rockville, MD: US Department of Health, Education, and Welfare.

HAMILTON, M. (1960) A rating scale for depression. *Journal of Neurology, Neurosurgery and Psychiatry*, **12**, 56–62.

—— (1967) Development of a rating scale for primary depressive illness. *British Journal of Social and Clinical Psychology*, **6**, 278–296.

HAYS, R. D., WELLS, K. B., SHERBOURNE, C. D., *et al* (1995) Functioning and well-being outcomes of patients with depression compared with chronic general medical illnesses. *Archives of General Psychiatry*, **52**, 11–19.

KATON, W. (1996) The impact of major depression on chronic medical illness. *General Hospital Psychiatry*, **18**, 215–219.

—— & SCHULBERG, H. (1992) Epidemiology of depression in primary care. *General Hospital Psychiatry*, **14**, 237–247.

——, VON KORFF, M., LIN, E., *et al* (1990) Distressed high utilizers of medical care: DSM–III–R diagnoses and treatment needs. *General Hospital Psychiatry*, **12**, 355–362.

——, ——, ——, *et al* (1992) Adequacy and duration of antidepressant treatment in primary care. *Medical Care*, **30**, 67–76.

—, —, —, *et al* (1995) Collaborative management to achieve treatment guidelines: impact on depression in primary care. *Journal of the American Medical Association*, **273**, 1026–1031.

—, Robinson, P., Von Korff, M., *et al* (1996) A multifaceted intervention to improve treatment of depression in primary care. *Archives of General Psychiatry*, **53**, 924–932.

Kessler, L. G., Burns, B. J., Shapiro, S., *et al* (1987) Psychiatric diagnoses of medical service users: evidence from the Epidemiologic Catchment Area program. *American Journal of Public Health*, **77**, 18–24.

—, Zhao, S., Katz, S. J., *et al* (1999) Past-year use of outpatient services for psychiatric problems in the National Comorbidity Survey. *American Journal of Psychiatry*, **156**, 115–123.

Lambert, M. J., Hatch, D. R., Kingston, M. D., *et al* (1986) Zung, Beck, and Hamilton rating scales as measures of treatment outcome: a meta-analytic comparison. *Journal of Consulting and Clinical Psychology*, **54**, 54–59.

Lefevre, F., Reifler, D., Lee, P., *et al* (1999) Screening for undetected mental disorders in high utilizers of primary care services. *Journal of General Internal Medicine*, **14**, 425–431.

Lin, E. H., Von Korff, M., Katon, W., *et al* (1995) The role of the primary care physician in patients' adherence to antidepressant therapy. *Medical Care*, **33**, 67–74.

—, Katon, W. J., Simon, G. E., *et al* (1997) Achieving guidelines for the treatment of depression in primary care: is physician education enough? *Medical Care*, **35**, 831–842.

Luborsky, L. (1962) Clinicians' judgements of mental health. *Archives of General Psychiatry*, **31**, 407–417.

McHorney, C. A., Ware, J. E., Lu, J. F. R., *et al* (1994) The MOS 36-item short form health survey (SF–36): III. Tests of data quality, scaling assumptions, and reliability across diverse patient groups. *Medical Care*, **32**, 40–66.

Moran, P. W. & Lambert, M. J. (1983) A review of current assessment tools for monitoring changes in depression. In *The Measurement of Psychotherapy Outcome in Research and Evaluation* (eds M. J. Lambert, E. R. Christensen & S. S. DeJulio), pp. 263–303. New York: Wiley.

Morgan, C. D., Wiederman, M. W. & Magnus, R. D. (1998) Discriminant validity of the SCL–90 dimensions of anxiety and depression. *Assessment*, **5**, 197–201.

Mossey, J. M. & Roos, L. L. (1987) Using insurance claims data to measure health status: the Illness Scale. *Journal of Chronic Diseases*, **40** (suppl. 1), 41S–50S.

Murray, C. J. L. & Lopez, A. D. (1996*a*) The global burden of disease in 1990: final results and their sensitivity to alternative epidemiological perspectives, discount rates, age-weights and disability weights. In *The Global Burden of Disease: A Comprehensive Assessment of Mortality and Disability from Diseases, Injuries, and Risk Factors in 1990 and Projected to 2020* (eds C. J. L. Murray & A. D. Lopez), pp. 247–293. Boston: Harvard School of Public Health.

— & — (1996*b*) Alternative visions of the future: projecting mortality and disability, 1990–2020. In *The Global Burden of Disease: A Comprehensive Assessment of Mortality and Disability from Diseases, Injuries, and Risk Factors in 1990 and Projected to 2020* (eds C. J. L. Murray & A. D. Lopez), pp. 325–395. Boston: Harvard School of Public Health.

Narrow, W. E., Regier, D. A., Rae, D. S., *et al* (1993) Use of services by persons with mental and addictive disorders: findings from the NIMH ECA program. *Archives of General Psychiatry*, **50**, 95–107.

Nordgren, J. C. (1995) Instruments for assessing depression in adults. In *Handbook of Depression* (eds E. E. Beckham & W. R. Leber), pp. 591–599. New York: Guilford Press.

Parkerson, G. R., Broadhead, W. E. & Chiu-kit, J. T. (1993) The Duke Severity of Illness Checklist (DUSOI) for measurement of severity and comorbidity. *Journal of Clinical Epidemiology*, **46**, 379–393.

—, Hammond, W. E. & Yarnall, K. S. H. (1994) Feasibility and potential clinical usefulness of a computerised severity of illness measure. *Archives of Family Medicine*, **3**, 968–973.

PEARSON, S. D., KATZELNICK, D. J., SIMON, G. E., *et al* (1999) Depression among high utilizers of medical care. *Journal of General Internal Medicine*, **14**, 461–468.

POTTS, M. K., DANIELS, M., BURNAM, M. A., *et al* (1990) A structured interview version of the Hamilton Depression Rating Scale: evidence of reliability and versatility of administration. *Journal of Psychiatric Research*, **24**, 335–350.

RADLOFF, L. S. (1977) The CES–D Scale: a self-report depression scale for research in the general population. *Applied Psychological Measurement*, **3**, 385–401.

—— & LOCKE, B. Z. (1986) The Community Mental Health Assessment Survey and the CES–D scale. In *Community Surveys of Psychiatric Disorders* (eds M. M. Weissman, J. D. Myers & C. E. Ross), pp. 177–189. New Brunswick, NJ: Rutgers University Press.

REGIER, D. A., BOYD, J. H., BURKE, J. D., *et al* (1988) One-month prevalence of mental disorders in the United States. *Archives of General Psychiatry*, **45**, 977–986.

——, NARROW, W. E., MANDERSCHEID, R. W., *et al* (1993) The DeFacto U.S. Mental and Addictive Disorders Service System: ECA prospective one-year rates of disorders and services. *Archives of General Psychiatry*, **50**, 85–94.

REHM, L. P. & O'HARA, M. W. (1985) Item characteristics of the Hamilton Rating Scale for Depression. *Journal of Psychiatric Research*, **19**, 31–41.

REVICKI, D. A., SIMON, G. E., CHAN, K., *et al* (1998) Depression, health-related quality of life, and medical cost outcomes of receiving recommended levels of antidepressant treatment. *Journal of Family Practice*, **47**, 446–452.

RICHTER, P., WERNER, J., BASTINE, R., *et al* (1997) Measuring treatment outcome by the Beck Depression Inventory. *Psychopathology*, **30**, 234–240.

ROBINS, L. N., WING, J., WITTCHEN, H-U., *et al* (1988) The Composite International Diagnostic Interview: an epidemiologic instrument suitable for use in conjunction with different diagnostic systems and in different cultures. *Archives of General Psychiatry*, **45**, 1069–1077.

ROST, K., ZHANG, M., FORTNEY, J., *et al* (1998) Persistently poor outcomes of undetected major depression in primary care. *General Hospital Psychiatry*, **20**, 12–20.

RUSH, A. J., GILES, D. E., SCHLESSER, M. A., *et al* (1986) The Inventory for Depressive Symptomatology (IDS): preliminary findings. *Psychiatry Research*, **18**, 65–87.

——, GULLION, C. M., BASCO, M. R., *et al* (1996) The Inventory of Depressive Symptomatology (IDS): psychometric properties. *Psychological Medicine*, **26**, 477–486.

SCHULBERG, H. C., BLOCK, M. R., MADONIA, M. J., *et al* (1996) Treating major depression in primary care practice: eight-month clinical outcomes. *Archives of General Psychiatry*, **53**, 913–919.

——, KATON, W., SIMON, G. E., *et al* (1998) Treating major depression in primary care practice: an update of the Agency for Health Care Policy and Research practice guidelines. *Archives of General Psychiatry*, **55**, 1121–1127.

SHIELS, C., ECCLES, M., HUTCHINSON, A., *et al* (1997) The inter-rater reliability of a generic measure of severity of illness. *Family Practice*, **14**, 466–471.

SIMON, G. E., VON KORFF, M., WAGNER, E. H., *et al* (1993) Patterns of antidepressant use in community practice. *General Hospital Psychiatry*, **15**, 399–408.

—— & —— (1995) Recognition, management, and outcomes of depression in primary care. *Archives of Family Medicine*, **4**, 99–105.

——, LIN, E. H., KATON, W., *et al* (1995*a*) Outcomes of 'inadequate' antidepressant treatment. *Journal of General Internal Medicine*, **10**, 663–670.

——, VON KORFF, M. & BARLOW, W. (1995*b*) Health care costs of primary care patients with recognized depression. *Archives of General Psychiatry*, **52**, 850–856.

—— & KATZELNICK, D. J. (1997) Depression, use of medical services and cost-offset effects. *Journal of Psychosomatic Research*, **42**, 333–344.

STEWART, A. L., HAYS, R. D. & WARE, J. E. (1988) The MOS short-form general health survey. Reliability and validity in a patient population. *Medical Care*, **26**, 724–735.

UNÜTZER, J., PATRICK, D. L., SIMON, G., *et al* (1997) Depressive symptoms and the cost of health services in HMO patients aged 65 years and older. *Journal of the American Medical Association*, **277**, 1618–1623.

ÜSTÜN, T. B., COOPER, J. E., VAN DUUREN-KRISTEN, S., *et al* (1995) Revision of the ICIDH: mental health aspects. WHO/MNH Disability Working Group. *Disability Rehabilitation*, **17**, 202–209.

—— & SARTORIUS, N. (eds) (1995) *Mental Illness in General Health Care: An International Study.* Chichester: Wiley.

VAN DER FELTZ-CORNELIS, C. M., LYONS, J. S., HUYSE, F. J., *et al* (1997) Health services research on mental health in primary care. *International Journal of Psychiatry in Medicine*, **27**, 1–21.

VON KORFF, M., WAGNER, E. H. & SAUNDERS, K. (1992) A chronic disease score from automated pharmacy data. *Journal of Clinical Epidemiology*, **45**, 197–203.

——, KATON, W., BUSH, T., *et al* (1998) Treatment costs, cost offset, and cost-effectiveness of collaborative management of depression. *Psychosomatic Medicine*, **60**, 143–149.

WARE, J. E. & SHERBOURNE, C. D. (1992) The MOS 36-item short form health survey (SF–36): I. Conceptual framework and item selection. *Medical Care*, **30**, 473–483.

——, KOSINSKI, M. & KELLER, S. D. (1996) A 12-item short-form health survey: construction of scales and preliminary tests of reliability and validity. *Medical Care*, **34**, 220–233.

WELLS, K. B., HAYS, R. D., BURNAM, M. A., *et al* (1989) Detection of depressive disorder for patients receiving prepaid or fee-for-service care. *Journal of the American Medical Association*, **262**, 3298–3302.

——, SHERBOURNE, C. D., SCHOENBAUM, M., *et al* (1999) *One-Year Impact of Disseminating Quality Improvement for Depression to Managed, Primary Care Practices: Results from a Randomized, Controlled Trial.* Working Paper Number P–143. Santa Monica, CA: RAND.

WILLIAMS, J. B. W. (1988) A structured interview guide for the Hamilton Depression Rating Scale. *Archives of General Psychiatry*, **45**, 742–747.

WORLD HEALTH ORGANIZATION (1997) *Composite International Diagnostic Interview (CIDI) Core Version 2.1.* Geneva: WHO.

—— (1999) *Disability Assessment Schedule WHO–DAS II. Draft for Reliability and Validity Field Trials.* Geneva: WHO.

ZITMAN, F. G., MENNEN, M. F. G., GRIEZ, E., *et al* (1990) The different version of the Hamilton Depression Rating Scale. *Psychopharmacology Series*, **9**, 28–34.

18 Measuring outcomes in mental health: implications for policy

RACHEL JENKINS and BRUCE SINGH

The activities and purposes of mental health services can be broadly described under four headings: needs assessment, inputs, processes and outcomes. Until the last few years, the focus of service development and evaluation was largely on input and process variables, and efforts on needs assessment and measuring outcomes (Jenkins, 1990, 1994) have been relatively recent. The strength of this book is that it illuminates the increasing number of possibilities to use outcome indicators as the main point of reference for measuring cost-effectiveness.

The approach that uses inputs of service adequacy has historically focused on the number of beds available, the type and ranges of buildings and places that are provided, the numbers of staff of different disciplines and their levels of training and the amount of money injected into the service system. Although this information is vital for assessing the performance of a mental health service, it is usually used in a very one-sided approach. Such information may be entirely misleading if the investment in a service, described in these terms, produces no actual benefits to patients. The input approach on its own, although frequently used and administratively convenient, can give no indication about whether services are actually achieving their goals.

The second and most common approach to assessing the performance of a mental health service is to use process measures. Examples of this approach are the determination of length of stay in hospital, bed occupancy rates, staffing levels, staff turnover rates, and the number and duration of community contacts for home treatment services. Again, this information is vital for understanding the dynamic way in which a variety of services operate, how the physical and human resource infrastructures are deployed in practice, and the distribution of these resources in different geographical and administrative sectors. This approach is the focus of performance management, which is increasingly emphasised as health services are run more and more on corporate lines. However, this can be compared to a detailed description of the functioning of an ocean liner without any reference as to whether the ship is sailing in the right direction. Auditing provides service process information, and service commissioning and the management of service provision are often based on such process information. As with input information, however, such process measures alone cannot shed any light on whether the intended aims of the service, both as a whole and in its components, are realised in practice.

The third approach, that of measuring outcome variables, is therefore the most important. In 1990, Jenkins called for a system of outcome indicators for mental health care:

> "In order to evaluate our health care system, we need to be able to measure the baseline health of the population, and then to measure the impact of health care on that baseline. We need to be able to monitor and evaluate progress towards more effective health care and better health, to evaluate the efficacy of health promotion and illness prevention programmes, and to improve resource allocation in health care. In order to do this effectively in a valid and reproducible manner, health indicators are required. Besides the more global indicators of general health, lifestyles, quality of life and health equity, we also need indicators relevant to the different categories of illness, and to specific strategies to prevent diseases, to alleviate disability, and to restore function."

Drawing on theoretical aspects of mental health care indicators and the various classes of outcome measures available, Jenkins drew up a preliminary system of indicators of health care input, process and outcome for the major categories of mental illness, including schizophrenia, affective disorders, neurosis, dementia, mental handicap, child psychiatry, forensic psychiatry, alcohol and drug misuse. The system was not intended to be definitive or exhaustive, but rather to form a basis for development by clinicians, researchers and planners for their own requirements.

A decade later, this book draws together much of the progress that has been made and illuminates the increasing number of possibilities of using outcome indicators as the main point of reference for measuring the cost-effectiveness of mental health services.

This decade has also seen revolutionary changes in the way governments approach health care, by setting health action targets, an approach initiated by the World Health Organization in its Health For All by the Year 2000 campaign.

England was one of the first countries to respond by establishing its "Health of the Nation" strategy, which set health outcome targets in five key areas, including mental health (Department of Health, 1994). Three targets were selected for mental health:

- to improve significantly the health and social functioning of mentally ill people
- to reduce the overall suicide rate by at least 15% by the year 2000 (from 11.0 per 100 000 population in 1990 to no more than 9.4)
- to reduce the suicide rate of severely mentally ill people by at least 33% by the year 2000 (from the lifetime estimate of 15% in 1990 to no more than 10%).

The first of these was a true mental health outcome target (as opposed to using inputs or process indicators as proxy measurements) and the second two targets were mortality outcome targets. In order to measure the mental health outcome target, the Royal College of Psychiatrists was commissioned to develop the Health of the Nation Outcome Scales (Wing *et al*, 1996), which are now widely used in the UK as well as in other countries such as Australia, and incorporated into the minimum data-set that will shortly become the common standard for mental health information (Glover, 2000).

With the recent change in government, England has now built on its earlier progress by establishing the "Our Healthier Nation" Strategy 1999, which has set a single target for each of the key areas (Department of Health, 1999):

- to reduce the death rate from suicide and undetermined injury by at least a fifth by 2010 – saving up to 4000 lives in total.

Similarly, over the last decade Australia set out its goals and targets (Commonwealth Department of Human Services and Health, 1994).

These developments have been inspired and motivated by a desire to be able to achieve and measure real health outcomes and health gains, and to move on from the rather static approach of using process indicators as a performance measure, which has the in-built risk that, in the attempt to produce an apparently good result with a process indicator, service providers may do too much of a relatively less useful activity at the expense of achieving good health outcomes.

However, these developments have happened in the course and context of an increasing need and drive to control rising costs, to deliver value for money and to audit services (Jenkins & Knapp, 1996). Management by objectives is an increasingly important tool in the development of health policy. The setting of objectives makes clear the intended outcomes of a national health strategy and it prompts attention to designing specific strategies that lead logically to the identification of component tasks and to the assignment of these tasks. Critical to this process is the consideration of the practicality of specific targets, timeline strategies and resource allocations. However, without clear means of assessing outcomes, a programme will have only expenditure of resources with no easily discernible accomplishments. Defining measurements makes it possible to organise the feedback from results and to review and revise objectives, roles, priorities and the allocation of resources systematically.

In several countries, measures of need have been constructed to guide the allocation of health care resources. The measurement of outcomes is clearly related to the measurement of need. The idea of shifting resources to where they can meet the greatest need or, more correctly, where they will lead to the best outcomes or do the most good is not difficult to grasp. If more good can be done than is being done, if more needs can be met with the same resources, then the argument is that is what should be done. This is the position that the development of evidence-based medicine attempts to establish. The concept of need incorporated into this planning framework is that of capacity to benefit. The move in a number of countries to plan health services with a focus on outcomes or health gain emphasises efficiency and equity in the context of needs.

Measurement of need is, in a sense, the gap between the current status and the best achievable outcomes. The national survey of psychiatric morbidity, which will be repeated in 2001, should become a rolling survey programme to ensure the government has continuing access to up-to-date national figures on mental health needs.

Another impetus for the development of a broader range of outcome measures in mental health has come from the pharmaceutical industry (Revicki, 1997). In order to gain approval for a drug, some countries (e.g. Australia) now require cost-effectiveness studies to show the value to the community of its introduction, particularly as, in the majority of cases, such new drugs are significantly more expensive. The evidence that the new antidepressants, the selective serotonin reuptake inhibitors, are no more effective than the established antidepressants in terms of their influence on symptom levels has forced a rethink of the outcomes that are being measured when treatment occurs to justify to sceptical governments the introduction of these agents (NHS Centre for Reviews and Disseminations, 1993). Quality of life and disability outcomes have thus received serious consideration for the evaluation of psychopharmacological treatments for severe psychiatric disorders.

The appearance of such measures in clinical outcome studies has been noted since the 1980s. Quality-of-life outcomes represent a patient-centred approach to evaluating the impact of both disease and treatment on functioning and well-being. Interest in quality-of-life outcomes and schizophrenia began with concerns about the functioning of chronically mentally ill patients following deinstitutionalisation during the 1970s. A number of instruments have now been developed to assess quality of life in patients with severe psychiatric disorder, despite criticisms that such patients are unable to provide valid and reliable assessments. The first generation of studies showed that such measures are useful for differentiating the therapeutic effects of the newer antidepressants and antipsychotic medications from the older ones. Nowadays, the majority of clinical outcome studies of new antidepressants and antipsychotics include quality-of-life measures, and these studies have shown significant improvements in patient outcome as measured by quality-of-life scales, despite the fact that the effect on symptom variables is usually no different from that of the older medications. In addition, a reduction in the number of adverse side-effects has come to be seen as an important outcome measure influencing compliance. However, it remains important to retain the distinction between quality of life and symptom severity and to retain symptom severity as a central outcome variable.

In the 1960s, the concept of justice entered the discussion of health care policy (Daniels, 1985). This was used in several different ways, sometimes to mean treating individual patients justly by observing their rights and sometimes that all patients were entitled to equal shares in the distribution of health care. In addition, discussions of public health have traditionally been concerned with the principle of utility – of maximising the total benefits for the populations involved. In fact, some would say that utility underlies all discussions of medical ethics. However, in recent years, utility has come to the fore because of the increasing importance, for public health medicine, of rationing scarce resources. Questions of the supply and fair distribution of health care resources are matters related to public policy and ones that are relevant for the principles of both utility and justice. Utility is the principle concerned with the maximising of outcomes and preferences. In its original formulation it concerned the greatest happiness of the greatest number. The question then arises of how one ensures the most effective use of limited resources to benefit the greatest number of people. A related question concerns which interventions will be both effective and affordable.

In many countries there has been a reassessment of the structure and organisation of mental health services to make them more effective and to achieve value for money. Many different models are being tried and common outcome measures are necessary to ensure that the lesson learnt in one country or part of a country can be used in others. Sharing information can also guide the way in which money can be invested in health in order to achieve the maximum health benefit. This book supports that process.

References

COMMONWEALTH DEPARTMENT OF HUMAN SERVICES AND HEALTH (1994) *Better Health Outcomes for Australians. National Goals, Targets and Strategies for Better Health Outcomes into the Next Century.* Canberra: Government Publishing Service.

DANIELS, N. (1985) *Just Health Care.* Cambridge: Cambridge University Press.

DEPARTMENT OF HEALTH (1994) *The Mental Illness Key Area Handbook* (2nd edn). London: The Stationery Office.

—— (1999) *Our Healthier Nation: Saving Lives,* cm4386. London: The Stationery Office.

GLOVER, G. R. (2000) A comprehensive clinical database for mental health care in England. *Social Psychiatry and Psychiatric Epidemiology,* **35,** 523–529.

JENKINS, R. (1990) Towards a system of outcome indicators for mental health care. *British Journal of Psychiatry,* **157,** 500–514.

—— (1994) Ageing in learning difficulties: the development of health care outcome indicators. *Journal of Intellectual Disability Research,* **38,** 257–264.

—— & KNAPP, M. (1996) Use of health economic data by health administrators in national health systems. In *The Handbook of Mental Health Economics and Health Policy, Vol. 1. Schizophrenia* (eds M. Moscarelli, A. Rapp & N. Sartorius), **44,** pp. 503–510. Chichester: Wiley & Son.

NHS CENTRE FOR REVIEWS AND DISSEMINATIONS (1993) The treatment of depression in primary care. *Effective Health Care Bulletin,* **1,** no. 5.

REVICKI, D. A. (1967) Methods of pharmaco-economic evaluation of therapies for patients with schizophrenia. *Journal of Psychiatry and Neuroscience,* **22,** 256–266.

WING, J. K., CURTIS, R. H. & BEEVOR, A. S. (1996) *HoNOS: Health of the Nation Outcome Scales. Report on Research and Development. July 1993 – December 1995.* London: Royal College of Psychiatrists.

Index